René Liechti

Hip Arthrodesis and Associated Problems

Foreword by M. E. Müller and B. G. Weber

Translated by Patrick A. Casey

With 266 Figures

Springer-Verlag
Berlin Heidelberg New York 1978

Dr. med. RENÉ LIECHTI
Hôpital du District de Nyon, CH-1260 Nyon

Translator: Dr. PATRICK A. CASEY
Oberwohlenstraße 45, CH-3033 Wohlen

Translation of the German edition:
Die Arthrodese des Hüftgelenkes und ihre Problematik

ISBN 3-540-06636-5 Springer-Verlag Berlin Heidelberg New York
ISBN 0-387-06636-5 Springer-Verlag New York Heidelberg Berlin

ISBN-13: 978-3-642-66875-3 e-ISBN-13: 978-3-642-66873-9
DOI: 10.1007/978-3-642-66873-9

Library of Congress Cataloging in Publication Data. Liechti, René, 1938– Hip arthrodesis and its problems. Translation of Die Arthrodese des Hüftgelenkes und ihre Problematik. Bibliography: p. Includes index. 1. Hip joint—Surgery. 2. Arthrodesis. I. Title. RD549.L513. 617'.58. 78-18778

Reproduction of the figures: Gustav Dreher GmbH, Stuttgart

Foreword to the German Edition

Until 10 years ago arthrodesis was considered the treatment of choice for the painful hip with unilaterally limited range of movement or for the severely incongruent hip. If the indication was right and the operation was correctly performed, a painless hip joint resulted which was capable of weight bearing and the majority of patients were very satisfied with the result.

Nowadays almost every hip patient and, unfortunately, the occasional orthopaedic surgeon, believes the total prosthesis (TP) to be perfectly suitable for the relatively young patient. However, they will rapidly become disillusioned, for patients under 50 years of age will surely ignore the warnings of their medical advisers and stress their painless hip prostheses to such a degree that a number of them will already have loosened within the first few years. An artificial joint can, of course, be replaced once or even twice, but what then?

In 1970, in a group survey conducted by the nine largest Swiss orthopaedic clinics, the effect of intertrochanteric osteotomy (IO) on pain, gait, mobility and fitness for work was carefully analysed. Guidelines were established in respect to indications, choice of procedure and operative technique. A group survey of the Swiss Orthopaedic Association is currently in progress in which the results 3–10 years following TP operation are being analysed, applying criteria similar to those in the IO survey.

Arthrodesis technique has changed radically over the last 15 years. In 1958 noone would have expected a hip arthrodesis (HA) to unite without the application of a cast. However, 6 years later double plates or cobra-head plates were being used in a number of clinics for the majority of arthrodeses with immediate postoperative mobilisation. Until now, however, no adequate survey of a large number of these novel arthrodeses existed. We therefore owe a considerable debt to Dr. Liechti for his painstaking investigation, assessment and analysis of such cases from the Orthopaedic Clinic at St. Gall. Dr. Liechti has systematically researched every case and was able to follow up no less than 525 of the 583 patients. The result of this extensive work is a surprise: who would have imagined that 90% of these HA patients would still be satisfied with the result of their operation 10–12 years afterwards? One is inclined to ask how many TP patients whose prosthesis has been implanted using the latest operative techniques would be equally satisfied over a similar period of time. Furthermore, one should not forget that an arthrodesis may be replaced by a total prosthesis if spinal or knee joint complaints arise following the former operation.

Dr. LIECHTI has not only surveyed the case material and analysed the results; he has furnished precise descriptions of the techniques used and has biomechanically investigated and assessed various methods in the laboratory using elastometric models. He was thus able to disprove certain current concepts. Indications and contraindications are extensively discussed in his work as are the complications and their management. The reader is thus presented with an excellent survey of hip joint arthrodesis. His attention is brought to the fact that the treatment of osteoarthrosis of the hip joint is difficult and has many facets and that more than one operative procedure is necessary. Indeed, in view of the broad range of hip joint diseases, the hip surgeon must be capable of performing several different procedures in order to ensure a perfect arthrodesis.

We are very grateful Dr. Dr. R. LIECHTI, our pupil, for writing this book which is directed at the hip surgeon, who, accepting the responsibility placed upon him, is dedicated to helping his patient.

M.W. MÜLLER
B.G. WEBER

Preface to the German Edition

In the last 10 years, total prosthetic replacement has become *the* hip operation for many but not all surgeons. In our clinic the increasing frequency of TP has been paralleled by a reduction in the frequency of IO and HA. For the experienced orthopaedic surgeon and hip surgeon, hip disease has so many facets that it could not possibly be tackled with one operation alone. Thus, HA seems recently to have won renewed recognition. It has once more become the procedure of choice in specific cases, possibly because of certain disadvantages and complications associated with TP which have somewhat tempered the original optimism. Currently, the risk of infection or loosening of the prosthesis is such that the operation cannot justifiably be recommended for patients under 55–60 years of age. In contrast with HA, in the majority of cases the results of TP or IO are not fully predictable. The loss of joint motion is offset by two important advantages:

– complete freedom from pain
– full weight bearing is possible on the arthrodesed hip.

On following up our HA operations from 1961 to 1971, we examined the development of the operative procedures in our clinic. We found that the range of indications had narrowed as stricter criteria were applied in choosing patients for operation. Adequate and precise operative techniques were developed. We studied the biomechanics of the hip joint extensively (effect of arthrodesis on the statics and dynamics of the hip joint and neighbouring joints).

Failures, particularly those resulting from inadequate bone union, have become rare as close attention is paid to the principles of stable internal fixation and also as a consequence of having a tested operative procedure for each individual case. We are able to draw on 11 years of experience involving 583 cases. We have deliberately omitted from our survey the HAs performed in 1972 since the follow-up period in these cases is too short, and because our views on the biomechanical and technical operative problems involved remain unchanged.

Because of the large number of cases involved and for the sake of simplicity, we have classified our HAs in five different types. Cases are included in which techniques were used which are now rare or which have been abandoned. We have tried to present a synopsis of our experience. On the basis of our results and observations we were able to confirm existing views and develop new concepts. Our operative techniques have withstood the test of time, i.e., a clinical follow-up period of 2–10 years.

In Part I (General Aspects) of this monograph, a short historical review is followed by a description of the effects of arthrodesis on the biomechanics of the arthrodesed and neighbouring joints. The general indications and operative techniques are extensively discussed. In Part II (Specific Problems and Case Material), an analysis of our results is presented and the indications and potentials of HA are illustrated using cases of osteoarthrosis of the hip, rheumatoid arthritis, hip dysplasia, posttraumatic hip conditions, joint infection, aseptic necrosis of the femoral head, Girdlestone hip (GH) and similar conditions.

The combination of HA with TP in bilateral hip disease is discussed, as is the possibility of performing these operations sequentially in the same hip if the first operation has failed.

Particular attention is paid to the prevention, recognition and treatment of complications following HA. This book is not intended to be a definitive survey of hip surgery; by summarising our experience and analysing the individual cases, both the successes and the failures, we simply wish to restore arthrodesis to the place which it rightly deserves in the hip surgeon's repertoire. I am particularly grateful to Prof. M. E. MÜLLER, who previously headed the Orthopaedic Clinic at St. Gall, and to Prof. B. G. WEBER, the present director of that clinic.

My interest in biomechanics and particularly in hip surgery was stimulated by my one-time chief, Prof. M. E. MÜLLER. I have been constantly impressed by his knowledge of the subject and by his dynamic approach. This work would have been impossible without the constant support, encouragement and advice of Prof. B. G. WEBER. His experience and valuable suggestions were a great help to me. I am also grateful to my friend and colleague Dr. O. ČECH, whose expert and comradely advice assisted me considerably.

Prof. W. HESS, Zürich, kindly read and corrected the manuscript.

The Saurer Company in Arbon generously offered me their laboratory facilities for the polarised light elastometry experiments.

The special AO plates for the latter experiments were made and donated by Dr. hc. R. MATHYS in Bettlach.

I am also grateful to all those persons who assisted in the preparation of the manuscript, in particular Mrs. E. WILD who patiently handled the considerable secretarial work involved; Miss V. JÖRG, who typed the manuscript with enthusiasm and understanding; the photographic technicians, Mrs. M. SCHAFFNER and Miss D. CLERICI, who were responsible for the excellent quality of the radiographs; and Miss K. SCHUMACHER, who drew the diagrams and pictures with artistic talent and cleverly translated my wishes into clear illustrations. Finally, I should like to thank Springer-Verlag in Heidelberg for the excellent quality of this book as finally published.

St. Gall R. LIECHTI

Table of Contents

Part I: General Aspects

Part II: Specific Problems and Case Material

Part I: General Aspects

List of Abbreviations

CDH	Congenital dislocation of the hip
GH	Girdlestone hip
HA	Hip arthrodesis
IO	Intertrochanteric osteotomy
LS	Lumbar spine
NHF	Necrosis of the femoral head
PA	Pseudarthrosis
PO	Pelvic osteotomy
SIJ	Sacroiliac joint
Tb	tuberculosis
TP	Total prothesis

I. Historical Review

The history of hip arthrodesis (HA) begins in the second half of the nineteenth century with the hip resection operations of MARGARY (1883, Italy), HEUSNER (1884, Germany) and LAMPUGNANI (1885, Italy) which were carried out in cases of congenital dislocation of the hip. However, the retention of a degree of mobility was intended in these procedures. This is in complete contrast to the procedure carried out by LAGRANGE (1886, France) who as far as is known was the first to attempt arthrodesis in a 16-year-old girl with dislocation and unspecific arthritis of the hip. The dislocated head was restored to the acetabulum and fixed with wires. Although the head of the femur did not redislocate, the desired ankylosis failed to occur and, one concludes from the case report, the procedure resulted in the first pseudarthrosis (PA) of an HA. In the English-speaking world, ALBEE (1908, United States) is regarded as the father of HA. In the German-speaking world this honor is accorded to ALBERT (1887, Austria), and in the French-speaking world, to DARAIGNEZ (1891, France) (Fig. 1).

DOLLINGER (1891, Hungary) furnished a precise description of the operative procedure. A lateral longitudinal incision 15 cm in length commences behind the tip of the greater trochanter. The muscle insertions are severed from the greater trochanter, the joint is opened and the femoral head is dislocated. The femoral head and the acetabulum are denuded of cartilage, the joint capsule is excised, and the head is fixed in the acetabulum with a screw (the latter was screwed into the pelvis from the trochanter under finger control) and the trochanter, femoral neck, femoral head and floor of the acetabulum are drilled through.

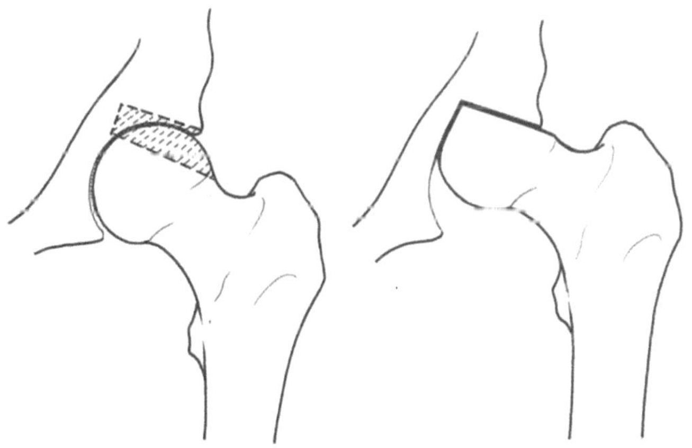

Fig. 1. *Intra-articular HA*. ALBEE (1908)

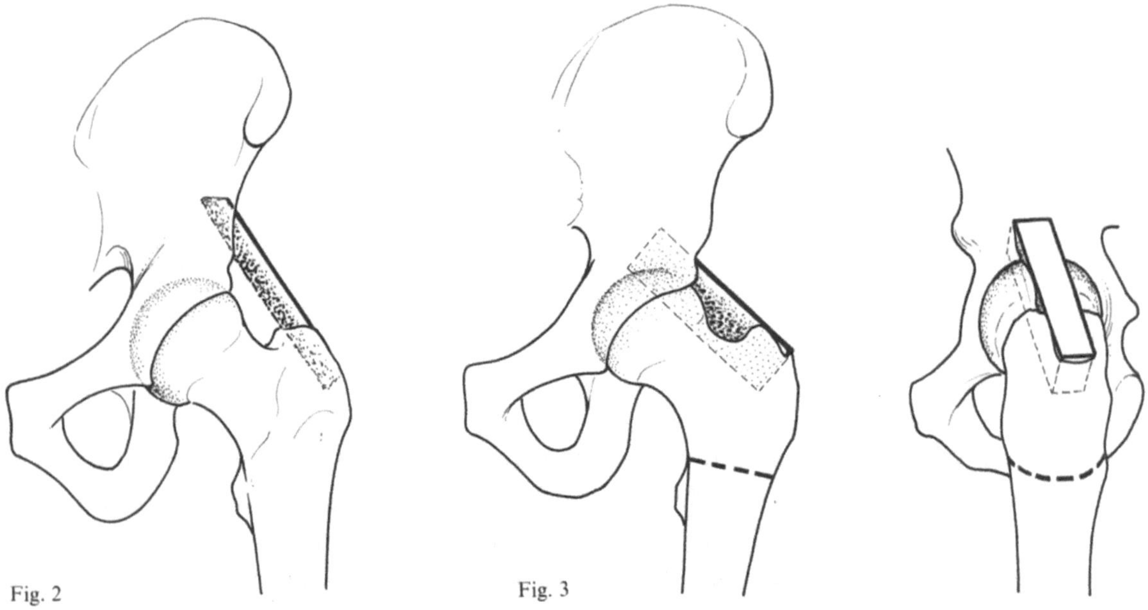
Fig. 2

Fig. 3

Figs. 2 and 3. *Iliofemoral HA*. (2) ALBEE (1915) – KAPPIS (1921); (3) HENDERSON (1933)

WINIWARTER (Germany) reported these cases again in 1892.

In the cases previously described, the procedure was always *intraarticular* with postoperative immobilisation of the joint, generally in abduction using a cast.

The first *extraarticular* HA operations in tuberculitic hips were described by ALBEE (1913), MARAGLIANO (1919, Italy) and SCHUMM (1929, United States). The procedures incorporated iliofemoral bone grafts (Figs. 2, 3).

Protagonists of *ischiofemoral bone grafting* were DE BEULE (1909, Belgium), MARAGLIANO (1921), CALVÉ (1931, France), TRUMBLE (1932, Australia), SPEED (1937, United States), BOSWORTH (1939, United States), BRITTAIN (1941, England), KNIGHT (1945, United States), FREIBERG (1946, Germany), VAN GORDER (1949, United States), KIRKALDY-WILLIS (1950, England), CHAPCHAL (1959, Switzerland) (Figs. 4, 5).

GHORMLEY (1931, United States) used the term *paraarticular* HA to describe the procedure in which the anterior joint capsule is opened but the head of the femur is not dislocated and broad resection of the joint surfaces is not carried out. This term was erroneously applied to a variety of HA operations which were in fact both intraarticular and extraarticular since the joint capsule is, of course, opened. Common to these operations is the application of an ileotrochanteric graft to the freshened femoral neck. This group includes the techniques described by KAPPIS (1921, Germany), HAAS (1922, United States) and HIBBS (1926, United States), MATHIEU and WILMOTH (1926, France), WILSON (1927, United States), GHORMLEY (1931, United States), CHANDLER (1933, United States), HENDERSON (1933, United States), BADGLEY (1947, United States), CATTANEO (1959, Italy). The bone grafts are taken from the iliac bone or from the greater trochanter or tibia.

DAVIS (1954, United States) described a bone graft taken from the iliac crest with retention of the muscular attachments. This has the advantage that the blood supply is retained with resulting improvement in bone formation (Fig. 6).

The *subtrochanteric osteotomy* first described by FARKAS (1939, Hungary) offers improved

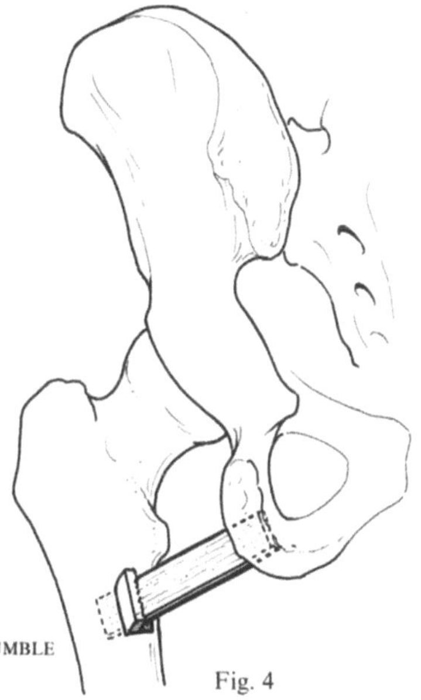

Fig. 4

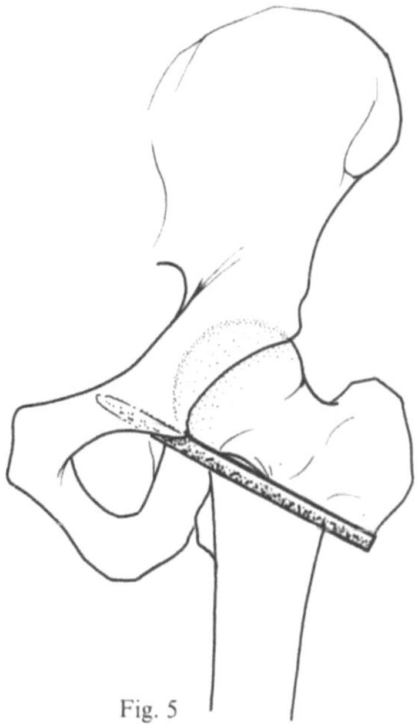

Fig. 5

Figs. 4 and 5. *Ischiofemoral HA*. (4) TRUMBLE (1922); (5) BRITTAIN (1941)

stability. It prevents direct transmission of disadvantageous movement from the long lever arm of the femur to the HA.

The era of application of internal fixation methods to HA begins with transarticular nailing. This method was made universally known by VAN NES (1922, The Netherlands), BURNS (1935/1939, England), WATSON-JONES (1934/1938, England), HARRIS (1943, United States), KÜNTSCHER (1953, Germany). HOWARD (1950, England) in cooperation with BRITTAIN (1952, England), added bone grafting to the transarticular nailing. APLEY and DENHAM (1955, England) performed intraarticular freshening and nailing followed by a subtrochanteric osteotomy (Figs. 7, 8).

However, all these methods required prolonged immobilisation in a cast. In order to avoid this, attempts to achieve greater stability by using new internal fixation techniques became more and more frequent.

MAY and MAUCK (1962, United States), DWYER (1964, Australia), ONJI, KURATA, KINDO (1965, Japan) were protagonists of *ischiofemoral nailing* using the Küntscher nail (Fig. 9).

CHARNLEY (1953, England) achieved greater bone contact and improved stability by *central dislocation* of the freshened femoral head into the medial pelvis and simultaneous internal compression fixation with a screw cranial to the femoral neck (Fig. 10).

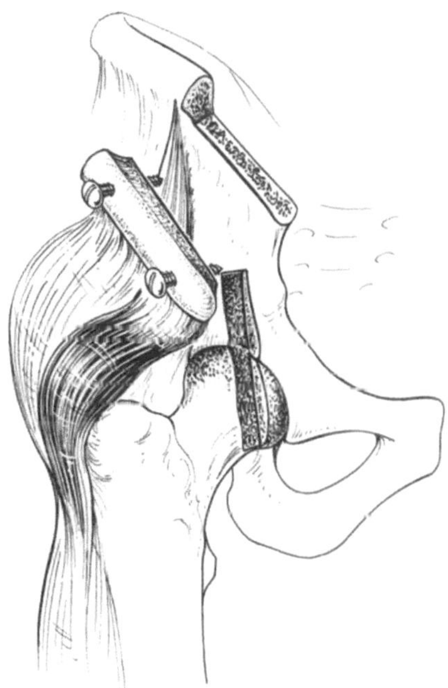

Fig. 6. *Iliac crest graft with muscle attachment*. DAVIS (1954)

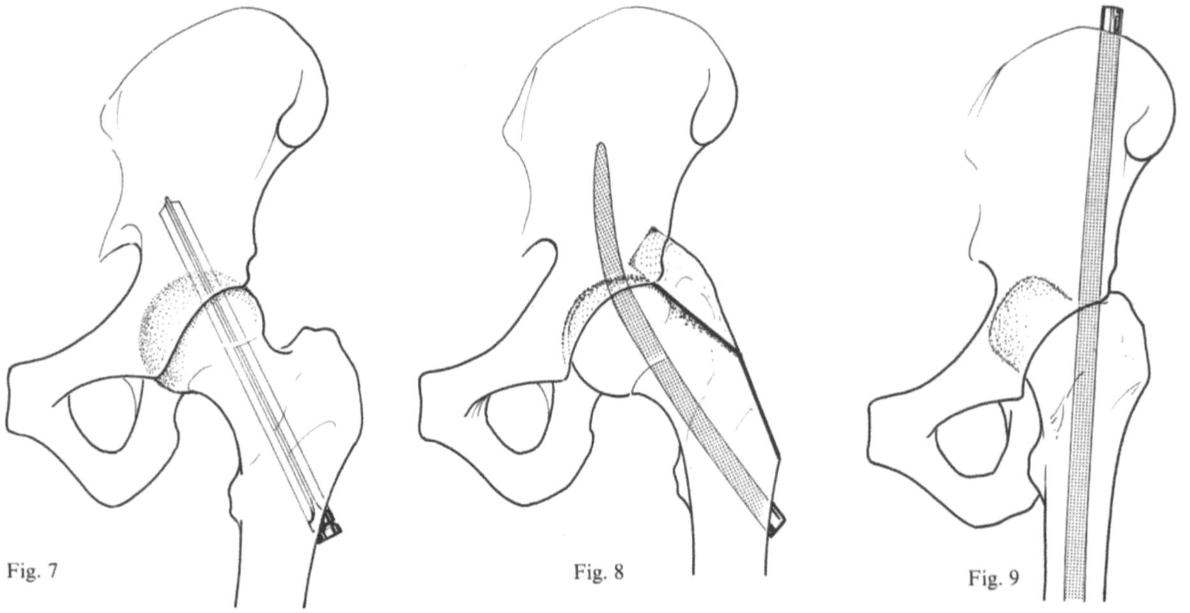

Fig. 7 Fig. 8 Fig. 9

Figs. 7–9. *Transarticular nail arthrodeses.* (7) WATSON-JONES (1939) using Smith-Peterson nail; (8) KÜNTSCHER (1953); (9) ONJI et al. (1965)

These principles were the starting point for the development of HA by means of *stable internal compression fixation.*

ALVIK (1962, Norway) used screw and plate internal fixation (Fig. 11). TEINTURIER (1966, France) described internal compression fixation using screws combined with a trochanteric bone graft with muscle attachment. MÜLLER (1967, Switzerland) achieved excellent stability by double-plate arthrodesis and recommends pelvic osteotomy (PO) in order to enlarge the contact surfaces.

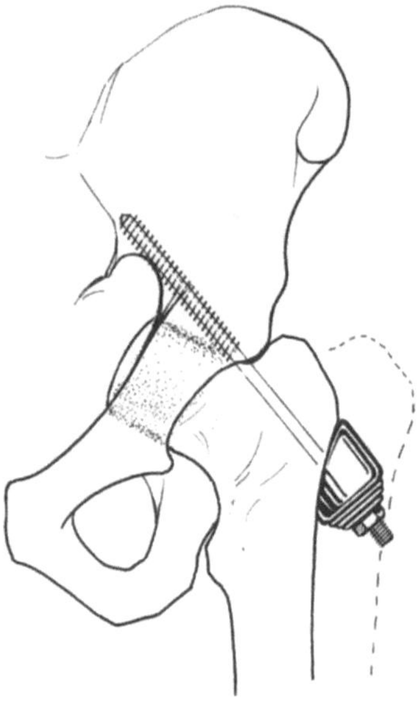

Fig. 10. *Central dislocation and internal compression fixation.* CHARNLEY (1953)

The method of AXER (1961, Israel), was modified by VIERNSTEIN and recommended by LANGE (1968, Germany). The femoral head is held in place by a rod which is anchored on the medial surface of the pelvis (Fig. 12).

Method and results of HA using the cobrahead plate developed by SCHNEIDER in Switzerland were published by GERTSCH (1966, Switzerland), MÜLLER (1967), DREYER and PINGEL (1969, Germany) and WIEDMER (1969, Switzerland) (Fig. 13). This technique amounts to a refinement of the double-plate arthrodesis and PO described by MÜLLER. The multiplicity of operative procedures is an indication of the difficulties encountered to date in solving two main problems. The first problem is an excessive rate of incomplete bone union (PA, fibrotic ankylosis) and the second is the necessity for

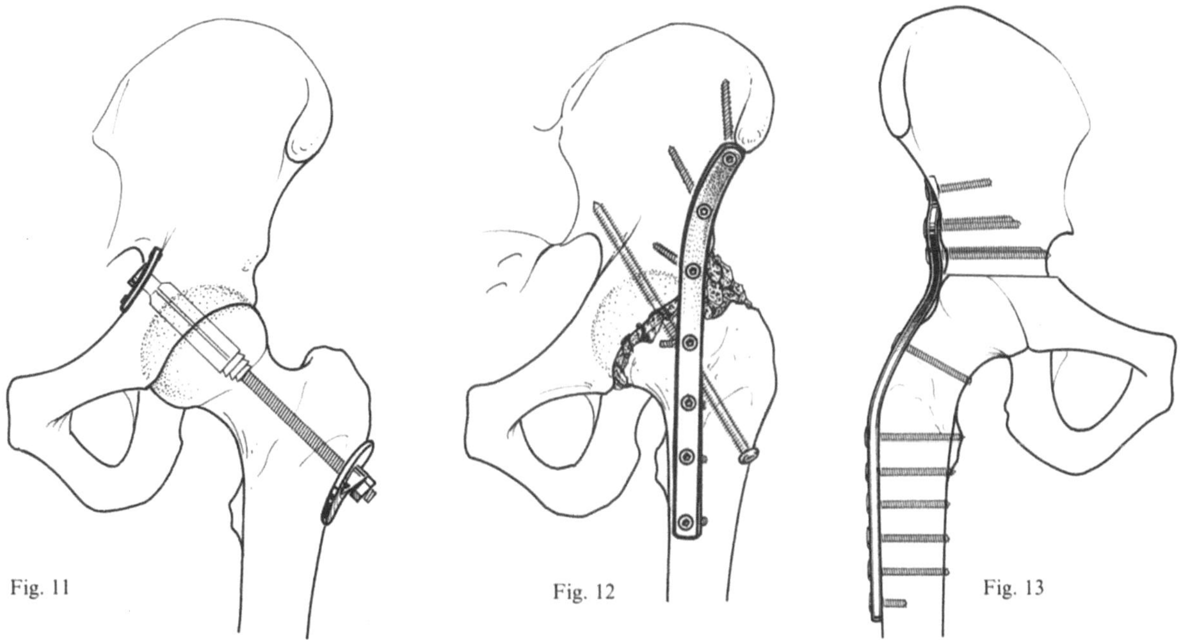

Figs. 11 – 13. *HA with rigid internal compression fixation.* (*11*) ALVIK (1962); (*12*) AXER (1961)—VIERNSTEIN; (*13*) SCHNEIDER'S cobra-head plate (1966)

prolonged cast immobilisation in bed. Optimal conditions for HA comprise adequate immobilisation of the ossifying joint components together with adequate bone-to-bone contact between those components and sufficient stability such that use of a cast is unnecessary and early mobilisation of the patient is possible.

Intraarticular, extraarticular and paraarticular fixation with or without internal fixation, subtrochanteric osteotomy or postoperative cast fixation all have one thing in common. In each case the aim is to prevent movement between the joint components. This stability is the most important prerequisite for rapid bone union in HA.

Summarising the history of HA one may differentiate the following techniques:

1. Extraarticular arthrodesis with cast fixation.
2. Paraarticular arthrodesis with cast fixation.
3. Intraarticular arthrodesis
   a) with cast fixation and with or without internal fixation
   b) without cast fixation and with stable internal fixation.

II. Anatomy of the Hip Joint

Thorough acquaintance with the anatomy of the hip joint is a prerequisite to hip surgery and the surgeon must be used to thinking in three dimensions. Only those basic principles and special features relevant to HA (including the operative risks) are dealt with in the following illustrations. Full descriptions of the anatomy of the hip joint may be found in anatomy text books (Figs. 14 – 17).

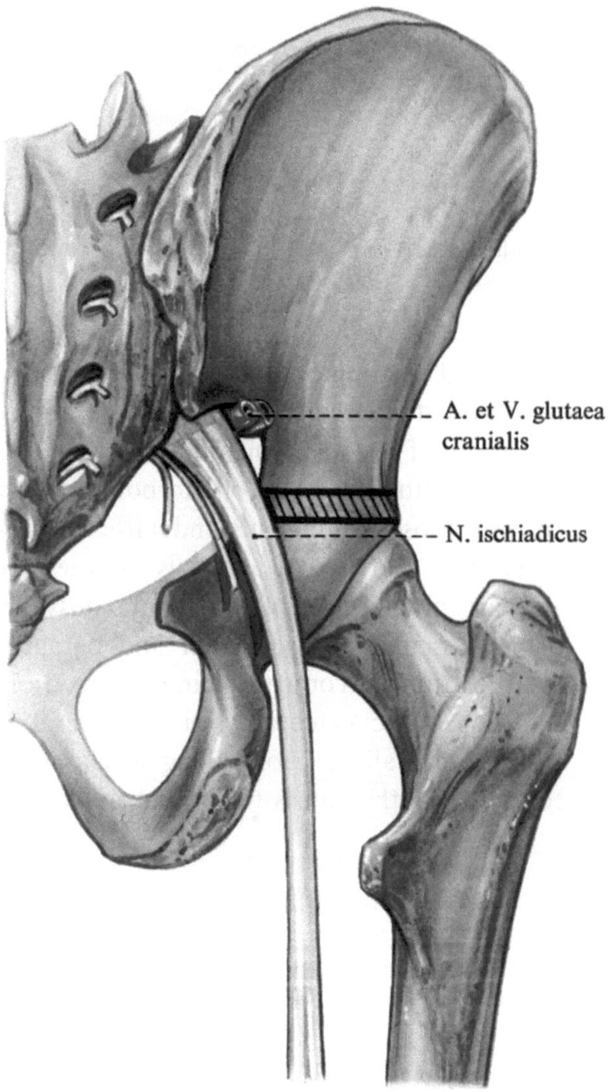

Fig. 14. *Arteries and nerves in the vicinity of the PO (dorsal aspect)*

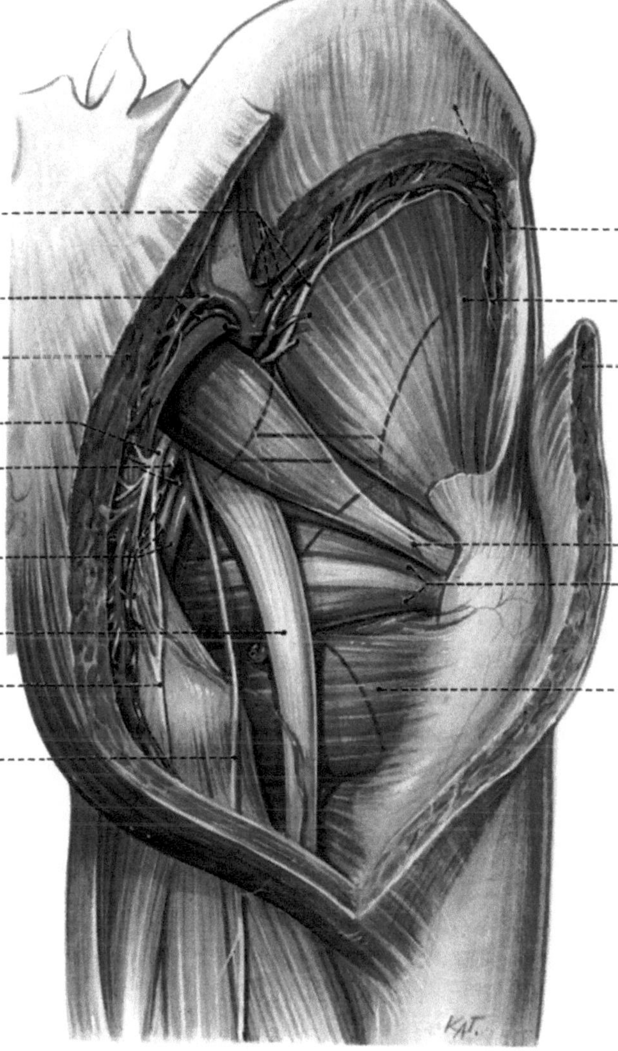

Fig. 15. *Vessels and nerves of the hip (dorsal aspect)*. The gluteus maximus and gluteus medius muscles have been divided. The vessels and nerves leave the pelvis through the greater sciatic notch above and below the piriformis muscle. The superior gluteal artery and the obturator nerve lie above the muscle and the inferior gluteal artery and the sciatic nerve below it (HAFFERL).

The sciatic nerve is covered by the gluteus maximus muscle. It passes distally between the ischial tuberosity on the medial side and the greater trochanter on the lateral side. It may be accompanied by one of the branches of the inferior gluteal artery. On passing out into the gluteal region it is already internally divided into tibial and common peroneal branches. The sciatic nerve may be injured during PO if it is insufficiently protected by HOHMANN retractors (injury caused by the osteotome or by the oscillating saw) or it may be directly injured by incorrect insertion of a pointed retractor. The nerve may be stretched by marked medial displacement of the distal pelvic component following osteotomy or it may be compressed by a bone fragment or a hematoma; injuries of this nature did not result during our HA.

The common peroneal branch of the sciatic nerve is much more frequently (if not exclusively) affected than the tibial branch. Injury to the whole sciatic nerve never occurred. This is explained by the fact that the sciatic nerve runs laterally and distally on leaving the sciatic notch below the piriform muscle, it lies very close to the acetabular margin and is only separated from the joint capsule by the thin external rotator muscle layer. The common peroneal part lies more laterally and is closest to the acetabular margin so that it is more prone to injury

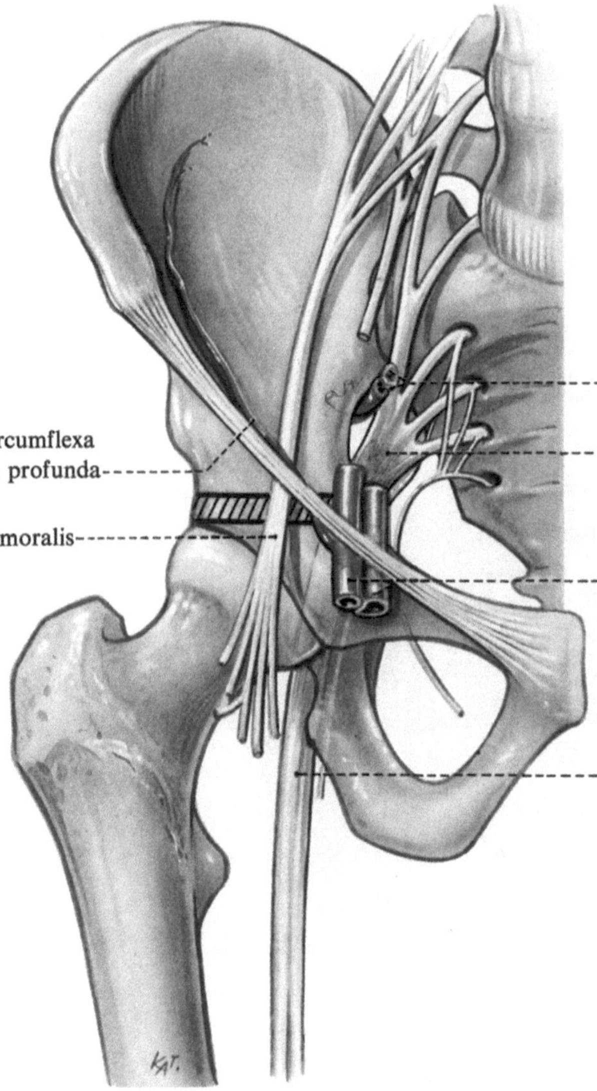

Fig. 16. *Arteries and nerves around the PO (ventral aspect)*

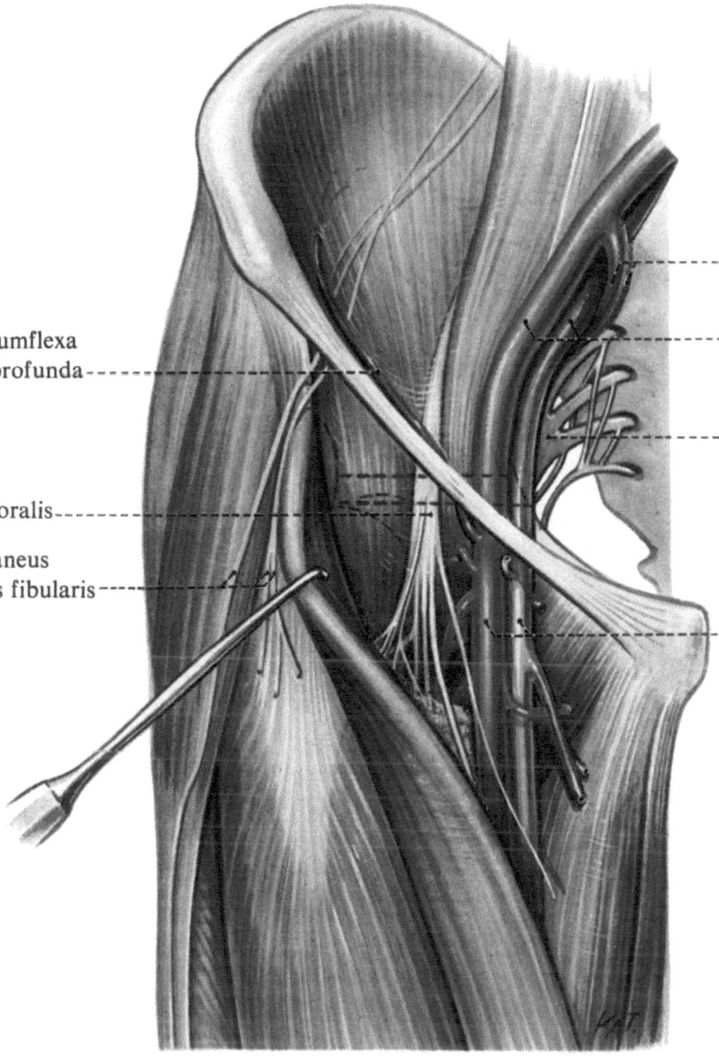

Fig. 17. *Inguinal region and anterior aspect of the upper leg; vessels and nerves of the femoral triangle.* The sartorius muscle has been retracted laterally.

On passing under the middle of the inguinal ligament, the artery lies lateral and the vein medial. The femoral nerve passes under the junction of the middle and the lateral thirds of the inguinal ligament lateral to the artery. It enters the thigh through the muscle hiatus.

The deep branch of the circumflex artery of the thigh leaves the external iliac artery under the inguinal ligament. Passing laterally, it first crosses the ventral aspect of the femoral nerve and follows the inguinal ligament as far as the anterior superior iliac spine, at which point it enters the fascia of the iliac muscle and runs along the iliac crest.

The deep branch of the circumflex artery of the thigh is endangered during PO and may be injured by a Hohmann retractor, particularly if the latter is inserted along the iliac crest too far laterally

III. Biomechanics of Hip Arthrodesis and Internal Fixation: Kinetics and Elastometry

1 Introduction

HA brings about radical changes in the statics and dynamics of the locomotor system. From a biomechanical point of view, the lumbar

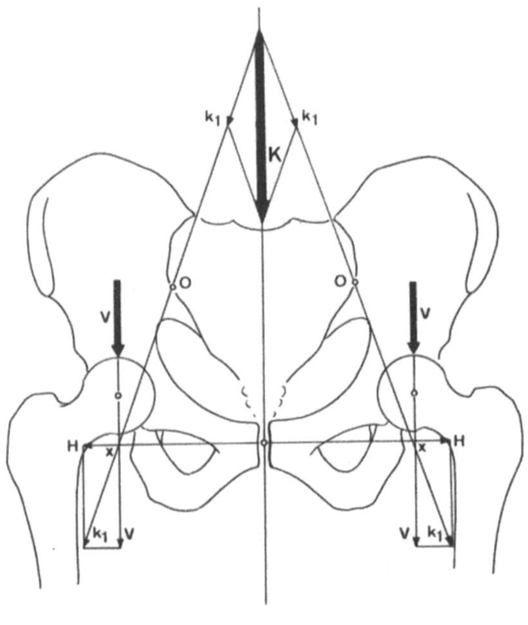

Fig. 18. *Distribution of forces during symmetrical standing on both legs* (Diagram by PAUWELS)

K Line of action of body weight;

O Centre of pressure of sacroiliac joint;

X Intersection of the vertical component V and the horizontal component *H*.

The action of the oblique components *k* 1 is given by the points *O* and *X*

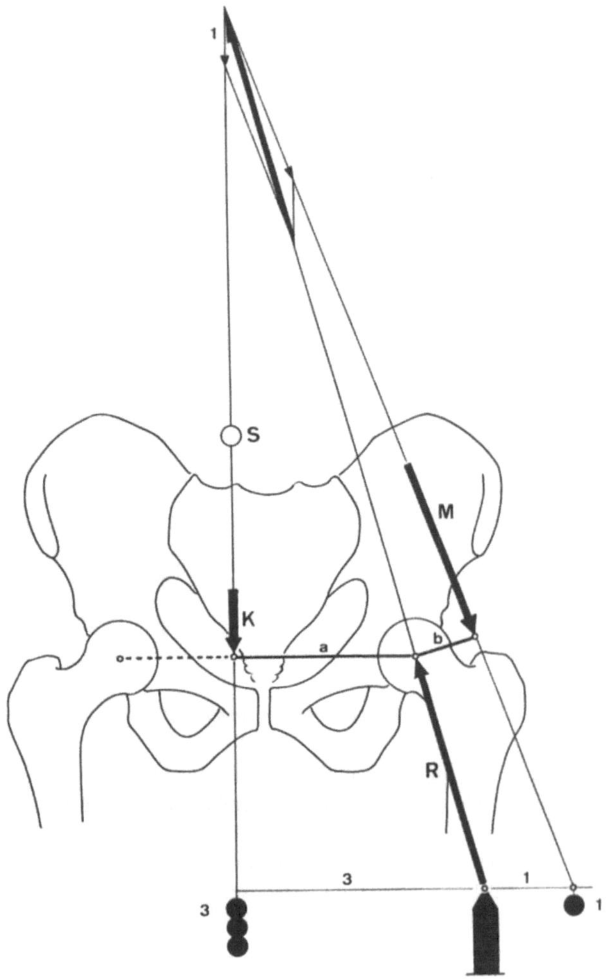

Fig. 19. *Resolution of forces during standing on one leg* (synthesised from diagrams by PAUWELS and MÜLLER).

S Resultant centre of weight of the nonloaded leg and upper body;

M Resultant of the abductor muscle forces;

R Resultant of the forces acting on the femoral head.

On standing on one leg under physiological conditions the leverage exerted by the muscles (*b*) is three times smaller than that exerted by the body weight (*a*).

K Line of action of the combined weights of the non-loaded leg and upper body

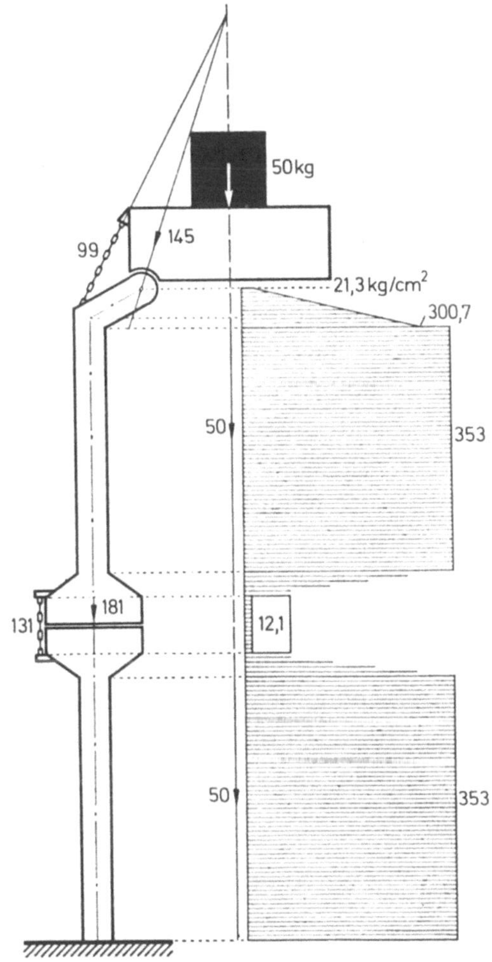

Fig. 20

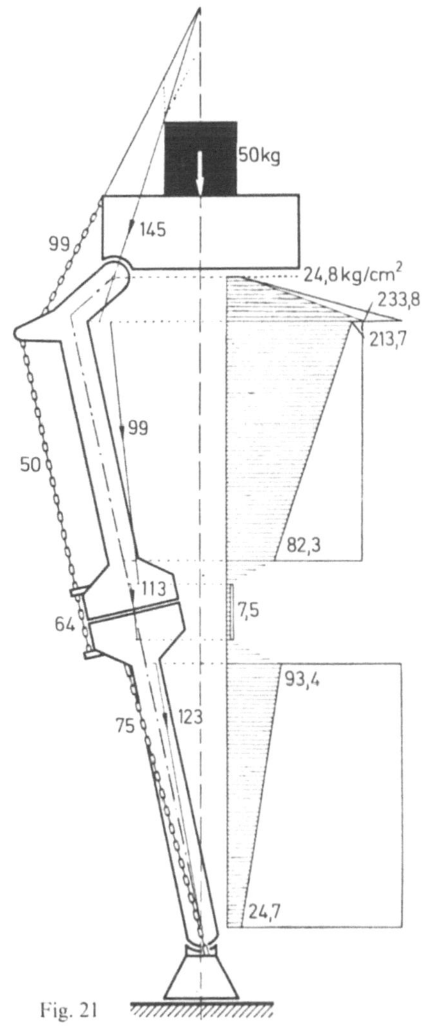

Fig. 21

Figs. 20 and 21. *Illustrations of the parts played by muscles, ligaments and axial deviation in reducing the predominant bending load on the skeleton.* (Taken from "Gesammelte Abhandlungen zur funktionellen Anatomie des Bewegungsapparates" by PAUWELS with kind permission of the author and publishers.)

The considerable load on the upper and lower segments of the column (20) is reduced in the upper segment by adding a chain (the iliotibial tract) (21). By tilting the axis and adding a final joint at the lower end of the column (ankle joint) the leverage exerted by the force acting on the column decreases progressively down the column

spine (LS), the sacroiliac joint (SIJ), the knee joint and the ankle joint on the same side as the arthrodesis and the hip joint on the opposite side should be regarded as a kinetic unit. Interruption of the chain by stiffening of one member necessarily results in a partial redistribution of the function of that member over the remaining elements or adaptation of those elements to the change in load.

Knowledge of the biomechanical principles is basic to an understanding of the adaptability of the joints mentioned to the compensatory changes in posture and movement.

2 Statics

2.1 Hip Joint and Lower Limb Skeleton

The principles enunciated by PAUWELS (1935, 1948 and 1950) remain valid for the hip joint and the lower limb skeleton.

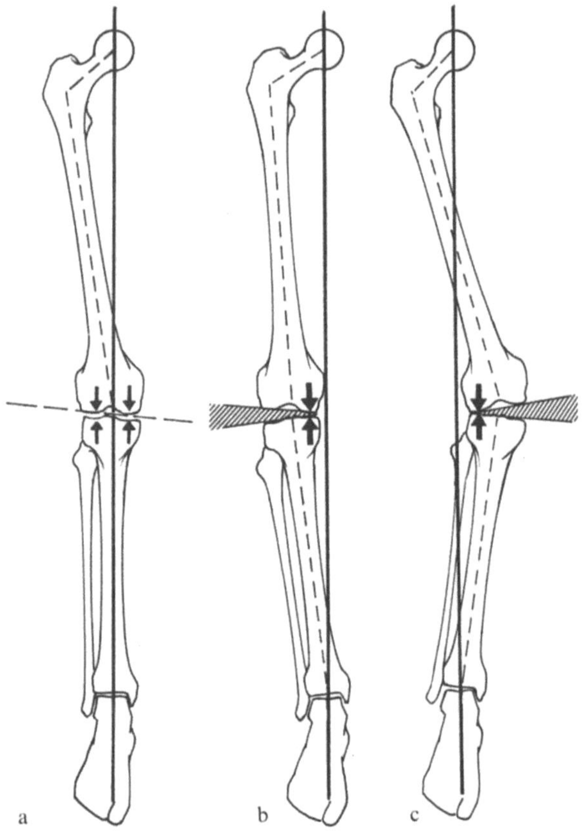

Fig. 22. *Relationship of the line of weight bearing to the axis of the knee joint.*

a) Under normal conditions the axis of the knee joint subtends an angle of 86° to the line of weight bearing. The lateral and medial segments of the joint are symmetrically loaded.

b) If the knee is in varus the line of weight bearing lies medial to the joint. There is correspondingly increased loading of the medial joint segment and lateral gaping.

c) The opposite obtains in the valgus knee. The line of weight bearing is lateral to the knee joint. The load on the lateral joint segment is increased and medial gaping occurs

2.1.1 Standing on Both Legs

All loads on the vertebral column are transmitted symmetrically to both SIJ, the pelvic girdle and both hip joints (Fig. 18).

The direction of the oblique component (K) is determined by the centre of pressure in the SIJ and by the point X (Pauwels).

2.1.2 Standing on One Leg

On standing on one leg, the biomechanics of loading are changed as follows (Fig. 19).

The resultant of body weight and that of the nonloaded leg is on the side of the nonloaded leg. While standing on one leg, the force acting on the head of the femur is directed downwards and laterally. Under normal conditions it subtends an angle of 16° to the vertical.

Body weight and muscle action (abductors of the hip) balance each other at the hip joint. The pressure in the hip joint is increased by the synergism of the adductors.

The mechanics and geometry of the locomotor system of the lower limb are better understood by studying the illustration published by Pauwels in 1950 (Figs. 20, 21).

It is important to notice that the bending moment to which the skeleton is subjected is markedly reduced by the *tension band action of the iliotibial tract* and by the physiological angulation at the level of the knee joint (physiological valgus). The *mechanical axis* passes through the centres of the femoral head, knee joint and ankle joint.

2.2 Knee Joint

Medial or lateral displacement of the centre of the femoral head results in medialisation or lateralisation of the load line in relation to the knee joint. This results in overloading of the tibial or fibular side of the knee joint, respectively. Corresponding situations occur on deviation of the knee-joint axis from normal as in the valgus or varus knee (Fig. 22).

3 Kinetics

3.1 Introduction

Pauwels' classic reflections on the dynamics of the lower limb skeleton deserve review.

a) Muscle action plays a relatively insignificant part in symmetrical standing on both legs since if the trunk is vertical only a small

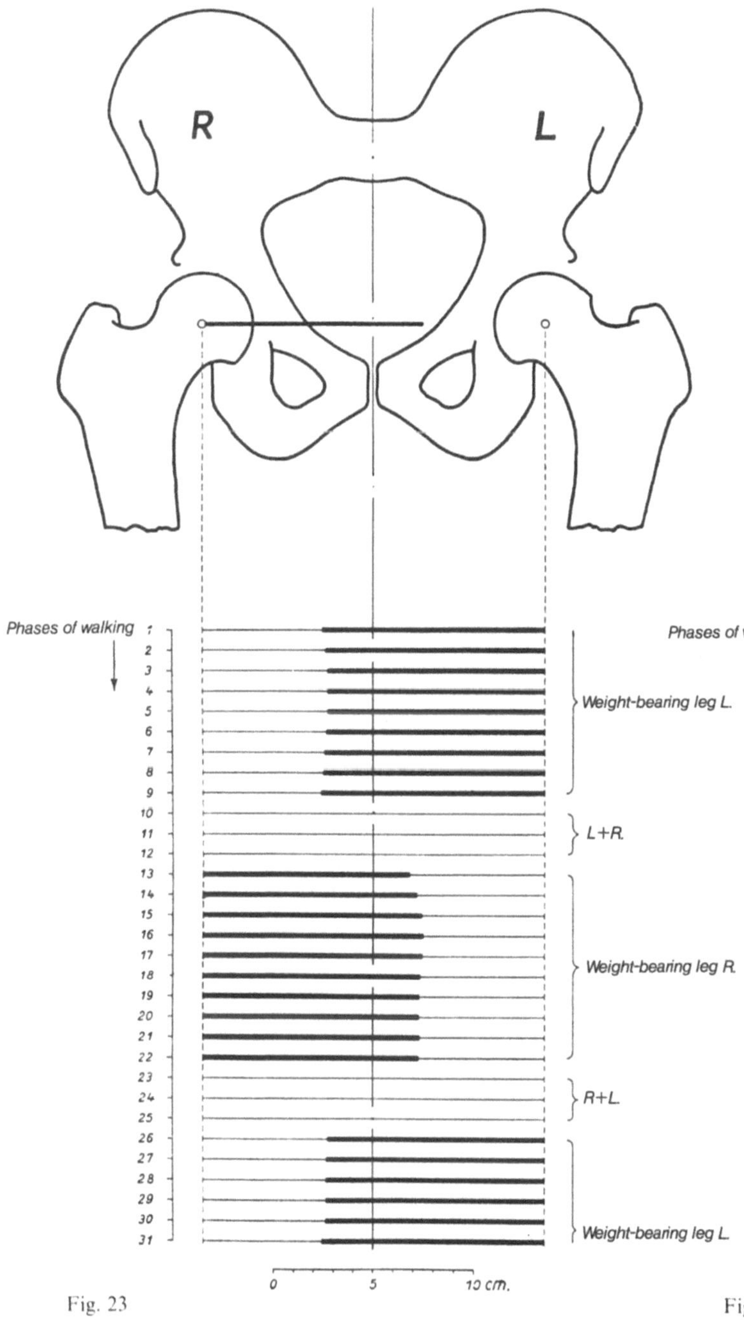

Fig. 23

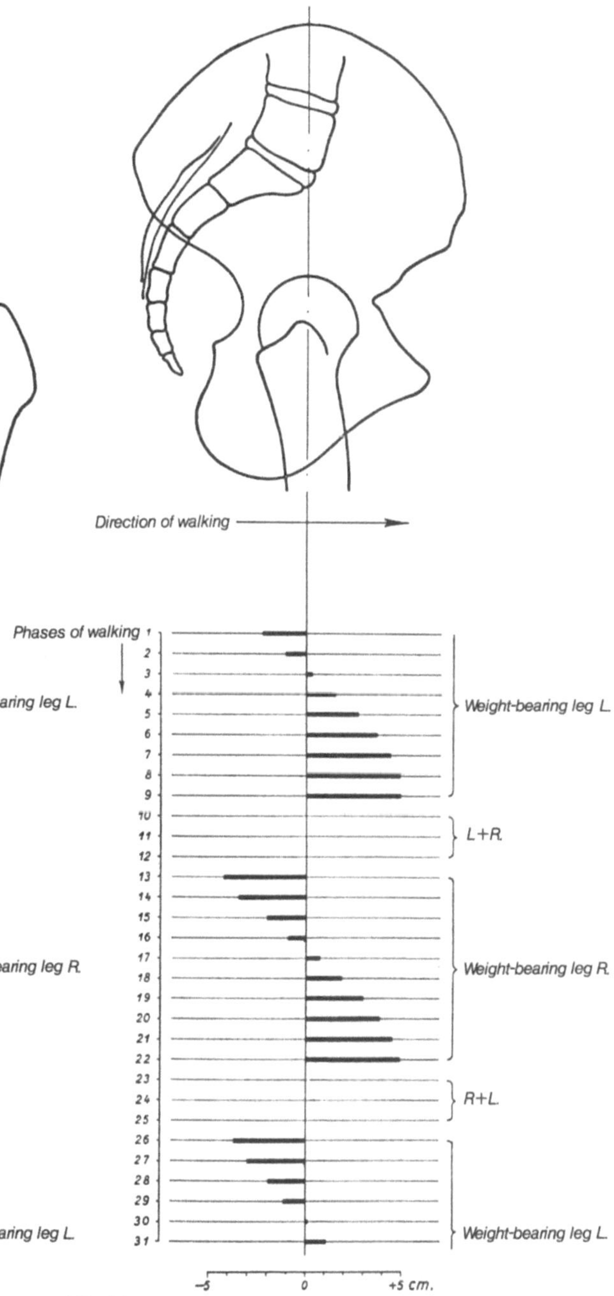

Fig. 24

Figs. 23 and 24. *Line of leverage of body weight viewed in the coronal plane (Fig. 23) and the sagittal plane (Fig. 24) during the weight-bearing phase of walking.* (From "Gesammelte Abhandlungen zur funktionellen Anatomie des Bewegungsapparates" by PAUWELS with kind permission of the author and publisher.)

component of the body weight acts in a torsional sense and very little muscular force is required to maintain the center of gravity over the axis of the hip joint.

b) Completely different conditions occur during walking since when one leg is swung forward the opposite hip takes the weight of the upper body as well as that of the leg which is off the ground. In addition, muscle force is required to prevent tilting of the pelvis to the side of the leg being lifted (abductors) and additional forces are dynamically generated during the sequence of movement.

The forces acting on the head of the femur are the body weight on the medial side and the forces of muscular contraction on the lateral side. PAUWELS took over and developed FISCHER'S work on center of mass by determining the length and direction of the line between the line of action of the body weight and the centre of rotation of the hip in the individual phases of walking.

In the following two illustrations the latter line is shown in the coronal and sagittal planes (Figs. 23, 24). It can be seen that the length of the line remains almost constant throughout the weight-bearing phase.

3.2 Hip Joint and Lower Limb Skeleton

Application of the above principles of action of freely mobile hips shows that on standing and walking there is a repetitive, even distribution of forces along the line of action which passes through the head of the femur, the knee and the ankle joint. There is balanced interplay between the forces acting on the skeleton of the leg (body weight, weight of the non-weight-bearing leg) and the forces of muscle action (adductors and abductors).

3.3 Pelvis and Lumbar Spine

3.3.1 Normal Conditions

If the conditions in the arthrodesed hip correspond to those in the exclusively weight-bearing leg, then the distribution of forces during standing and walking hardly differs from normal. However, correct positioning of the arthrodesed hip is a prerequisite (Fig. 25).

In this case, the pelvis and spine are straight. Symmetrical leg length is, of course, a precondition. For this reason, leg shortening following HA should be corrected by orthotic measures.

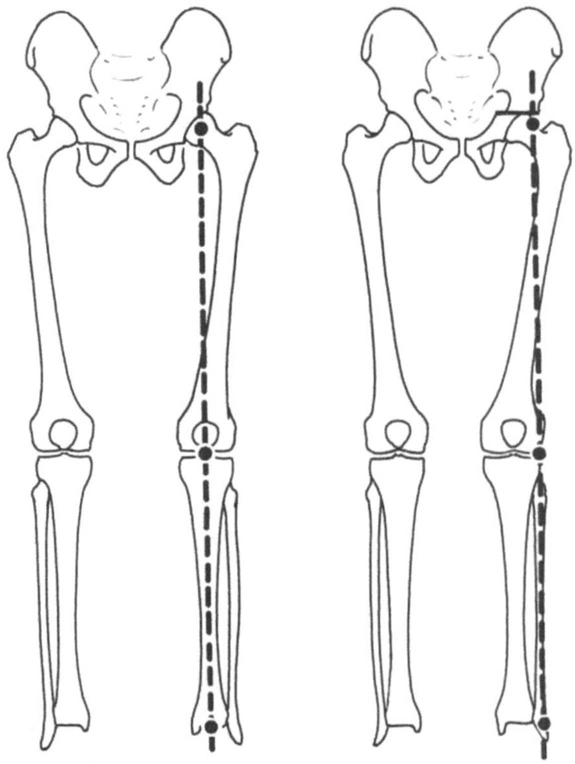

Fig. 25. *Effect of HA on the axis of weight bearing and the leverage exerted by body weight.*

a) The physiological line of weight bearing passes through the centres of the hip, knee and ankle joints.

b) Following HA the axis is displaced somewhat laterally. The leverage exerted by the body weight is reduced on account of the medial displacement following PO

3.3.2 Differences in the Coronal Plane

Differences from normal, whether abduction or adduction, result in tilting of the pelvis which is compensated for by corresponding curvature of the vertebral column (Fig. 26).

3.3.3 Differences in the Sagittal Plane

If the individual stands on both legs and the hip is arthrodesed at the correct angle, there is in the sagittal plane an almost symmetrical distribution of the resultants of body weight and muscle force. The resultants of weight and muscle force increase in proportion to the distance between the joint and the line of loading. An increase in adduction leads to medial displacement of the line of leg loading which may be particularly detrimental in cases of varus knee.

A change in hip position, whether it be flexion or extension, results in tilting of the pelvis. This is detrimental to the lumbar spine since the unphysiological position must be compensated for by an increase or decrease in lordosis (Figs. 27 – 29*).

For this reason, HA is compatible with a gait of normal appearance only if there is *adequate flexibility of the lumbar spine*. This is particularly important in young female patients who obviously have psychological difficulty in adapting to a limp (Fig. 30).

An ideal case of HA requires a lordosis of 20° for maintenance of upright trunk posture. An optimal functional result cannot be expected unless the freedom of movement in relation to the neutral position of the pelvis is distributed in the ratio of one-third lordosis to two-thirds kyphosis (OTTE) (Figs. 31, 32).

Failure to fulfil these conditions (a usual occurrence in older patients) reduces the chances of achieving a gait of normal appearance with comfortable sitting.

* Figs. 27 – 29: From R. MERLE D'AUBIGNÉ et al., "L'arthrodese dans les luxations congenitales de la hanche chez l'adulte" with kind permission of the author.

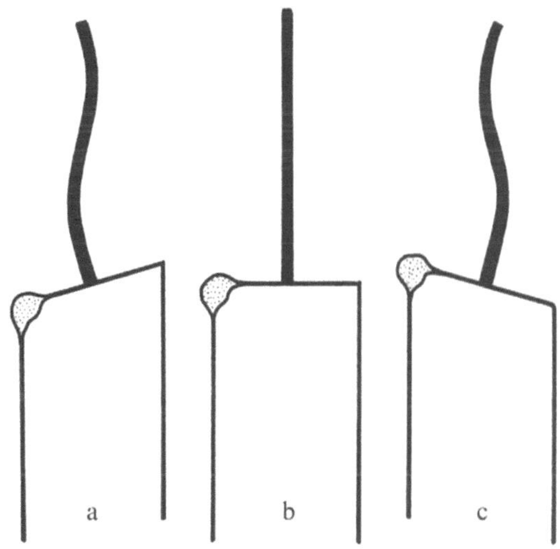

Fig. 26. *Effect of tilting in the coronal plane on the vertebral column.*
a) Stiff hip in abduction.
b) HA correctly performed.
c) Stiff hip in adduction.

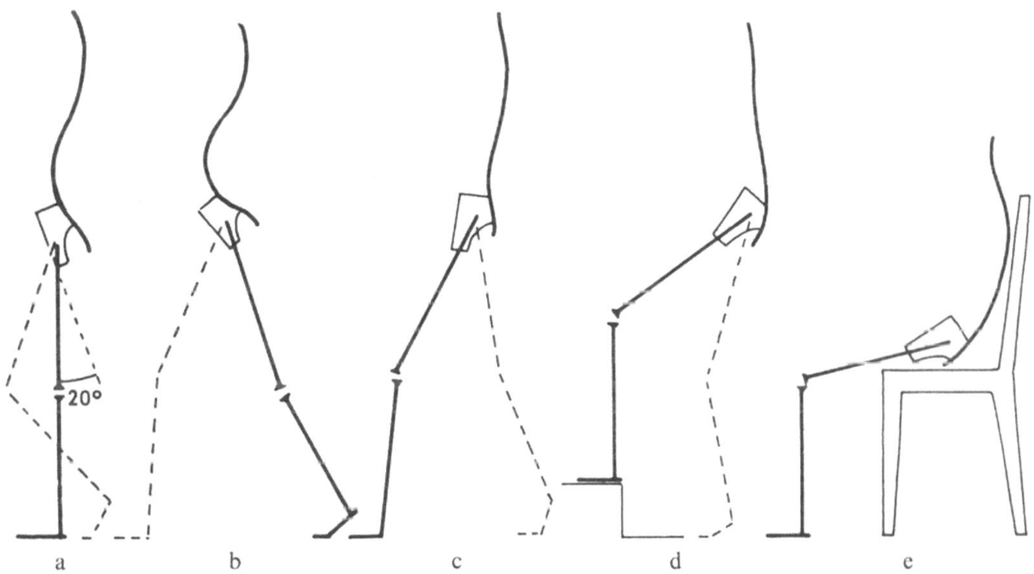

Fig. 27. *HA with 20°* of flexion.*
a) Moderate lordosis when standing on the arthrodesed leg.
b) Marked lordosis on stepping forward with the opposite leg.
c) Physiological lordosis on commencing weight bearing on the arthrodesed leg.
d) Climbing stairs facilitated by reduction of lordosis.
e) Comfortable sitting if adequate kyphosis possible

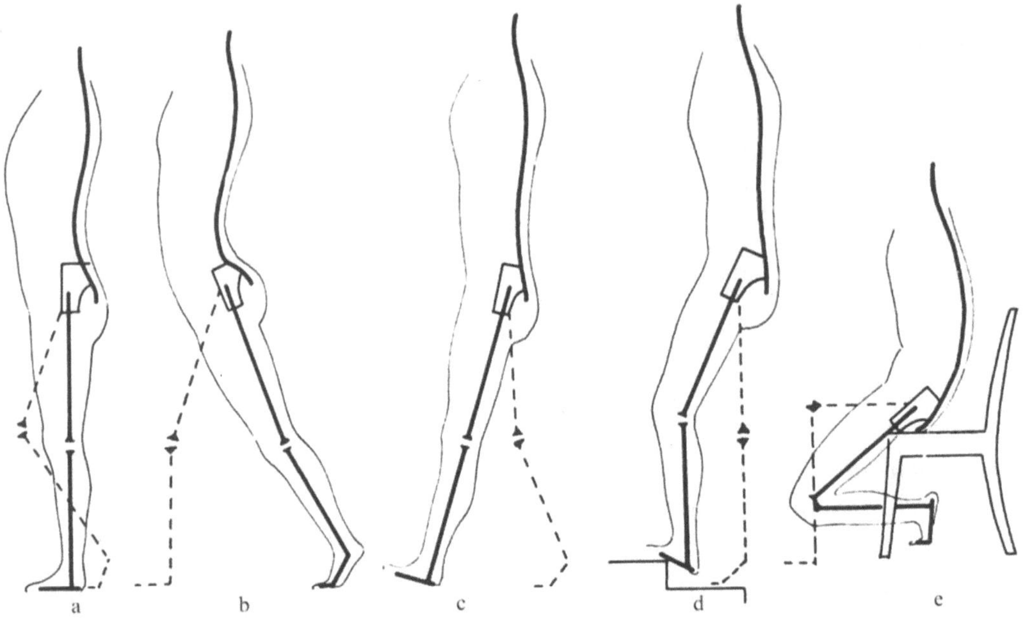

Fig. 28. *HA with 0° of flexion.**

a) Ideal standing on the arthrodesed leg.

b) Lumbar lordosis reserve suffices to allow adequate step forward with opposite leg.

c) Reduced length of pace on arthrodesed side since further pelvic reclination is impossible.

d) Climbing stairs with arthrodesed leg difficult.

e) Sitting uncomfortable

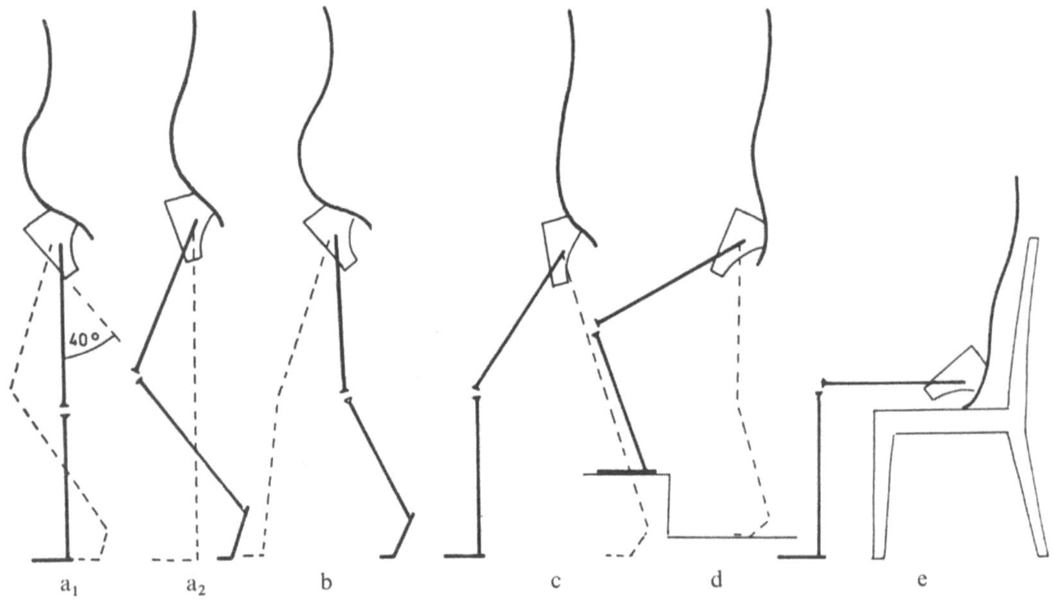

Fig. 29. *HA with 40° of flexion.**

a_1) Standing alone on arthrodesed leg almost impossible because of severe lordosis.

a_2) . . . resulting in increased load on the non-arthrodesed side.

b) Very short non-weight-bearing phase of walking with main action at knee level.

c) Lordosis still present on stepping on to arthrodesed leg.

d) No problems on climbing stairs.

e) Comfortable sitting without severe kyphosis

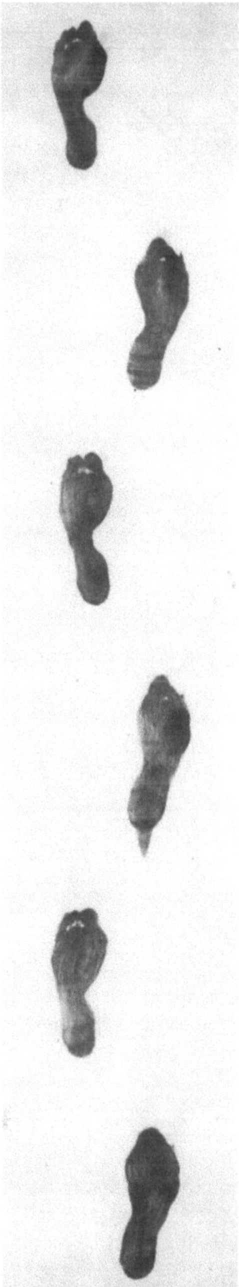

Fig. 30. *Gait following HA*. L. H., ♂, aged 59, No. 153488. Length of pace same on arthrodesed and nonarthrodesed sides

3.3.4 Knee Joint

An intact knee joint on the arthrodesed side is necessary for a good functional result. Total ankylosis or arthrodesis of the ipsilateral knee joint is an *absolute contraindication to HA*. Inadequate flexion of the knee joint is particularly disadvantageous to the patient with an arthrodesis since it renders walking over uneven surfaces more difficult and the patient becomes dependent on others (putting on shoes and tying shoe laces) (Fig. 33).

The significance of valgus or varus angulation also requires explanation. Valgus deformity of the knee joint is particularly disadvantageous since it is almost always increased by HA and particularly by medial displacement (following central dislocation or PO).

A corrective supracondylar osteotomy is indicated if symptoms arise as a result of deformity. This restores symmetrical loading of the condyles.

3.3.5 The Contralateral Hip

This is the last important component to be considered in a discussion of the kinetics of HA. During walking, the total range of movement on the arthrodesed side is concentrated in the form of rotatory motion in the contralateral hip thus severely increasing the functional load on that joint. According to AHLDAUCK and LINDAHL a forward angle of 40° is necessary for a normal step forwards following HA.

With a normal hip extension of 20°, flexion of 20° (measured from the zero position and equal to 40° measured against the fully extended normal hip joint) is necessary for a stride of adequate length (OTTE). A functionally perfect result following HA can therefore be expected only if there is a full range of motion in the contralateral hip.

If flexion is reduced in the contralateral hip, the degree of flexion must be increased in the arthrodesed hip in order to obtain an adequate length of stride. However this is only possible within the already mentioned limits of extension of the lumbar spine.

If the degree of flexion of the arthrodesed hip is inadequate, circumduction occurs and results in increased and frequently painful rotational loading of the mobile hip.

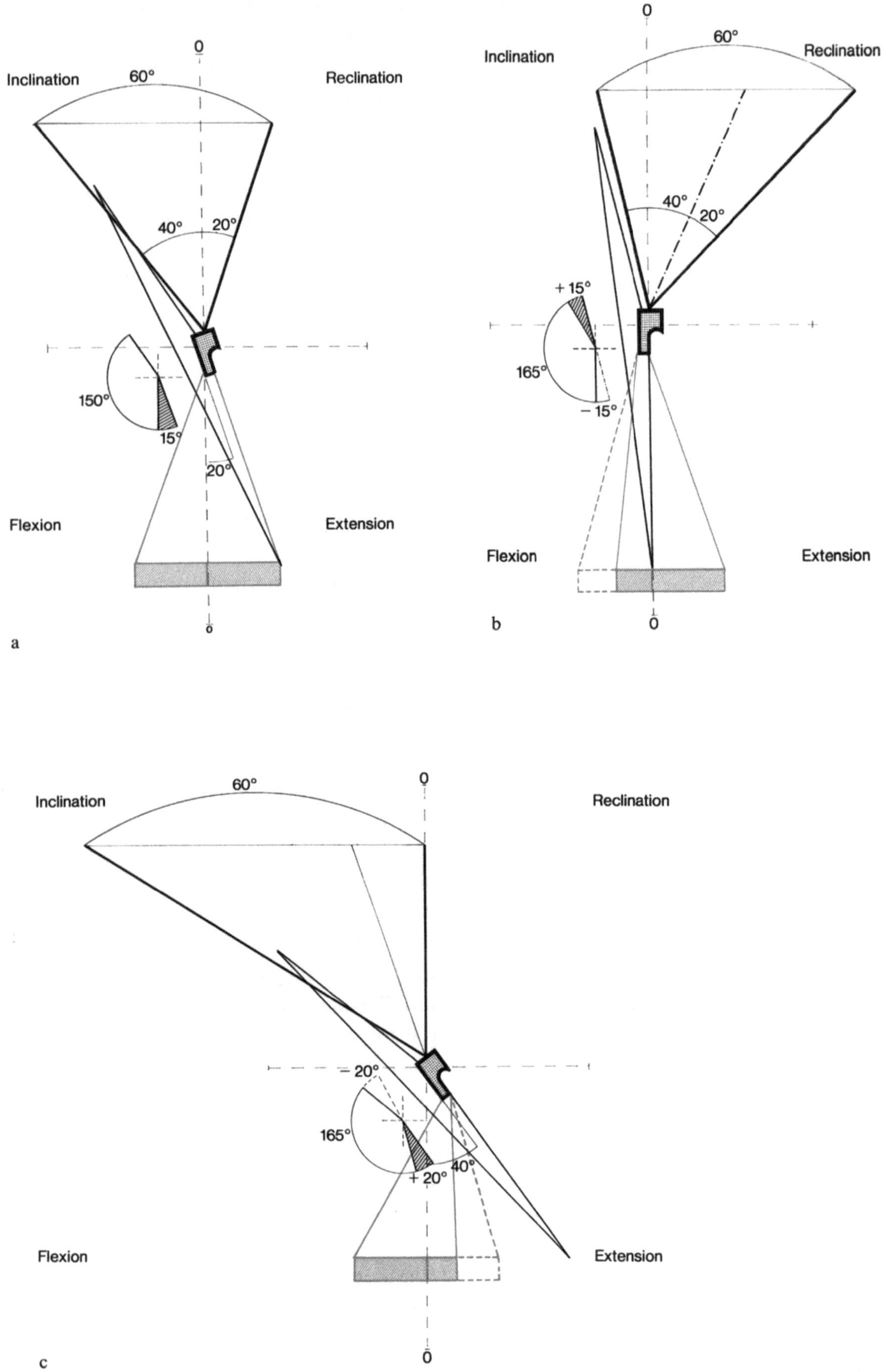
0
Inclination
60°
Reclination
40°
20°
150°
15°
20°
Flexion
Extension
0
a
0
Inclination
60°
Reclination
40°
20°
+15°
165°
−15°
Flexion
Extension
b
0
0
60°
Inclination
Reclination
−20°
165°
+20°
40°
Flexion
Extension
c
0

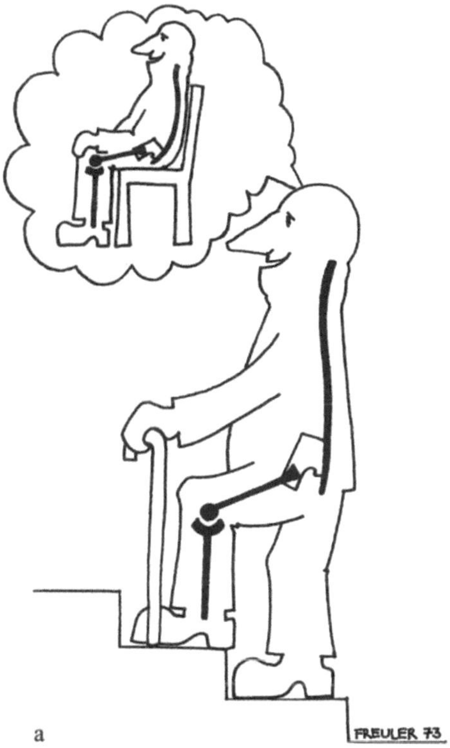

a

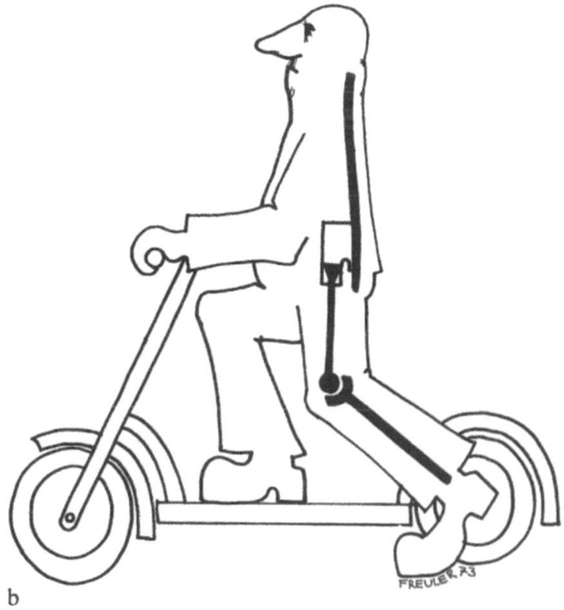

b

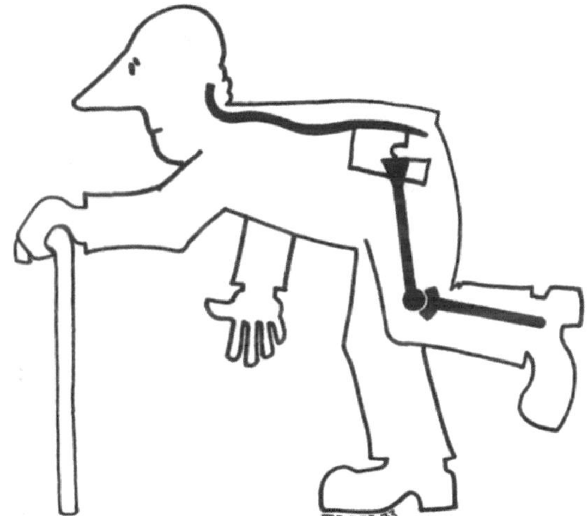

c

Fig. 32. *Effect of arthrodesing the hip in different degrees of flexion.*

a) Correct position (up to 25° flexion). Climbing stairs, walking and sitting with little difficulty.

b) Flexion = 0°. The improved push-off is particularly noticeable when riding a scooter. The forced upright position allows a good view of the traffic.

c) Excessive flexion (greater than 30°). Only for patients who move directly from the sitting position to their target without stopping to stand on the arthrodesed leg

Fig. 31. *Diagrammatic representation of the effects of HA on the spine and on walking (sagittal plane).*

Above: theoretical range of movement between inclination and reclination.

Below (black): theoretical range of flexion/extension (with freely mobile hip).

Below (red): Non-weight-bearing phase of walking following arthrodesis.

a) Flexion = 20°; inclination: reclination = $^2/_3$:$^1/_3$; normal non-weight-bearing phase of walking.

b) Flexion = 0°; pushing off on arthrodesed leg satisfactory but shortened non-weight-bearing phase since further reclination impossible.

c) Flexion = 40°; reverse of above. Short pushing-off phase, stepping on to arthrodesed leg good. Duration of non-weight-bearing phase similarly reduced since further inclination is impossible

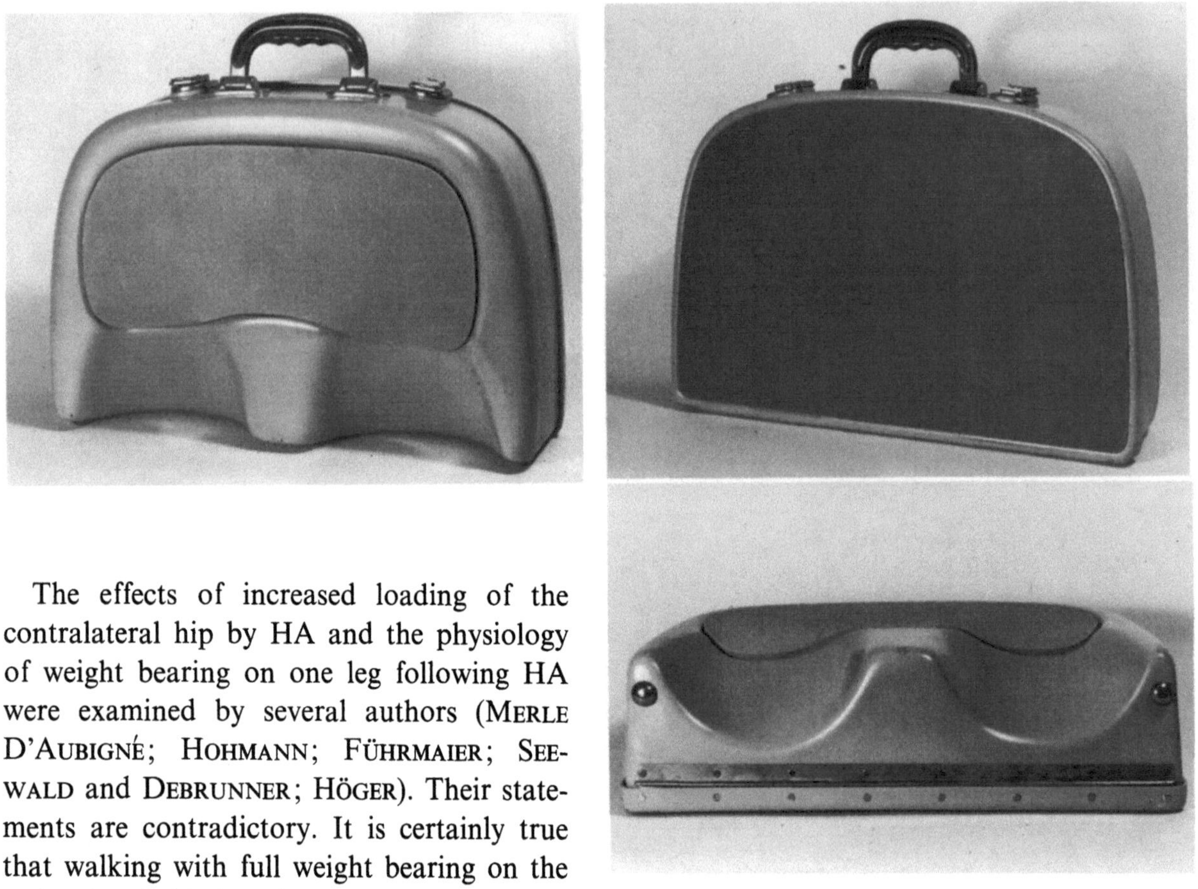

The effects of increased loading of the contralateral hip by HA and the physiology of weight bearing on one leg following HA were examined by several authors (MERLE D'AUBIGNÉ; HOHMANN; FÜHRMAIER; SEEWALD and DEBRUNNER; HÖGER). Their statements are contradictory. It is certainly true that walking with full weight bearing on the arthrodesed side is only possible if there is no pain and full stability. It is also indisputable that HA results in prolongation of the non-weight-bearing phase of locomotion on the operated side.

Fig. 33. *Aids for arthrodesis patients*

a) Portable "suitcase-seat". This facilitates sitting on low chairs.

b) Suspenders attached to tapes facilitate pulling on stockings in the upright position.

c) Objects can be easily picked up from the floor with extended tongs

4 Biomechanics of Individual Hip Arthrodeses

4.1 Introduction

Countless methods of HA have been described subsequent to that of ALBERT (1886) and new methods are still being described. Up to the present, no one method has prevailed, which proves that the associated problems have not yet been definitively solved.

The first HA operations were carried out by simple freshening of the joint surface and frequently failed, mainly because complete ankylosis failed to occur. For this reason, a biomechanical solution was looked for which would create a biological environment more conducive to ossification in the hip. Two approaches were taken:

a) changes in hip geometry (by IO, CHARNLEY's "central dislocation" or the PO described by MÜLLER).
b) stabilisation by internal fixation (ranging from adaptation osteosynthesis to stable internal fixation).

A discussion of the biomechanics of individual arthrodesis procedures now follows.

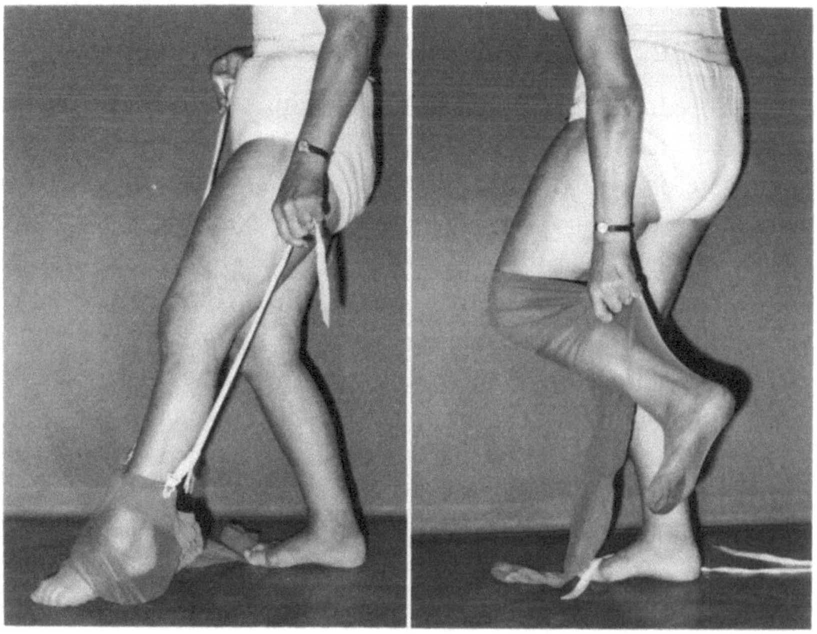

b

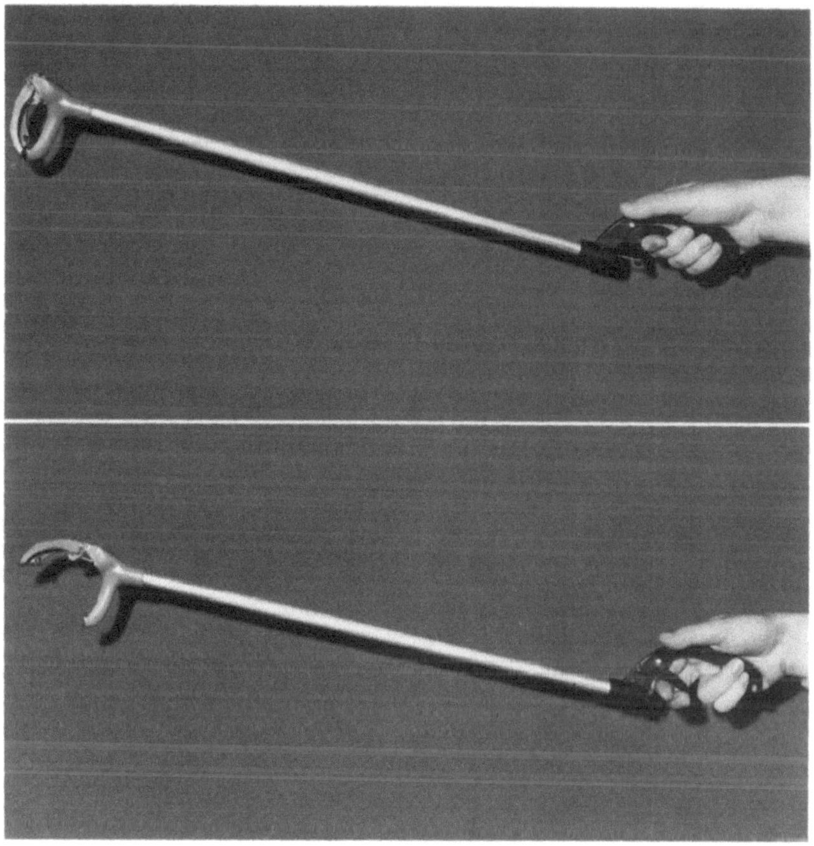

c

Fig. 33 b, c Legend on page 22

4.2 Arthrodesis by Resection of the Joint Surfaces

In this procedure the anatomical relationships are largely retained. The frequent failures (inadequate or totally absent bone union) are due to the absence of stabilising factors.

Adequate immobilisation of the head of the femur is prevented by the forces generated by the excessive leverage of the long femur.

IO reduces the leverage on the head of the femur and thus isolates it from the greater part of the forces which would otherwise act on it. In this manner, adequate immobilisation can be obtained by a simple internal fixation (Fig. 34).

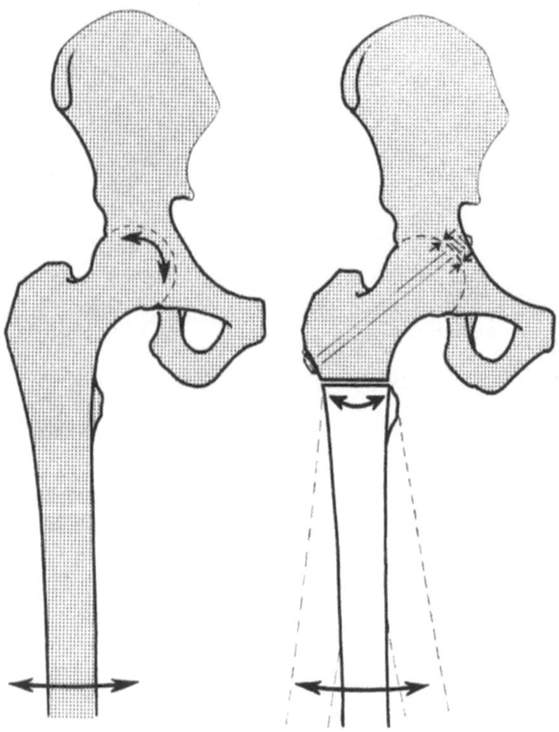

Fig. 34. *Effect of IO on HA*. Less movement is transmitted to the joint from the distal femur

4.3 Extra-articular Hip Arthrodeses

A bridge graft between the femur and the pelvis is the basis of these HA procedures. The aim of the graft is to bring about extra-articular bone union between the pelvis and the femur. The graft is placed either proximally (ALBEE and modifications) or distally (TRUMBLE, BRITTAIN and others) (Fig. 35). The graft placed proximally to the joint is mainly under tension and that distal to the joint is mainly under compression. The latter is surely more advantageous from a biomechanical point of view.

4.4 Hip Arthrodeses with Central Dislocation

Central dislocation increases the contact area, brings about a more intimate union between femoral head and pelvis and results in medial displacement. Thus, with the exception of flexion-extension movement, a degree of intrinsic stability is achieved. However, detrimental loading of the neck of the femur occurs which in practice leads to fatigue fractures (Fig. 36).

4.5 Hip Arthrodesis with Pelvic Osteotomy

PO and medial displacement also ensure a large area of contact in cancellous bone which increases stability and promotes bone union. Usually the proximal end of the femur is remoulded to such an extent that the femur and the pelvis form a single column (Fig. 37).

Thus, on loading, the forces are transmitted directly from the pelvis to the femoral diaphysis. It is largely on account of this that early postoperative partial weight bearing is possible.

Medial displacement results in static and kinetic changes in the skeleton of the lower limb. These have already been discussed (Pp. 14, 16).

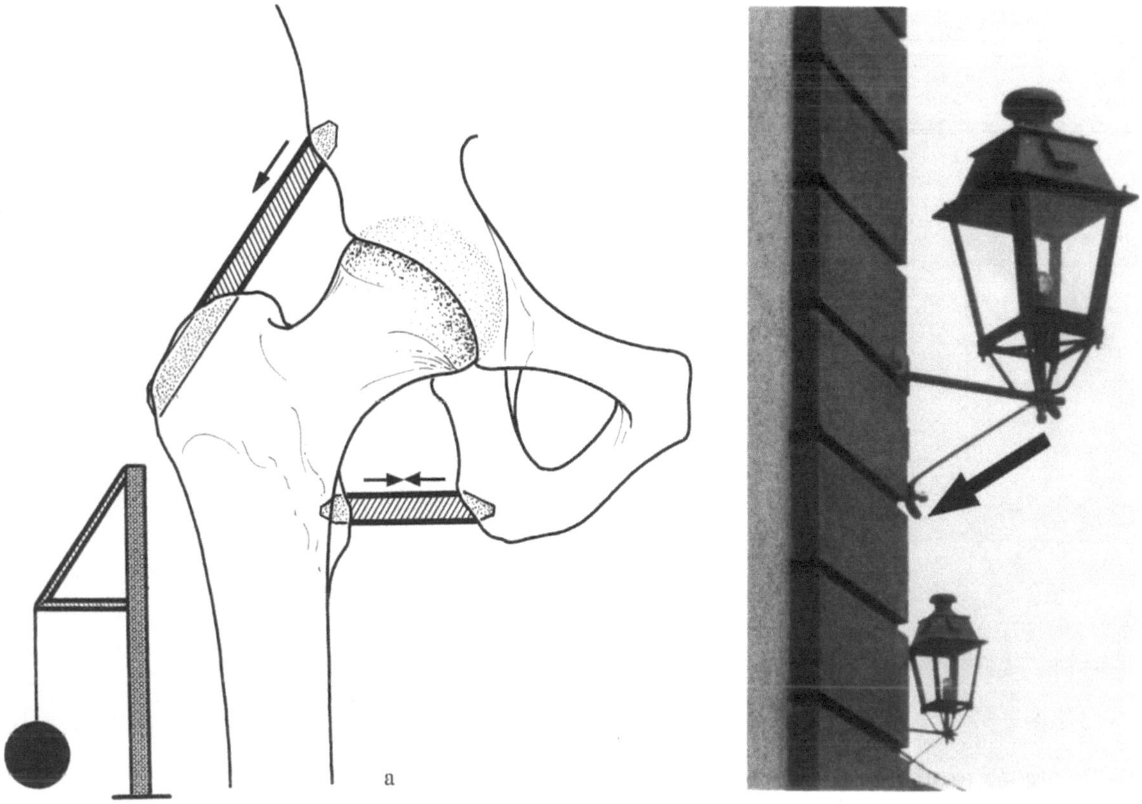

a

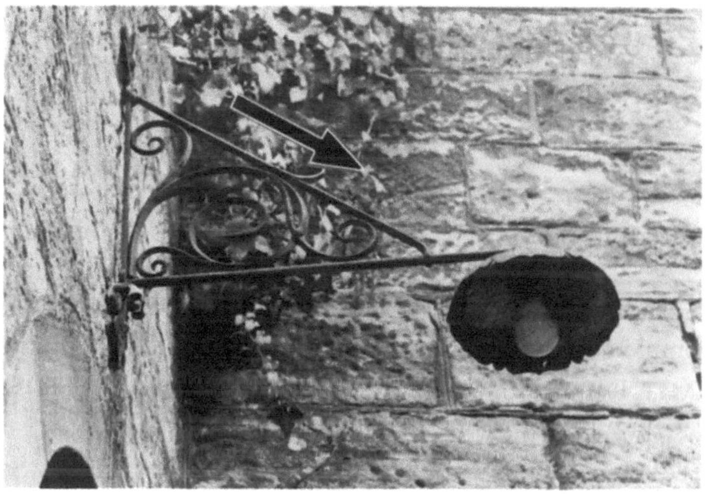

c

Fig. 35. *Extra-articular HA*. The iliofemoral graft is mainly under tension (cf. Fig. 35c). The ischio-femoral graft is mainly under compression (cf. Fig. 35b)

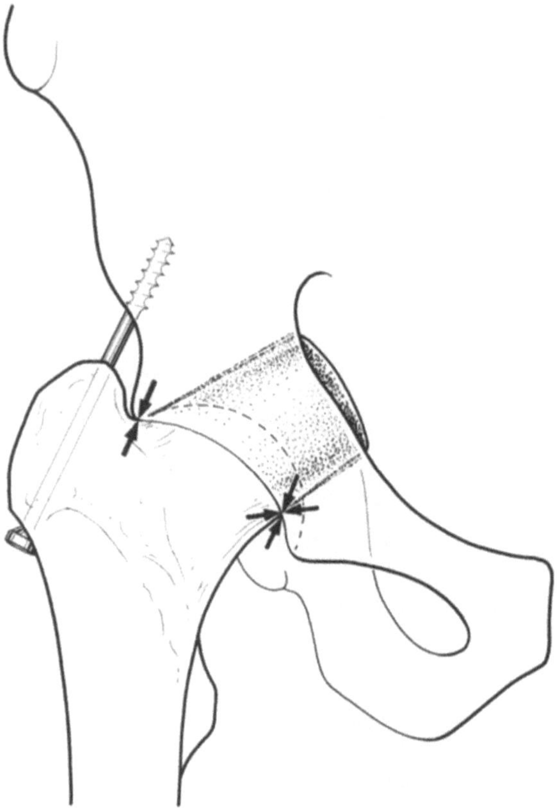

Fig. 36. *The Charnley technique: HA with central dislocation.* The stress concentration at the point shown explains the fatigue fractures which are frequently observed

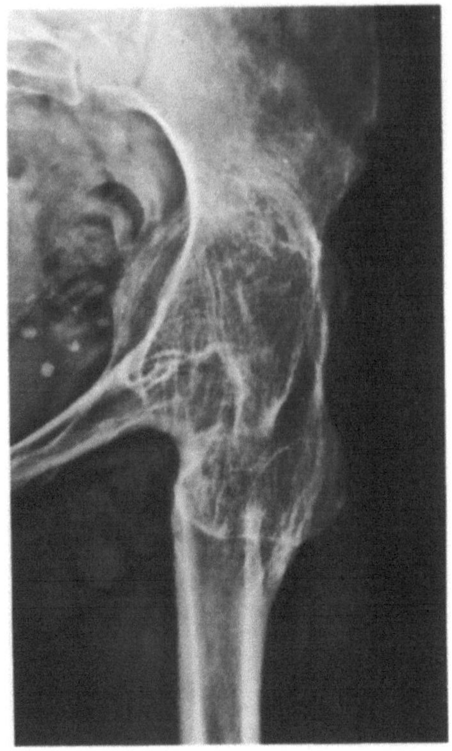

Fig. 37. *Example of column formation following HA.* R. A., ♂ aged 64, No. 125163. Three years following HA

5 Biomechanics and Technique of Internal Fixation in Hip Arthrodesis

5.1 Introduction

Nowadays, practically all HA procedures are complemented by stable internal fixation. Every internal fixation involves stabilisation and, in addition, compression adaptation of the contact surfaces between femur and pelvis. Minimal internal fixation (HA in infected cases) must also provide adequate rigidity.

Precise attention to the internal fixation technique required for each type of HA should always result in a successful operation (complete bone union with correct positioning of leg) (Figs. 38, 39).

Internal fixation almost always involves compression. The operative techniques used in the different types of arthrodesis which we have carried out will now be individually discussed.

5.2 Type I Hip Arthrodesis

Freshening of the joint surfaces, fixation of the greater trochanter as an iliofemoral bridge graft, IO).

Internal fixation is carried out using compression screws.

5.2.1 Screw Fixation of the Iliofemoral Bridge Graft

(Greater trochanter applied to the pelvis). A cancellous bone compression screw is used with a washer. The screw thread must be entirely buried in bone. The screw obtains an optimum hold if the thread passes through the medial cortex of the pelvis. It is placed at a right angle to the pelvic bone (Figs. 40 – 42).

a

c

d

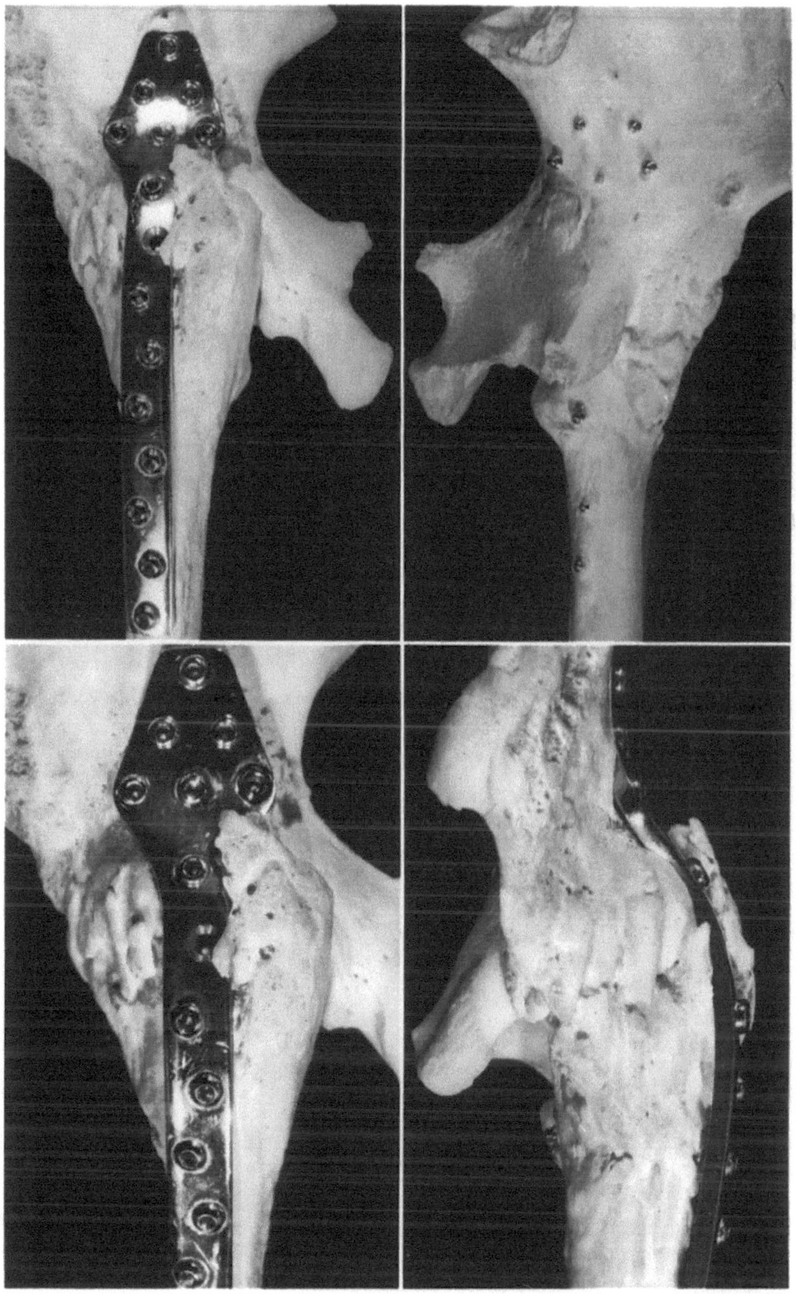

Figs. 38 and 39. *Complete bone union following cobra-head plate arthrodesis,*

Figs. 38a – 38d. *Without pelvic osteotomy.* Original joint no longer recognisable. Excessive callus formation around the proximal part of the plate

a b

c d

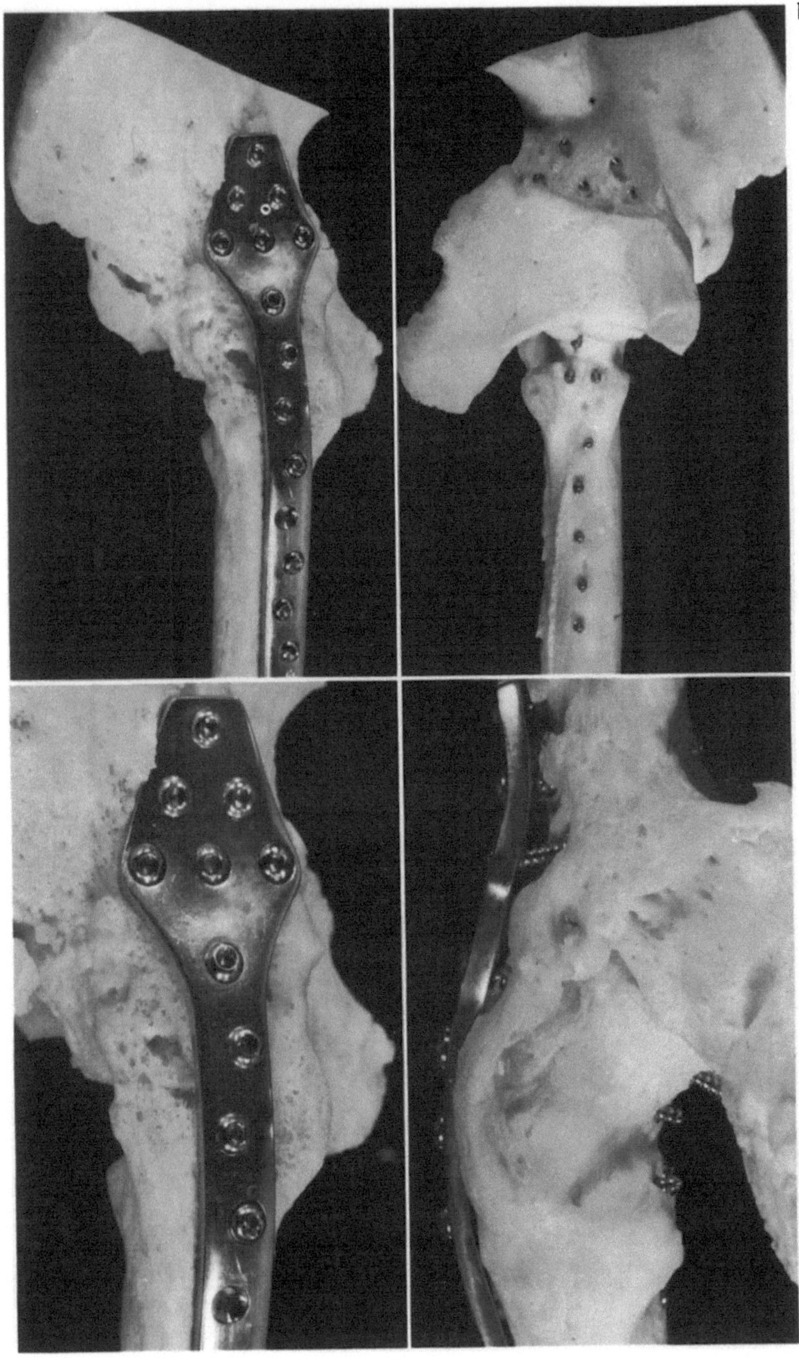

Figs. 39a – 39d. *With pelvic osteotomy.* The space between the plate and the head of the femur has been completely filled with bone (trochanteric graft and formation of a bone bridge between the pelvis and the proximal femur)

Fig. 41. *Type I HA.* L. B., ♀, aged 56, No. 84869

a) Before operation

b) Immediately following operation

c) 10 months later. Bone union has occurred

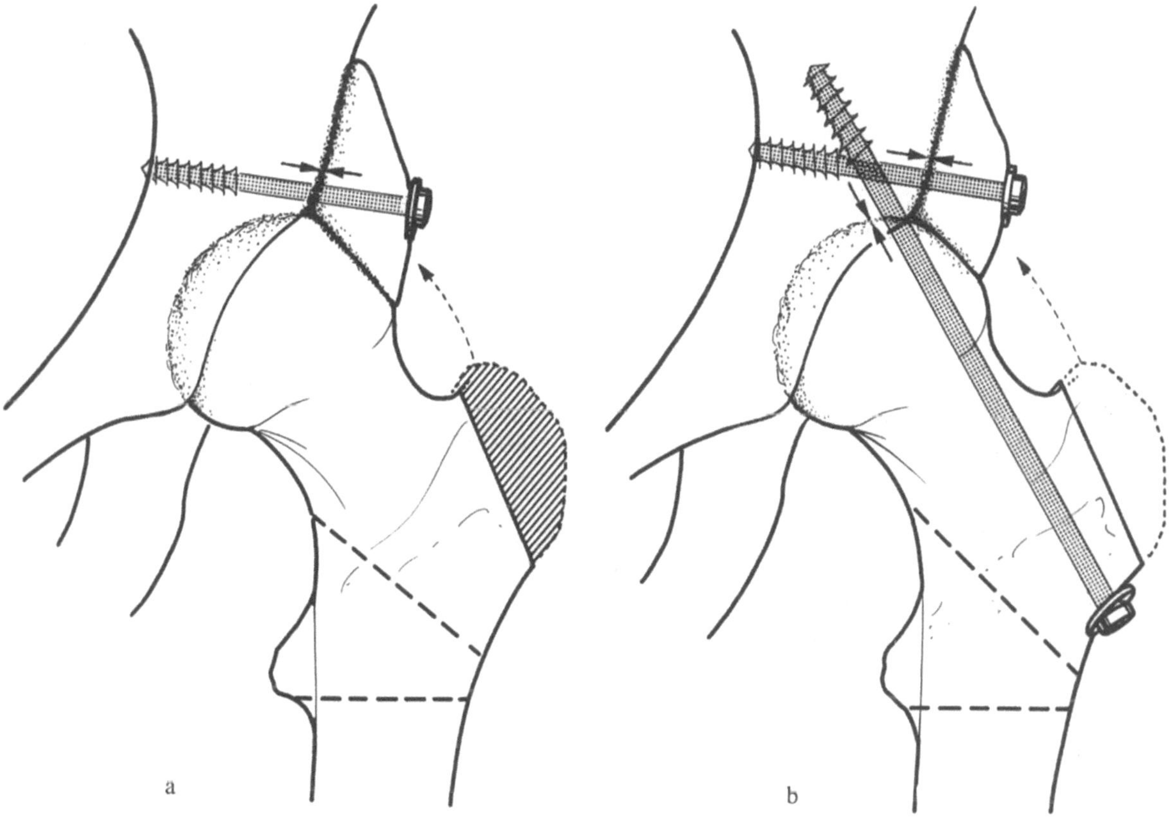

Fig. 40. *Type I HA.*

a) The iliofemoral trochanteric bridge graft is fixed to the pelvis with a cortex screw. The previous high IO and the subsequent intertrochanteric/subtrochanteric osteotomy are shown with interrupted lines.

b) Additional fixation of the proximal femur to the pelvis using a cancellous bone screw

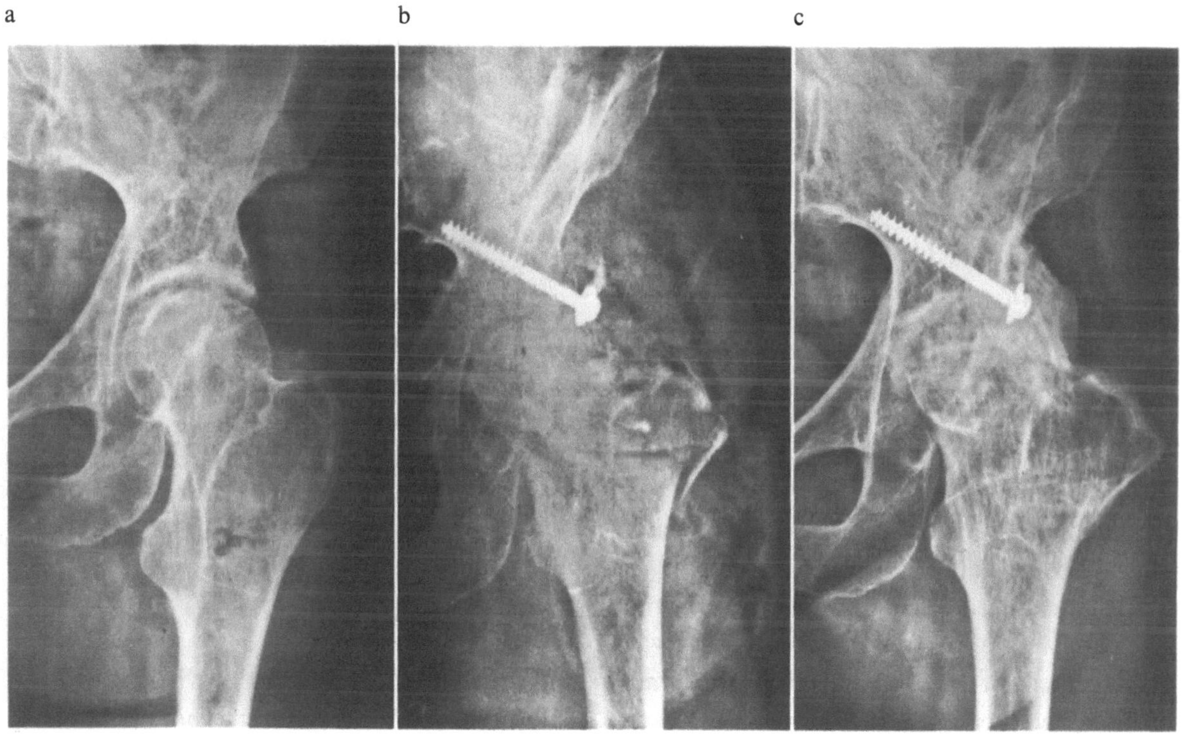

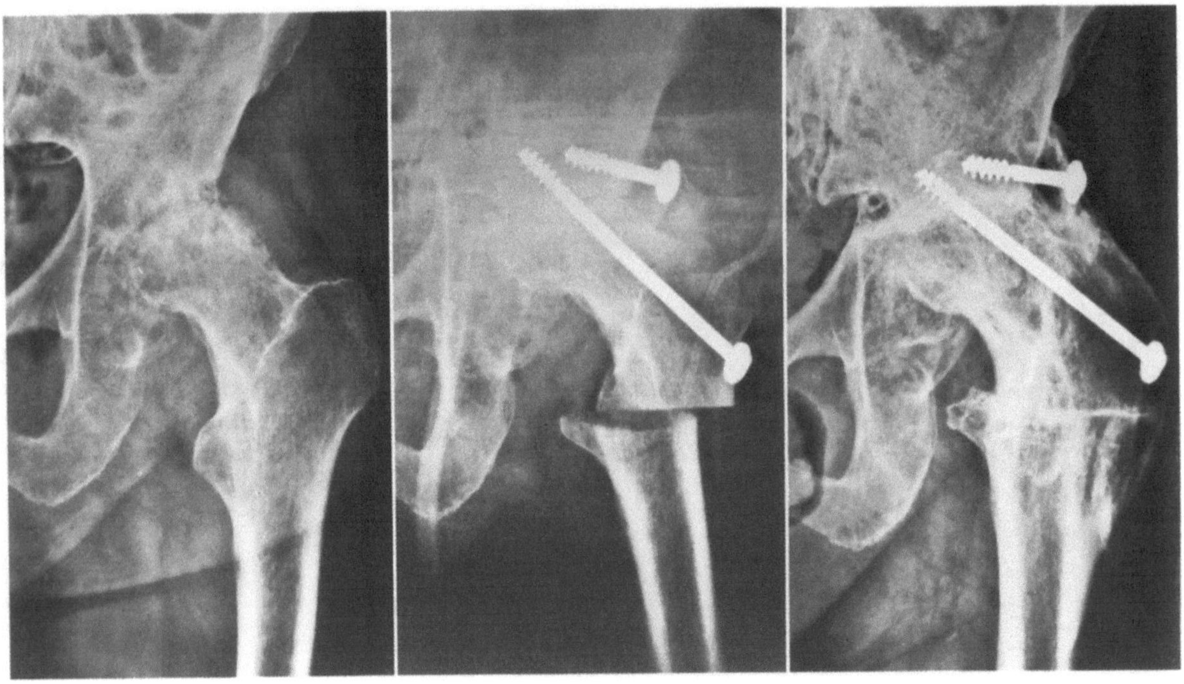

a b c

Fig. 42. *Type I HA*. S. A., ♀, aged 78, No. 142927
a) Before operation
b) Immediately following operation
c) Two years later. Complete union

5.2.2 Screw Fixation of the Proximal End of the Femur to the Pelvis

Both joint surfaces are freshened or resected and a cancellous bone compression screw with a short thread is inserted in the direction of the femoral neck. This screw should also be screwed into the medial cortex of the pelvis (Fig. 43). Both cases described involve pure compression internal fixations.

5.3 Type II Hip Arthrodesis

(Freshening or resection of the joint surfaces, internal plate fixation; IO.)

A plate is used for internal fixation. It may act purely as a buttress, preventing upward displacement of the proximal end of the femur, or it may be used to exert compression.

5.3.1 Buttress Plate

A plate which is to function purely as a buttress is fixed only to the pelvis. Generally, three cortex screws are used in conjuction with a broad six-hole plate. Since the plate is to prevent upward displacement of the proximal end of the femur, it should be bent so that its distal part exerts lateral compression on the latter (Figs. 44, 45).

This technique is seldom indicated and only in cases when later correction of leg length is required, e.g., following GIRDLESTONE hips (GH) which are first fixed in slight abduction and then a few weeks later compressed by adduction.

5.3.2 Compression Plate

This technique is indicated when improved stability is required or severe changes in pelvic

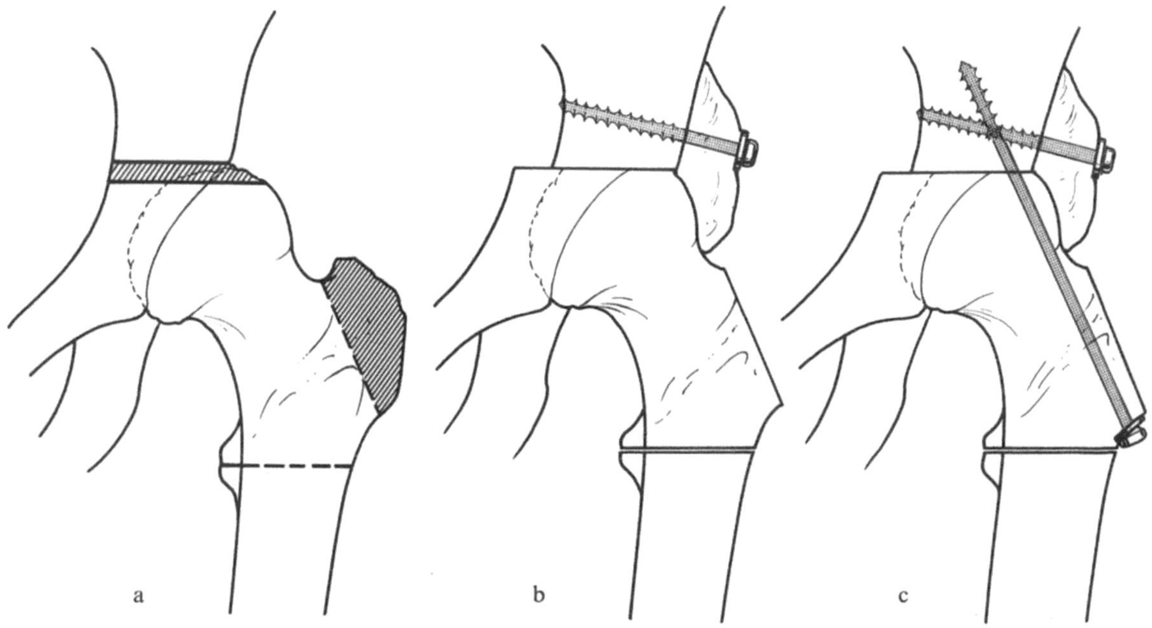

Fig. 43. *Type I HA* with *PO*.

a) The cross hatching indicates the PO and the greater trochanter which is to be removed.

b) Following PO and screw fixation of the iliofemoral trochanteric graft.

c) Further screw fixation of the proximal femur to the pelvis

anatomy render the use of the cobra-head plate impossible. An IO is always carried out at the same time.

First the proximal part of the plate is fixed to the pelvis with three cortex screws. During this procedure the leg should be maintained in slight adduction in order to position the femoral neck more vertically. The special compressor is then placed in position across the angle. The screw which is used to fix the compressor should subtend an angle of 15° to an imaginary line which is at 90° to the long axis of the femur. The plate is then tensioned and fixed with screws. The IO is then carried out (Fig. 46).

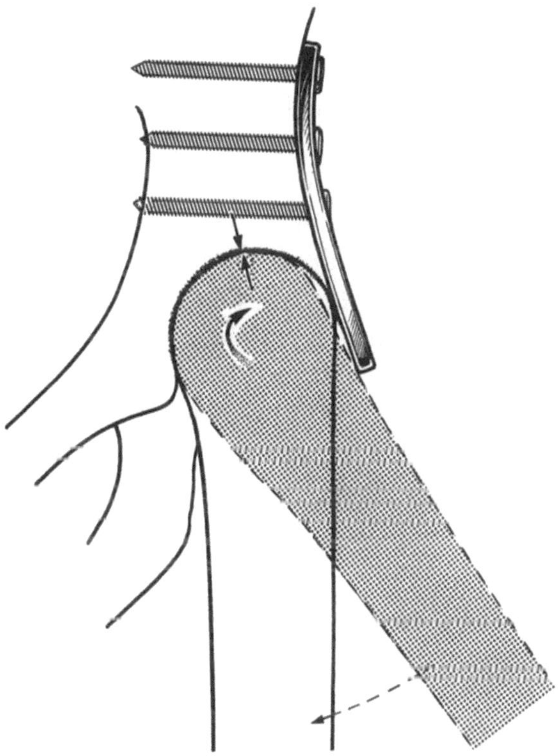

Fig. 44. *Type II HA with buttress plate*. The final leg position is adjusted a few weeks later. The plate keeps the head of the femur in the acetabulum. Adduction increases the pressure on the arthrodesis

5.4 Type III Hip Arthrodesis

(Freshening or resection of the joint surfaces, stable internal fixation with two plates.)

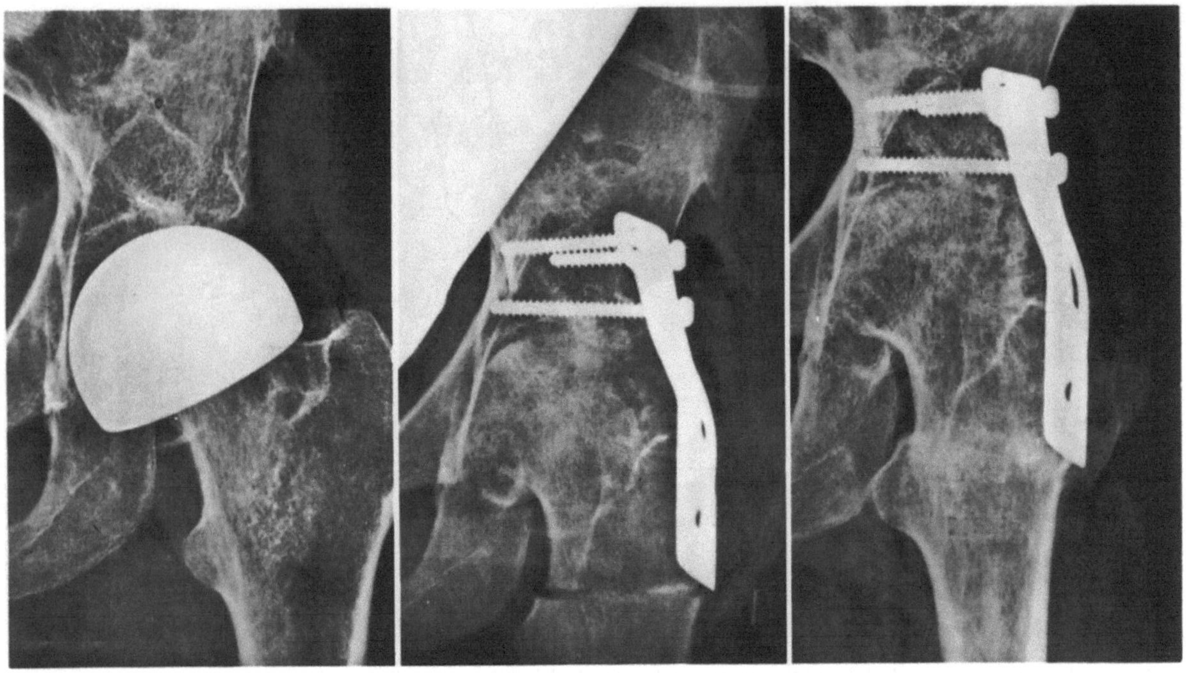

Fig. 45. *Type II HA with buttress plate following cup arthroplasty.* M. M., ♀, aged 21, No. 89399.

a) Before arthrodesis

b) The proximal femur is compressed by appropriate bending of the distal plate.

c) Three months later. IO union complete, HA union almost complete

The internal fixation comprises two plates which are at right angles to each other in two planes. This was the first completely stable internal fixation performed by us which allowed immediate mobilisation of the patient without postoperative cast fixation. In 1966 it was replaced by the cobra-head plate. Nowadays it is only occasionally used in the treatment of PA.

Following PO, the broad lateral 10-hole or 12-hole plate is screwed to the pelvis, placed under compression and fixed with screws. The anterior plate is then screwed into place in a similar manner. In the majority of cases, the broad (usually 8-hole) plate suffices (Figs. 47, 48).

5.5 Type IV Hip Arthrodesis

(Freshening or resection of the joint surfaces; usually pelvic osteotomy; stable internal fixation with a cobra-head plate.)

5.5.1 Correct Technique

Of all the methods with which we are familiar, arthrodesis using a cobra-head plate provides the greatest stability. However, correct application of a well contoured plate is a prerequisite. This is carried out as follows. Following PO and bending of the plate to fit the bone contours, the plate is temporarily fixed with the central screw 5 – 10 mm above and parallel to the osteotomy. The use of a single screw allows simple adjustment of leg flexion. The plate is then gently tensioned with the plate tensioner and the desired position of the extremity is checked with the special device. At this point, one should bear in mind that subsequent tensioning of the plate will produce abduction of 10°. *This implies that the leg should be in 15° of adduction before the plate is tensioned* (Fig. 49). The remaining screws are inserted in the head of the plate. The plate is then tensioned. Frequently the tensioning is overdone, thus

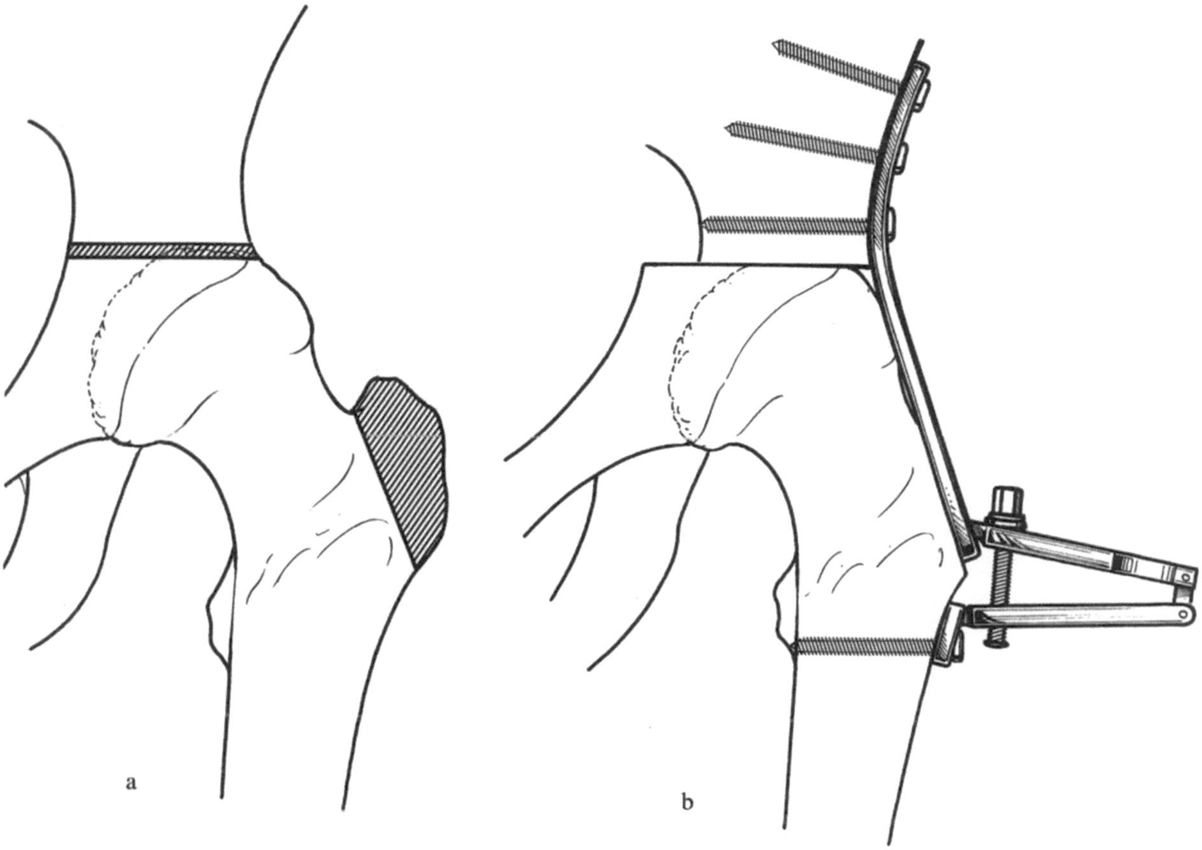

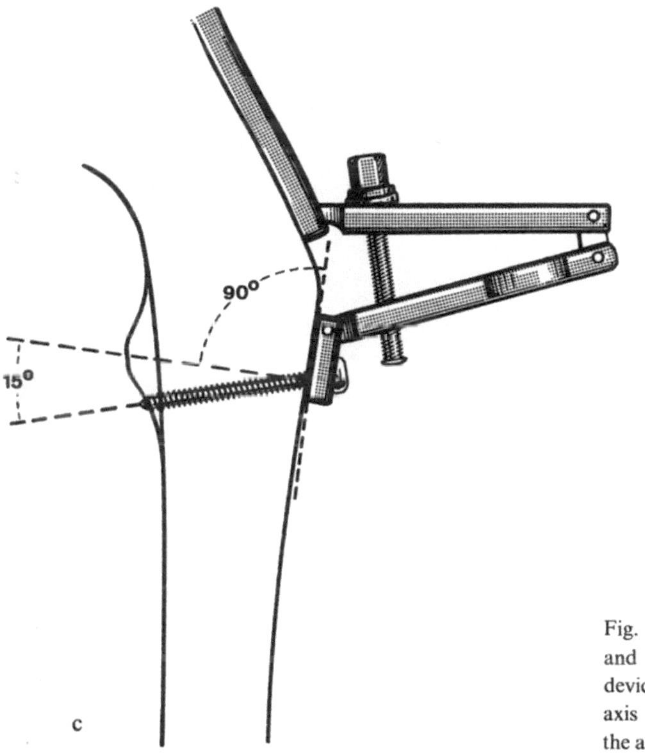

Fig. 46. *Type II HA*. The proximal plate is fixed to the pelvis and the plate is then tensioned. Using the special tensioning device which is fixed with a screw which is at 75° to the long axis of the femur, considerable tension can be applied despite the angulation

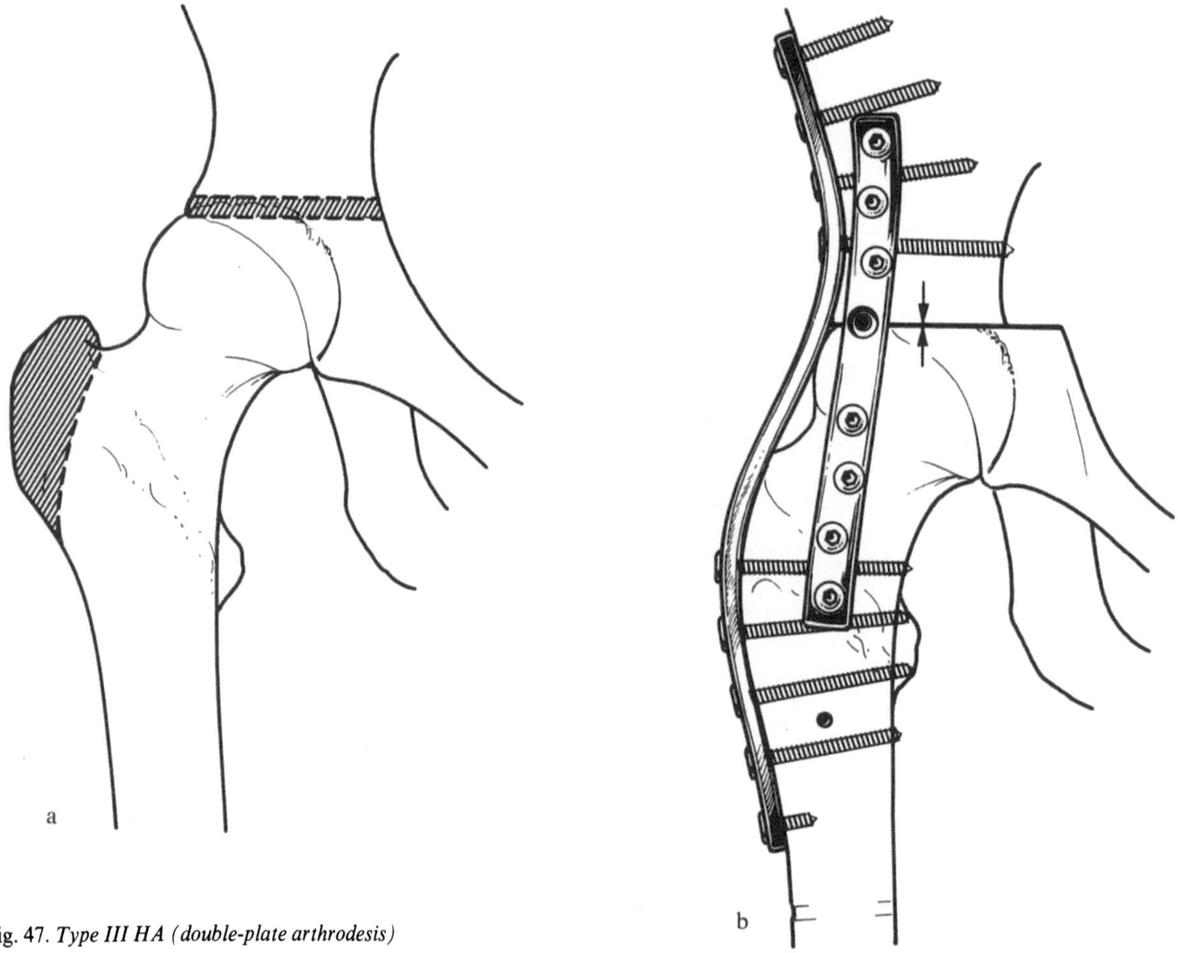

Fig. 47. *Type III HA (double-plate arthrodesis)*

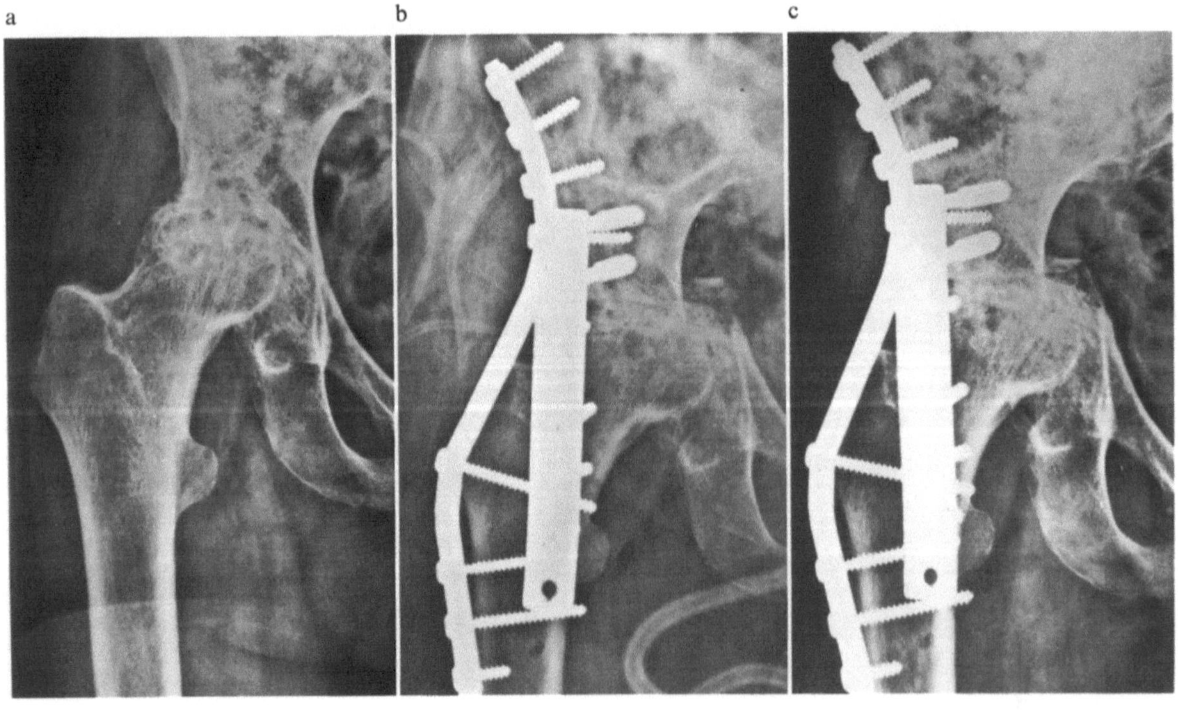

Fig. 49. *Correct leg position*

a) Before tensioning the cobra-head plate. On tensioning the plate abduction of at least 10° occurs. The leg should therefore be placed in 10° – 15° adduction before tensioning.

b) Following tensioning of the plate the gap no longer gapes laterally

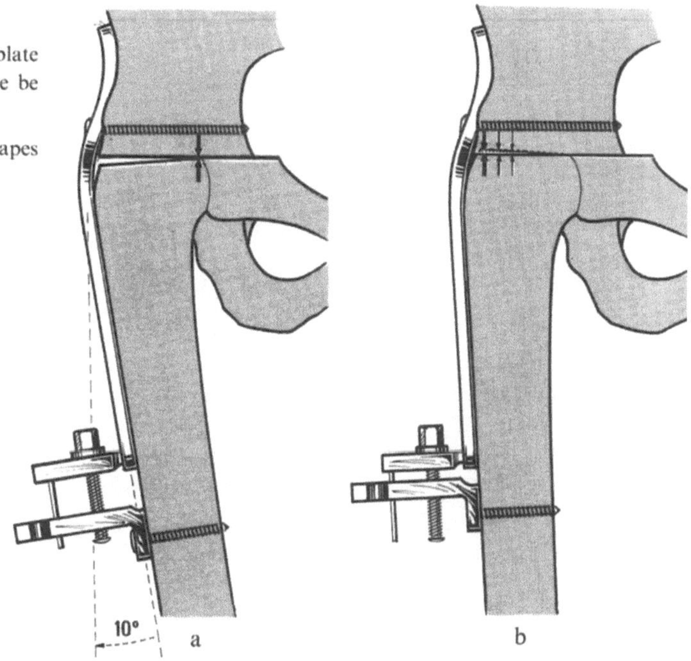

causing gaping of the osteotomy when the plate is fixed.

5.5.2 Incorrect Technique

Failure to bend the plate correctly so that it fits snugly against the bone or incorrect application of the plate are both biomechanically detrimental and result in unstable internal fixation. This in turn leads to failure of the arthrodesis (loosening of the metal or PA). The cobra-head plate should not be placed too high up. The dense pelvic bone (i.e., the roof of the acetabulum) proffers the best anchorage.

Inadequate or poor contouring of the cobra-head plate reduces the tension-band effect of the plate. The best of tried and tested surgical or orthopaedic techniques may fail if the operator has failed to understand its principles or to perform the operation correctly. For example, the strongest of implant material used in the operative treatment of fractures is bound to fail if instability causes it to be subjected to severe tension, compression or shear forces. If, on the other hand, the biomechanical circumstances are correctly assessed and adequate account is taken of the prevailing skeletal geometry and the correct operation is then carried out, the implant material which would otherwise have failed will prove adequate to the task. Depending on the culinary ability of the cook, a well-hung tender piece of meat may be converted into a tasty delicacy or into an indigestible piece of leather. In a similar manner, the stability of an internal fixation depends not only on the quality of the implant material used but also on the appropriateness of its use and the skill with which it is implanted. The best of tools is useless in the hands of a bad workman. The biomechanically beneficial factors in cobra-head plate arthrodesis are discussed in detail on pp. 77, 82–84.

Fig. 48. *Example of a Type III HA*. N. D., ♂, aged 28, No. 100637.

a) Before operation.

b) Immediately following double-plate arthrodesis.

c) Eight months later. Clinical and radiological HA union

KALÉN (1968) published an extensive work on the dependence of the immediate postoperative stability of HA on the type of internal fixation used. The results derived from his experiments on cobra-head plate arthrodesis

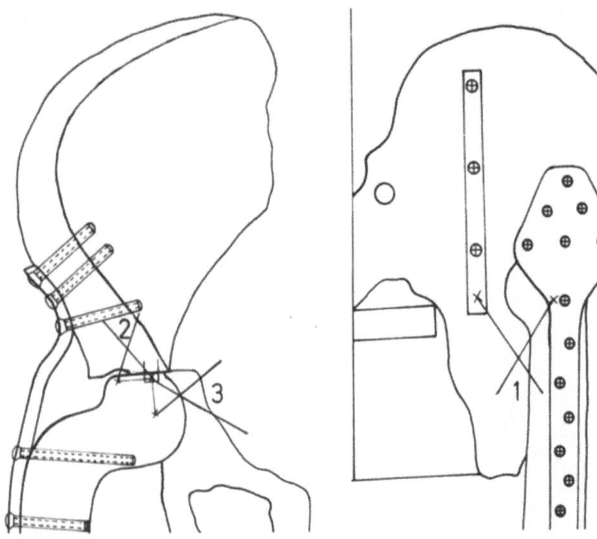

Fig. 50. *Original diagram of the experimental set-up used by* KALÉN

cannot be evaluated since the plates were incorrectly applied. KALÉN's original drawings of his experimental setup (Fig. 50) show the cobra-head plate anchored too high up. The lower row of three parallel screws in the cobra head should lie approximately 5 mm above and parallel to the PO. In addition, the plate was incorrectly bent to fit the bone so that there was inadequate direct contact between the implant and the bone, particularly at the iliofemoral junction. Finally, there is inadequate contact between the osteotomy surfaces (see Fig. 51). This is a result of excessive medial displacement of the distal pelvic component. One may also assume that it was morphologically impossible to apply adequate compression across the contact surfaces by tensioning the plate since this would have resulted in abduction deformity. The biomechanical situation in the case shown must be regarded as disadvantageous. In order to obtain worthwhile experimental results, the fit of the cobra-head plate and the PO should be as illustrated in Figures 95–97. Elastometric investigations have shown that correct contouring of the plate results in good distribution of the prevailing forces over the whole contact surface, especially if there is moderate medial displacement following PO and pretensioning of the plate.

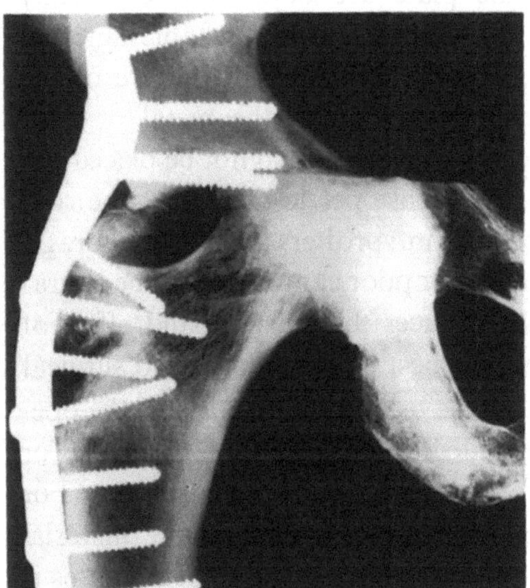

Fig. 51. *Example of a cobra-head plate arthrodesis taken from the publication by* KALÉN. Inadequate contact between the osteotomy surfaces.
Plate inadequately bent to fit the bone. (Figs. 50 and 51 are reproduced with kind permission of the author.)

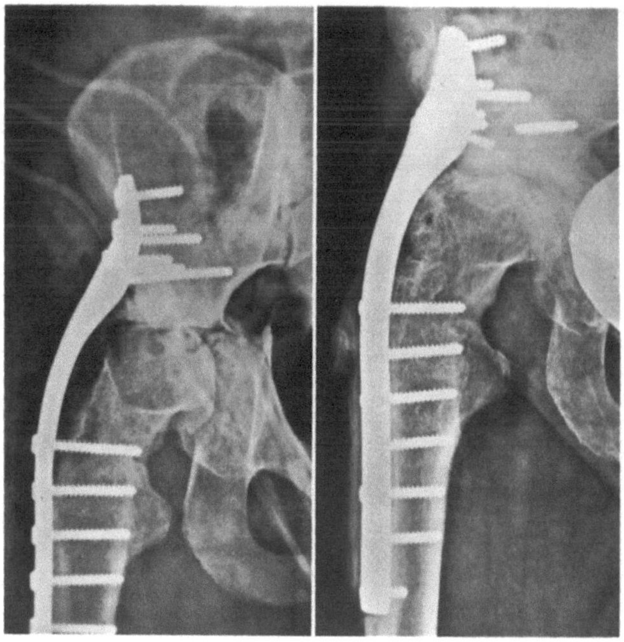

Fig. 52. *Pseudarthrosis as a result of incorrect cobra-head plate arthrodesis technique*. F. R., ♀, aged 28, No. 64572.

a) The cobra-head plate has been applied too far above the osteotomy. In addition to pure compression, shear forces are generated at the level of the arthrodesis. Inadequate rigidity.

b) Two years later. Pseudarthrosis of the HA. Screw fracture. Bone resorption around all the screws which pass through the head of the plate

In addition, the cobra-head plate arthrodesis seen on the radiograph published by KALÉN does not comply with our criteria. In the case shown, the greater trochanter should have been removed and inserted as a graft into the wedgeshaped space between the lateral acetabular roof, the freshened neck of the femur and the plate. Further, at least one of the screws passing through the distal cobra head seems to be fixed in the head of the femur rather than in the pelvis.

It is clear that a Type IV arthrodesis performed incorrectly will not be sufficiently rigid (increased shear forces) and may result in PA (Fig. 52).

5.6 Hip Arthrodesis in the Presence of Infection

(Freshening of the adjacent bone surfaces; fixation of the proximal part of the femur to the pelvis by means of two cancellous bone screws; IO). In this arthrodesis two cancellous bone screws are used. One exerts compression and the other functions more as a positioning screw.

The compression screw is screwed into the pelvis along the axis of the femoral neck just above the innominate tubercle. The short thread of this cancellous bone screw should take hold in the medial pelvic cortex and thus be completely buried in pelvic bone.

In a similar manner, the positioning screw is inserted just above the compression screw and is driven into the pubic ramus at right angles to the axis of the femur. If the screws are inserted with the leg abducted, bringing the femoral neck into a vertical position following IO results in an increase in leg length (Figs. 53, 54).

6 Elastometry

6.1 Introduction

Elastometry allows visualisation of the lines of mechanical force in a body and has been used for many years for the investigation of biomechanical processes. With the aid of this

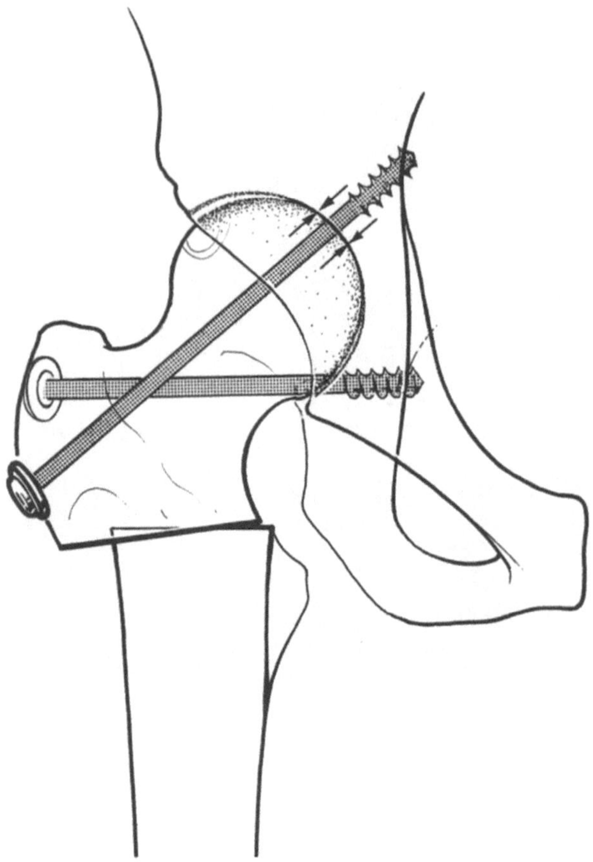

Fig. 53. *HA with minimal but rigid internal fixation*

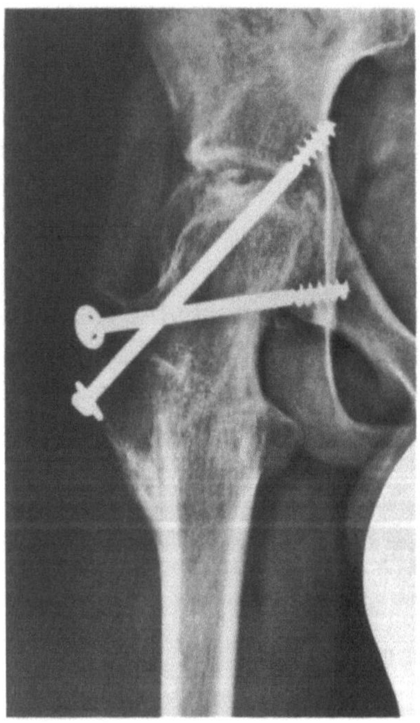

Fig. 54. *HA by internal screw fixation in a case of hip joint infection.* H. H., ♂, aged 17, No. 142572.

Bone union 4 months following HA

method, we have attempted to find solutions to a number of our working hypotheses.

Our series of cases comprises a total of 583 HA operations. In 258 cases, the cobra-head plate was used and was almost always combined with PO. This arthrodesis (Type IV) has been our method of choice since 1967. In the course of clinical and radiological follow-up, the following questions have arisen and, in some cases, have remained unanswered:

a) What degree of medial displacement following PO results in optimum distribution of forces across the whole contact surface?
b) To what degree should the cobra-head plate be pretensioned?
c) How can one explain the occurrence of fatigue fracture following cobra-head plate arthrodesis (always at the distal end of the plate)? The last distal screw in the plate only passes through one femoral cortex, the intention being to prevent an abrupt transition in the forces transmitted from the plate to the bone in this region. Is this measure effective?

In the literature on HA by means of central dislocation (the CHARNLEY method), fractures of the femoral neck have been repeatedly reported. In our series, this technique was used only twice and we are therefore unable to present clinical data on this complication. However, with the aid of a model, we have attempted to demonstrate the factors responsible for this complication.

6.2 Experimental Method

The models were cut out of Araldite sheet and are precise reproductions taken from the radiographs (pelvis-proximal femur; magnification 1:1) of four operated patients. The following arthrodesis types are represented:

Model 1: HA with central dislocation (Fig. 55)

Model 2: Cobra-head plate arthrodesis with PO and small medial displacement (Fig. 56)

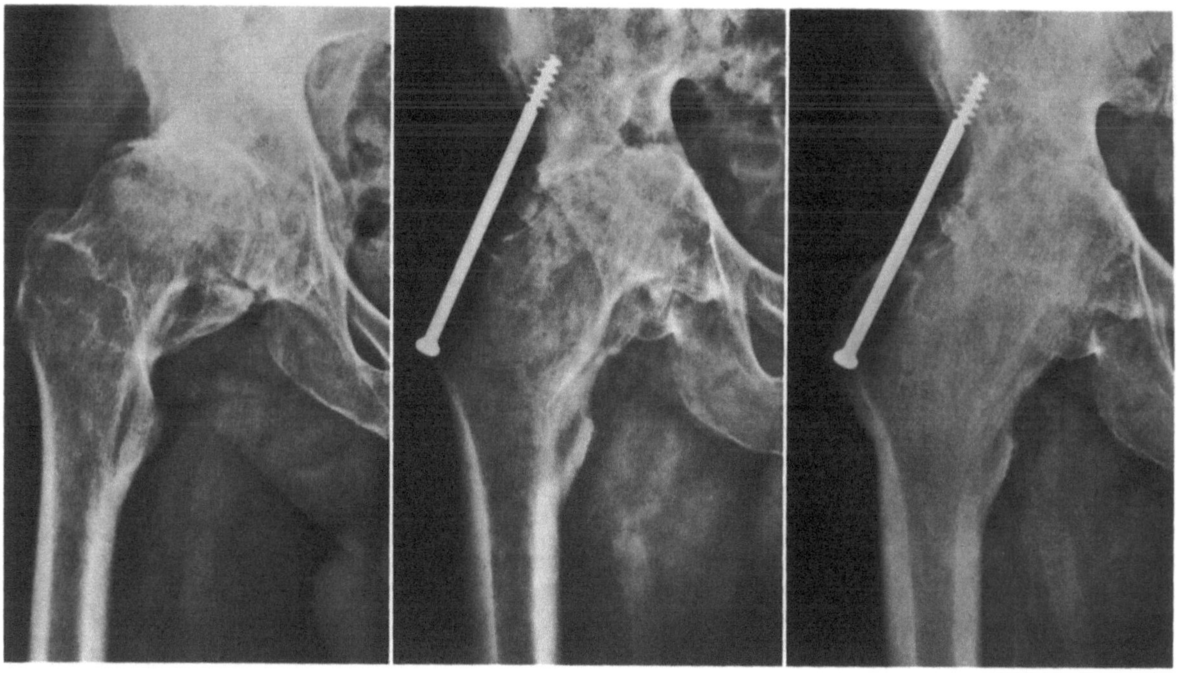

a b c

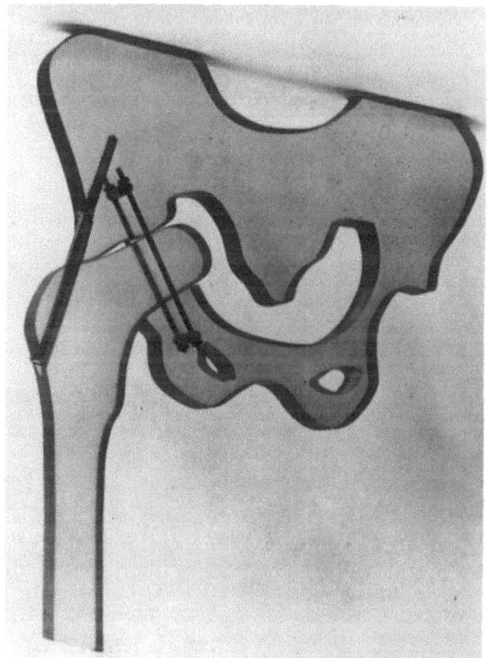

d

Figs. 55 – 58. *Cases and models used for elastometry experiments*

Fig. 55. *HA with central dislocation.*

K. F., ♂, aged 47, No. 66008.

a) Before operation.

b) One month following operation.

c) Follow-up 17 months later; perfect HA.

d) Corresponding model cut from Araldite sheet

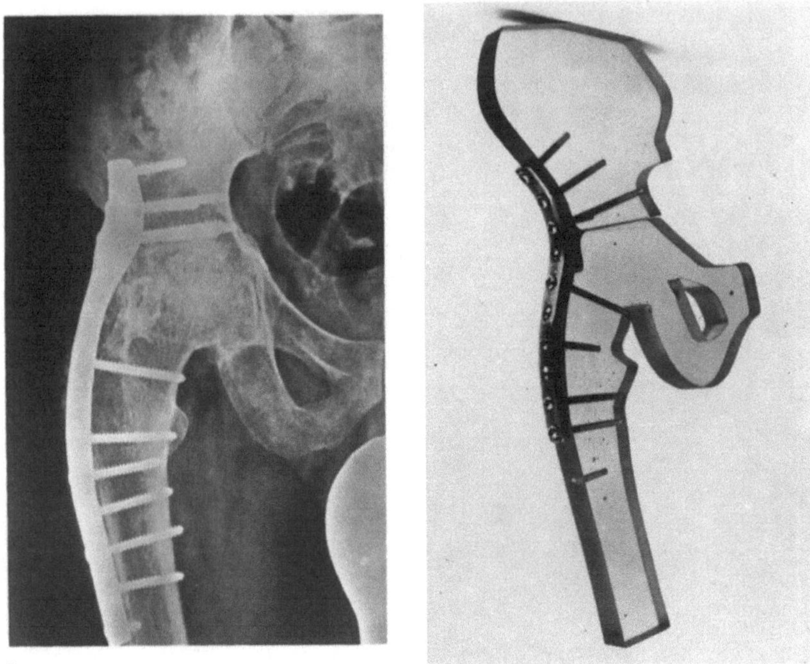

a b

Fig. 56. *Type IV HA with small degree of medial displacement following pelvic osteotomy*. B. R., ♂, aged 31 years, No. 111670.

a) HA united 7 months following operation.

b) Corresponding model

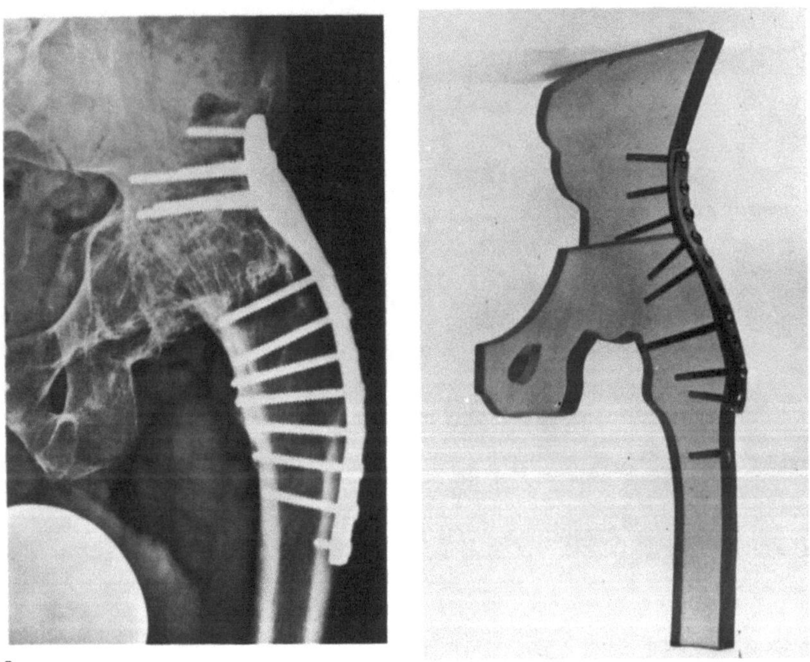

a b

Fig. 57. *Type IV HA with moderate degree of medial displacement following PO*. M. F., ♂, aged 54 years, No. 109081.

a) Follow-up 5 years following HA; perfect result.

b) Corresponding model

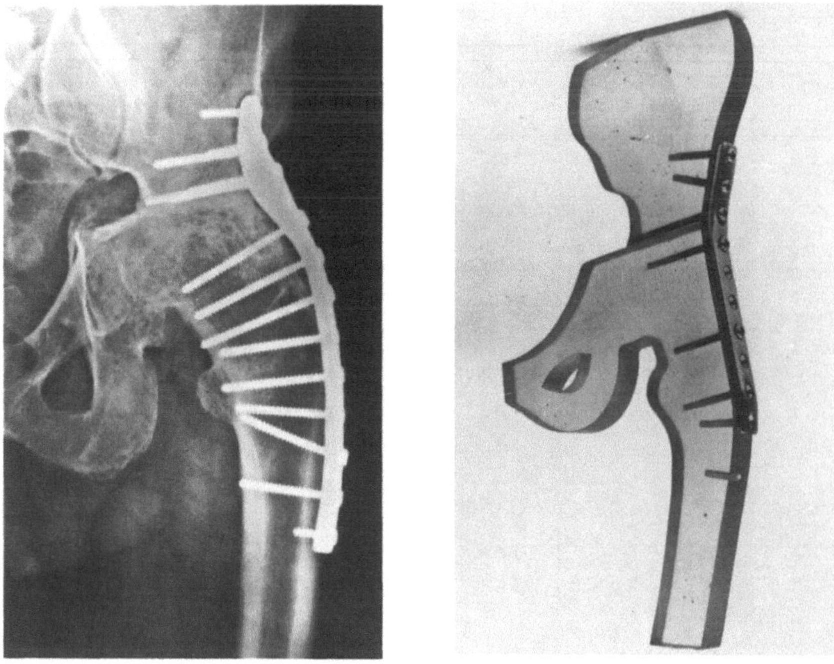

a b

Fig. 58. *Type IV HA with large degree of medial displacement following PO.* L. F., ♂, aged 56 years, No. 119126.

a) HA clinically and radiologically united 10 months following operation. Bone resorption around the proximal part of the plate.

b) Corresponding model

Model 3: Cobra-head plate arthrodesis with PO and moderate medial displacement (Fig. 57)

Model 4: Cobra-head plate arthrodesis with PO and extensive medial displacement (Fig. 58)

Three-dimensional models were not constructed. They present technical problems, require considerable time to prepare and, last but not least, they are expensive. Furthermore, the arthrodesed hip is no longer a ball joint and can be adequately represented in two dimensions so that the expense of three dimensional models is unjustified*.

For technical reasons, Araldite sheet cannot be made sufficiently thick such that it will support a cobra-head plate (impurities in the material and a high level of intrinsic stress). For this reason, broad straight plates with central holes were used. Bending and contouring of the plate, drilling and tapping of the screw holes and tensioning and fixation of the plates with screws were all carried out with the internal fixation instruments and materials used in our clinic. Internal stresses generated by screwing the plates to the models could largely be abolished by warming the Araldite.

Using the angle of 16° which had been established by PAUWELS (Fig. 59), the model was loaded and the resulting strains were visualised with the polarimeter (Fig. 59b).

* In contrast, when investigating problems associated with TP it would be advantageous to be able to work three dimensionally).

Figs. 59a and b. *Experimental rig*

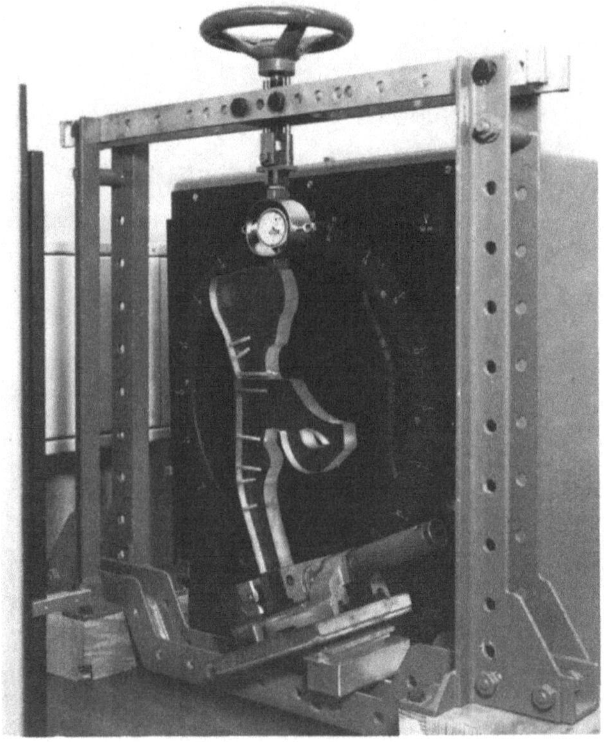

a

b

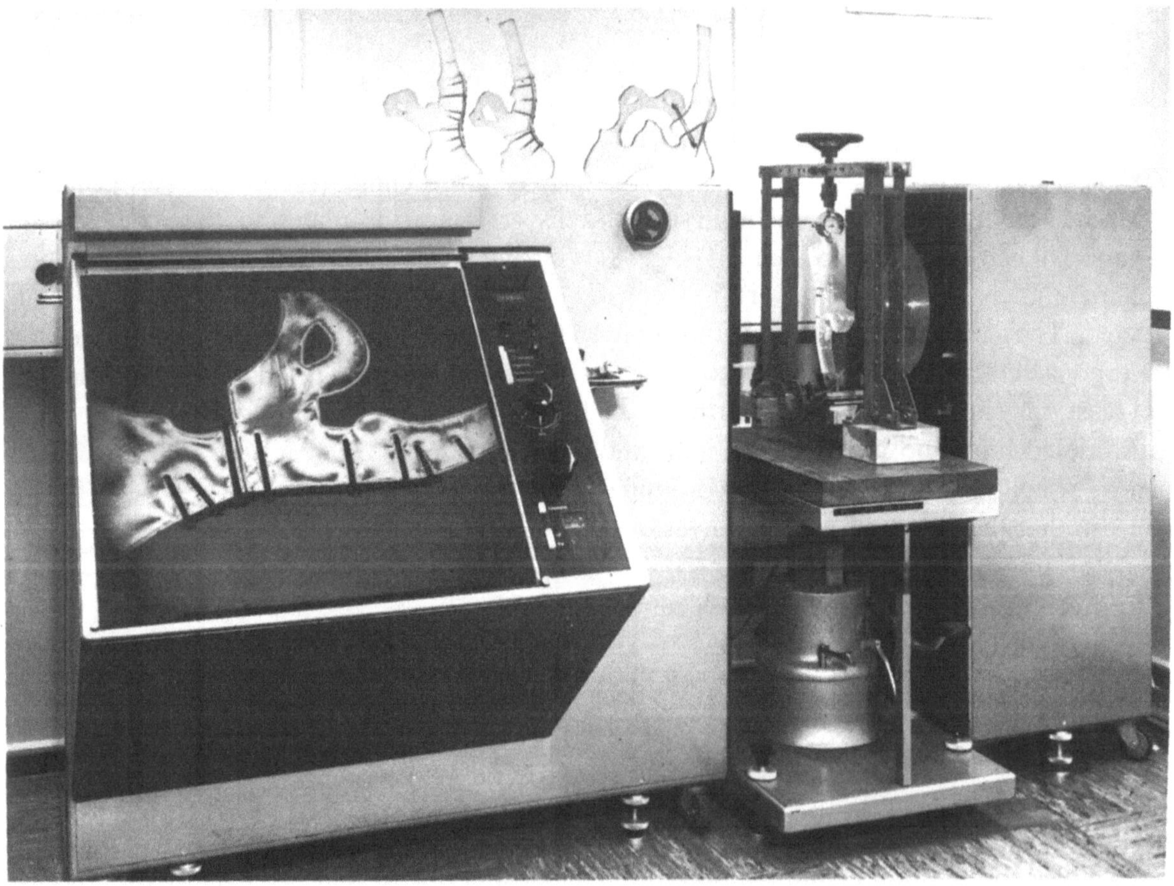

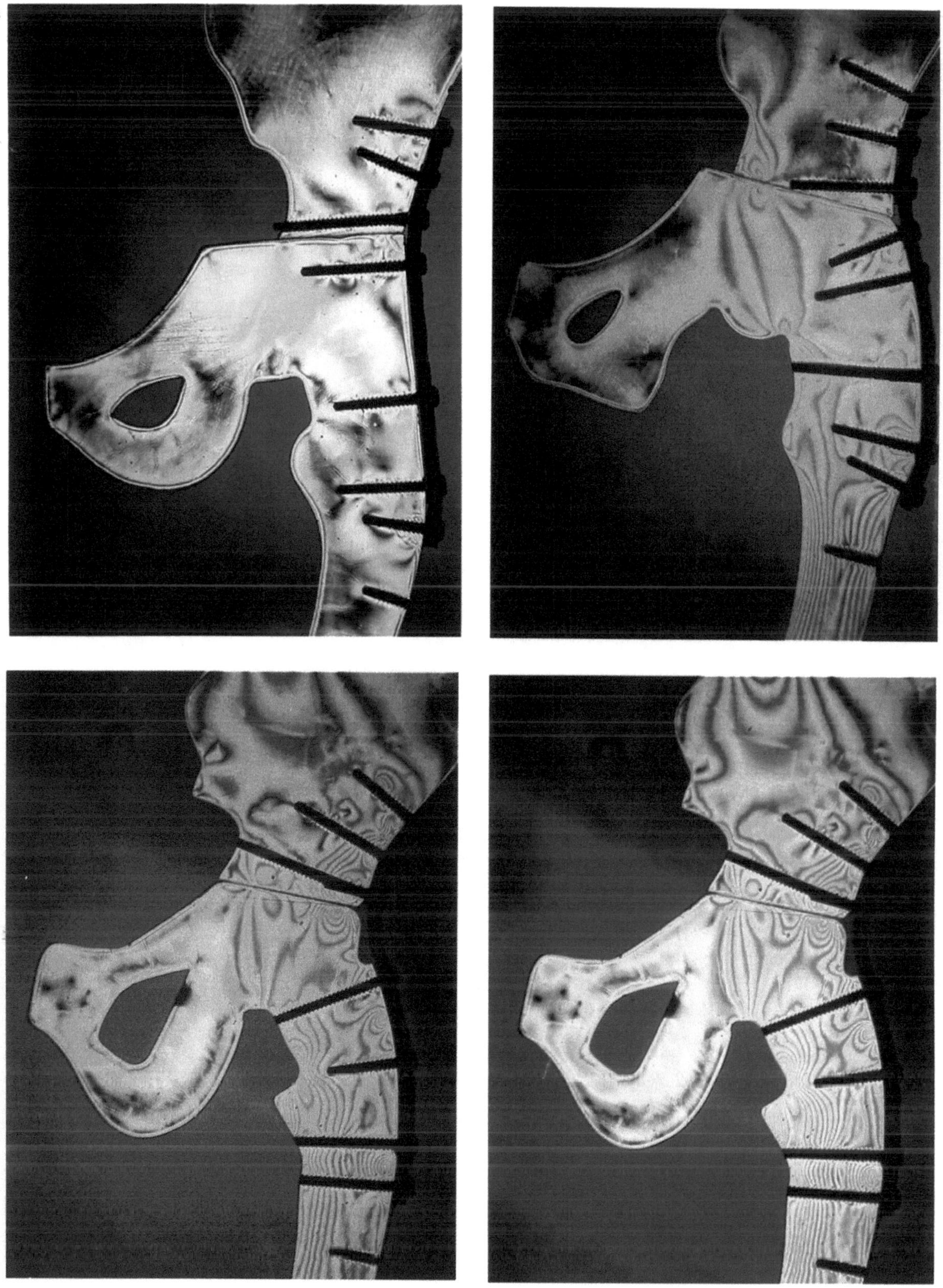

Fig. 60. *Relationship of stress distribution to medial displacement of the distal pelvic component following PO. Minimal medial displacement.*

a) Without load c) 80 kg load

b) 60 kg load d) 100 kg load

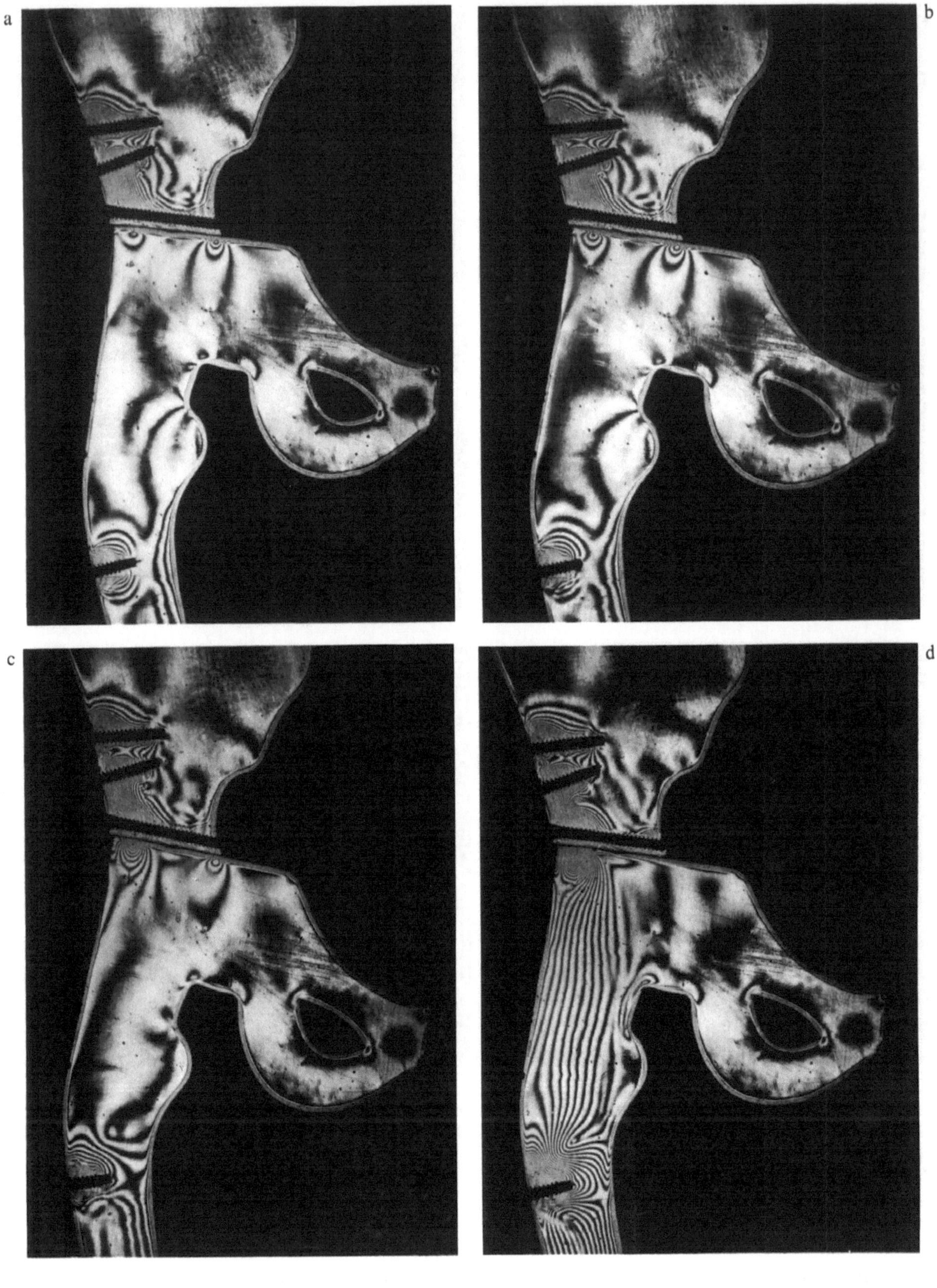

Fig. 61. *Relationship of stress distribution to medial displacement of the distal pelvic component following PO. Moderate medial displacement.*

a) Without load c) 80 kg load

b) 60 kg load d) 100 kg load

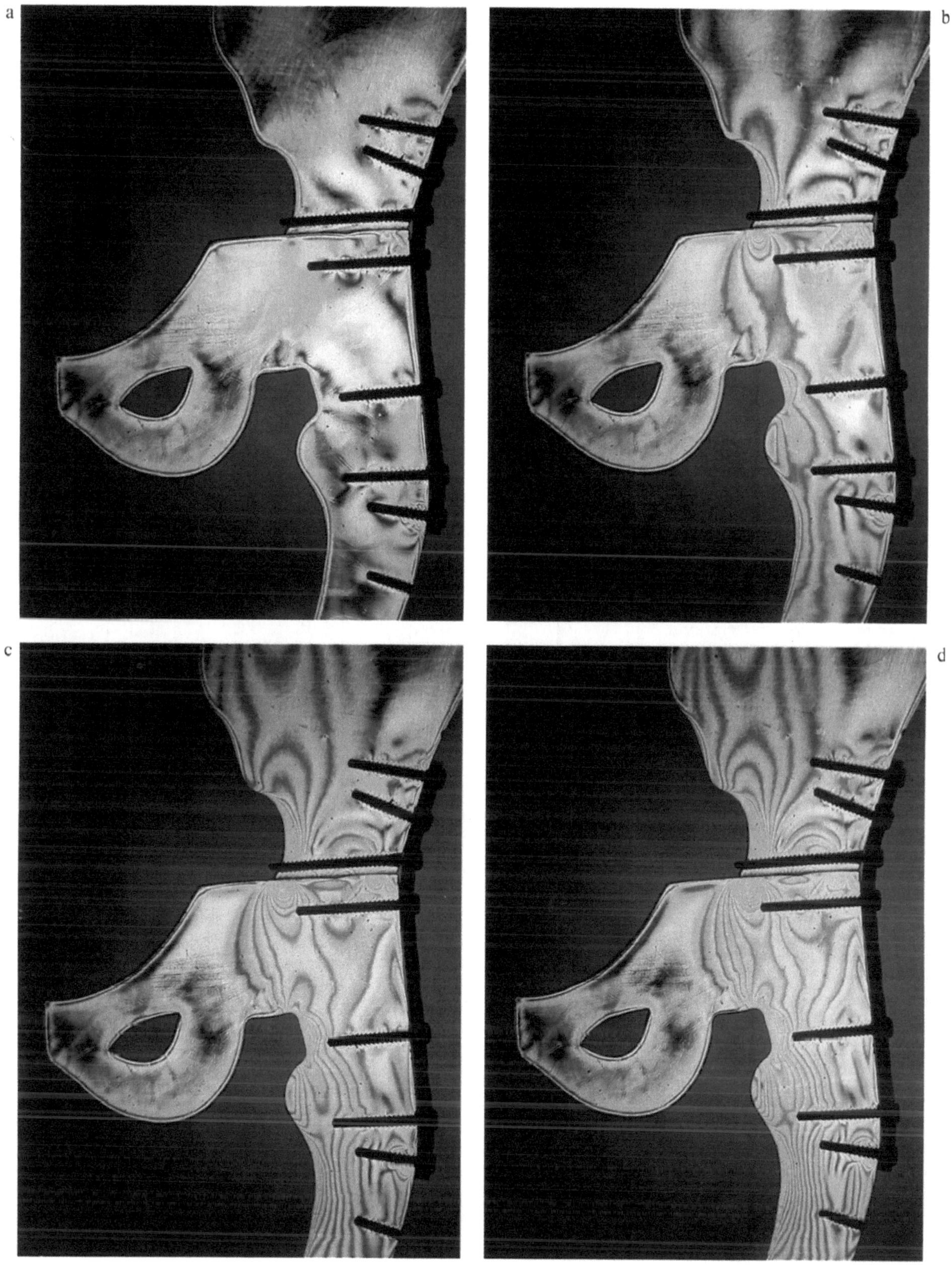

Fig. 62. Relationship of stress distribution to medial displacement of the distal pelvic component following PO. Large degree of medial displacement.

a) Without load c) 80 kg load

b) 60 kg load d) 100 kg load

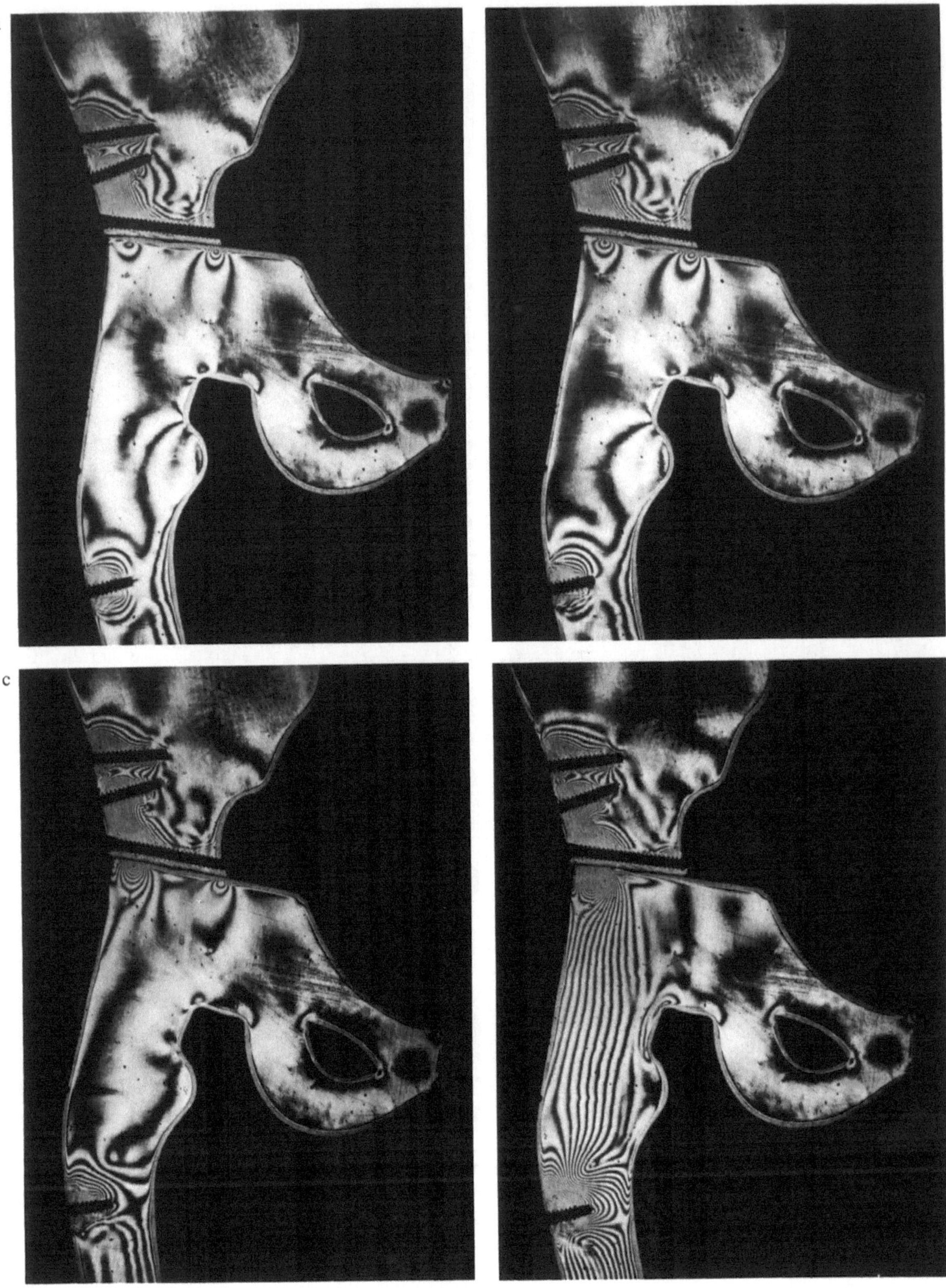

Fig. 63. *Relation between stress distribution and pretensioning.*

a) With a 60 kg load; plate fixed proximally; tensioning device applied (no pre-tension).

b) Slight pretensioning. The lateral part of the osteotomy is also compressed.

c) Moderate pretensioning. Ide

d) Excessive pretensioning. Exc ny

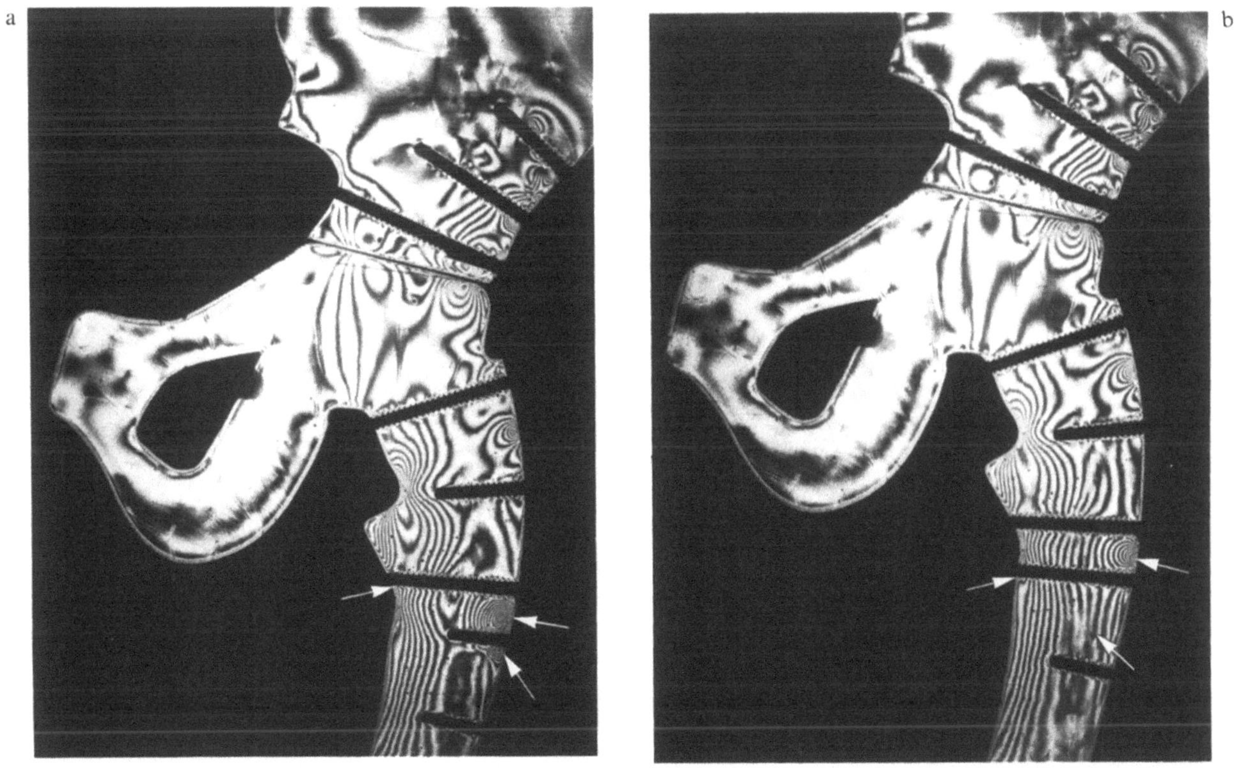

Fig. 64. *Relationship between stress distribution and length of the distal screw.*
a) Short screw b) Long screw

6.3 Results

6.3.1 Effects of Medial Displacement

The following pictures show the distribution of forces during different phases of loading with small, moderate and large degrees of medial displacement (Figs. 60 – 62).

6.3.2 Effects of Pretensioning of the Plate

The changes in the lines of tension with increasing pretensioning of the plate are visible in the following photographs (Figs. 63a – 63d).

6.3.3 Influence of the Length of the Distal Screw

It should be emphasised that these experiments are purely mechanical and do not take into account the biomechanical factors in bone (Fig. 64).

6.3.4 Hip Arthrodesis with Central Dislocation (Charnley) (Figs. 65, 66).

6.4 Evaluation of Experimental Results

With small or moderate degrees of medialisation, the tension forces are evenly distributed over the whole contact surface. A large degree of medial displacement results in asymmetrically increased loading of the medial side of the femoral diaphysis.

The forces are also concentrated on the medial side of the osteotomy; the lateral side is hardly compressed. This maldistribution of compression is abolished by slight pretensioning of the plate. Moderate pretensioning suffices to ensure optimum distribution of forces over the contact surfaces; on standing on the leg the weight of the upper body and that of the nonloaded leg combine to even out the compression of the osteotomy. Further tension is detrimental for two reasons:

a b

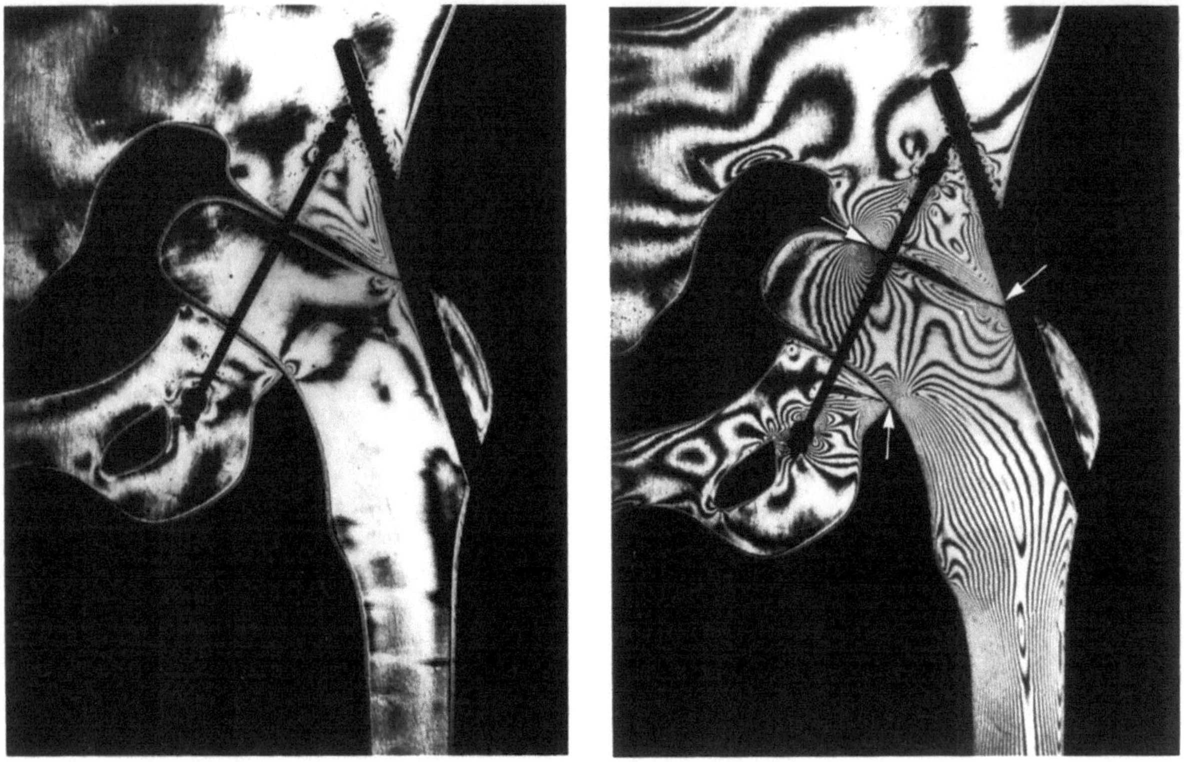

Figs. 65 and 66. *Distribution of forces following HA with central dislocation (Charnley method)*

Fig. 65. *Model without cancellous screw.*

a) No load b) With a 100 kg load (point concentration of forces)

a b

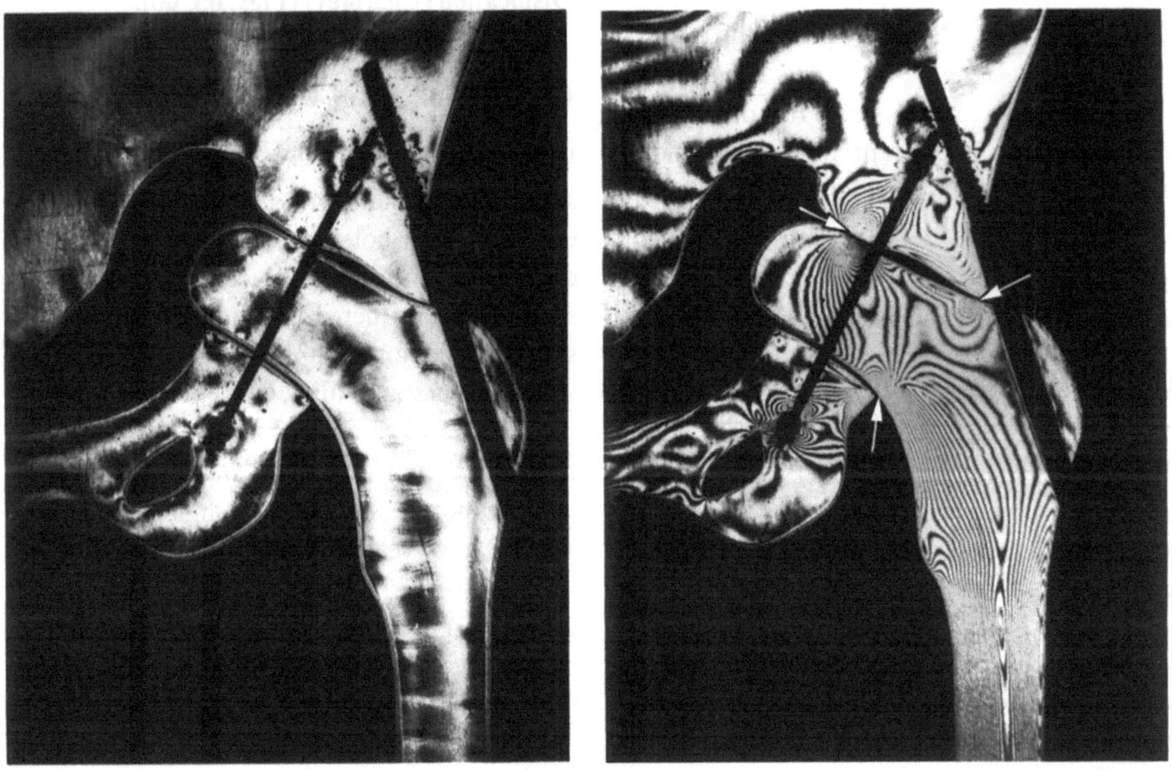

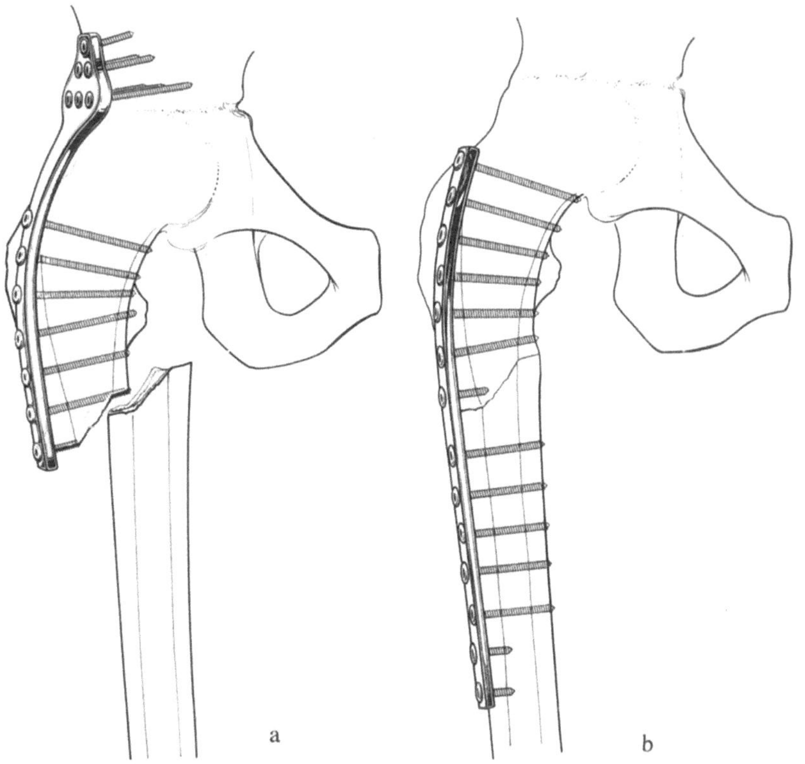

Figs. 67 – 68. *Fatigue fractures at the distal end of the plate*

Fig. 67. (See also Fig. 258.)

a) Fracture line with short distal screw.

b) Rigid internal fixation of the fracture

1. The proximal end of the femur is driven into the pelvis on the lateral side.
2. The osteotomy gapes on the medial side and, since this area is not subjected to much pressure, the condition is detrimental to rapid bone union.

As far as the length of the distal cortex screw is concerned, a long distal screw seems to be better. The distribution of the tension forces is improved despite the fact that the use of the long screw also results in a significant concentration of forces on the lateral side between the two final screws. Use of a short final screw causes significantly increased concentration of forces around that screw and also, to a lesser degree, around the tip of the screw immediately proximal to it. This corresponds precisely to the course of the fracture lines seen in our fatigue fractures (Figs. 67, 68).

It should be noted, however, that a relatively short plate was used in our model. If the plate extends further down the femoral diaphysis, the peak tensions around the final screw are significantly reduced. A short screw is used in the final hole in order to render the change in stress level at the lower end of the plate (where high peak tension forces occur) more gradual (WEBER).

In the HA model with central dislocation there is almost total stress concentration at the points of contact between the femoral neck and the pelvis. These points lie proximally on the lateral aspect of the femoral neck and distally on the medial aspect. The proximal medial point of contact is also highly stressed but to a significantly lesser degree than the lateral point of contact. This localised overloading easily explains the occurrence of fatigue fracture of the femoral neck along the line joining the proximal lateral and distal medial

Fig. 66. *Model with additional fixation of the greater trochanter to the pelvis using a cancellous screw.*

a) No load

b) With a 100 kg load (not significantly different from Fig. 65b)

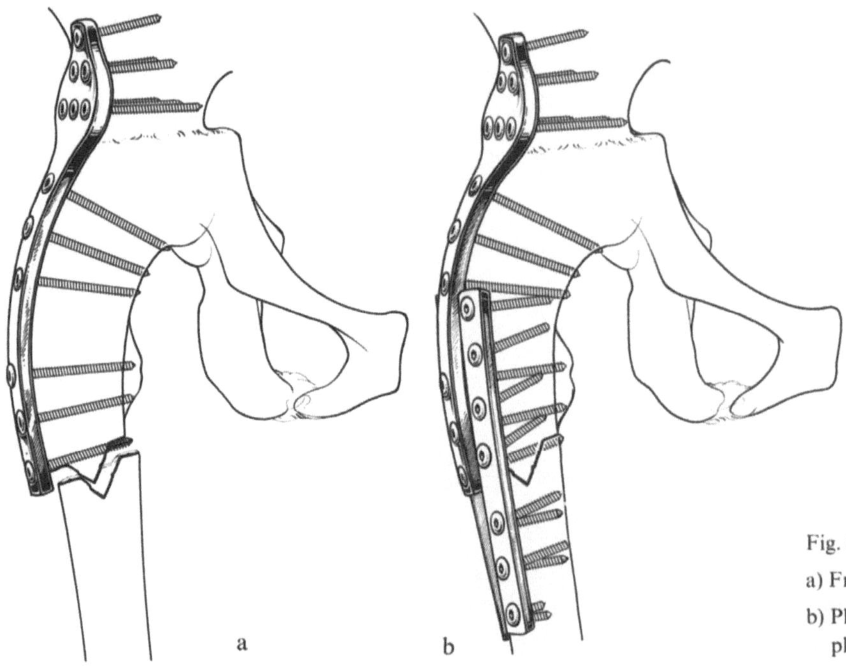

Fig. 68. (See also Fig. 260.)
a) Fracture line with long distal screw.
b) Plate fixation; a single neutralising plate would have sufficed

points of contact between femoral neck and pelvis. The pressure distribution is hardly changed by additional iliofemoral screw fixation by means of a cancellous bone screw through the greater trochanter.

6.5 Summary

Our elastometric investigations have shown that:

- A small or moderate degree of medial displacement is mechanically better than a very large degree of medial displacement.
- Moderate pretensioning of the plate produces an ideally even distribution of compression over the whole contact surface.
- Depending on the length of the last screw, different patterns of stress concentration at the distal end of the plate occur. The two typical fatigue fracture lines correspond to the varieties of stress concentration.
- The femoral neck fracture which is known to occur in HA with central dislocation is a result of detrimental concentration of stress at the point of contact between femoral neck and pelvis.

7 SUMMARY

The biomechanical effects of the static and dynamic changes induced by HA and the effects of the arthrodesis on the neighbouring centres of movement and on the contralateral hip were discussed.

An adequate capacity for static and dynamic compensation is a prerequisite for an optimal HA. Inadequate capacity to compensate constitutes a relative or absolute contraindication for HA.

A stiff ipsilateral knee joint or almost complete absence of lumbar spinal flexibility are *absolute contraindications*.

On the other hand, slight lumbar pain or moderate degenerative changes in the lumbar spine or in the ipsilateral knee or contralateral hip joint are only relative contraindications.

The angle of the hip following arthrodesis is determined by the structural principles of the pelvic and lower limb skeleton. Thus:

Flexion: 15° – 20°

Ab-/adduction: zero position or slight adduction (up to 5°)

Rotation: zero position or slight external rotation (5° – 10°)

A significant difference in leg length must always be corrected orthotically (wedged shoes) or by surgery since the resulting pelvic tilt may cause compensatory scoliosis. Generally speaking, one should not attempt to correct a difference in leg length by putting the HA in abduction.

Excessive medial displacement following PO should be avoided since this is biomechanically detrimental and, in addition, it should be avoided in young women since it may narrow the birth canal and present difficulties during delivery. Knowledge of the structural principles of the pelvic and lower limb skeleton and close attention to the internal fixation method applicable to the arthrodesis in question are prerequisites for a successful HA.

IV. General Indications for Hip Arthrodesis

1 Introduction

Operations for treatment of partial or total destruction of the hip joint may be divided into three basic types:

- Intertrochanteric osteotomies
- Prosthetic replacements
- Hip arthrodeses

The beneficial effect of IO is usually temporary and the latter operation is frequently followed by one of the other types. In contrast, TP and HA are intended as final solutions. The enormous increase in TP in recent years has been paralleled by a decrease in the frequency of IO and an even greater reduction in the number of HA operations performed. Several authors have rejected HA in favour of prosthetic replacement (JONES, JUDET, STINCHFIELD and CAVALLARO; STOFFEL). NEFF (1956) was in illustrious company (CHARNLEY, MCKEE, BUCHHOLZ, COVENTRY) when he went so far as to say "Arthrodesis of the hip is a declaration of surgical bankruptcy comparable to the amputation of a limb." Although our case material is now dominated by TP, HA has retained a valid place. The types of operation in the last 11 years were 47% IO, 15% HA, 38% TP (Fig. 69, Table 1).

Table 1 shows particularly well the marked increase in TP which parallels the decrease in IO. The peak frequency of HA occurred in 1965 – 1967 at the time of introduction of stable internal fixation with double plates and particularly using the cobra-head plate.

A trough occurred in 1969 when only 20 HA were performed. In recent years there has been a more precise redefinition of the type of

Table 1. Operations for primary or secondary arthrosis of the hip (1961 – 1971)

Year	Inter-trochanteric osteotomy	%	Arthrodesis	%	Total prosthesis	%	Total
1961	193	74	30	11	39	15	262
1962	175	67	63	24	23	9	261
1963	214	73	47	16	33	11	294
1964	290	69	60	14	71	17	421
1965	219	55	80	20	98	25	397
1966	201	45	110	24	138	31	449
1967	128	34	67	18	177	48	372
1968	141	41	44	13	155	46	340
1969	105	24	20	5	310	71	435
1970	88	26	28	8	221	66	337
1971	79	22	34	9	247	69	360
Total	1833	47	583	15	1512	38	3928

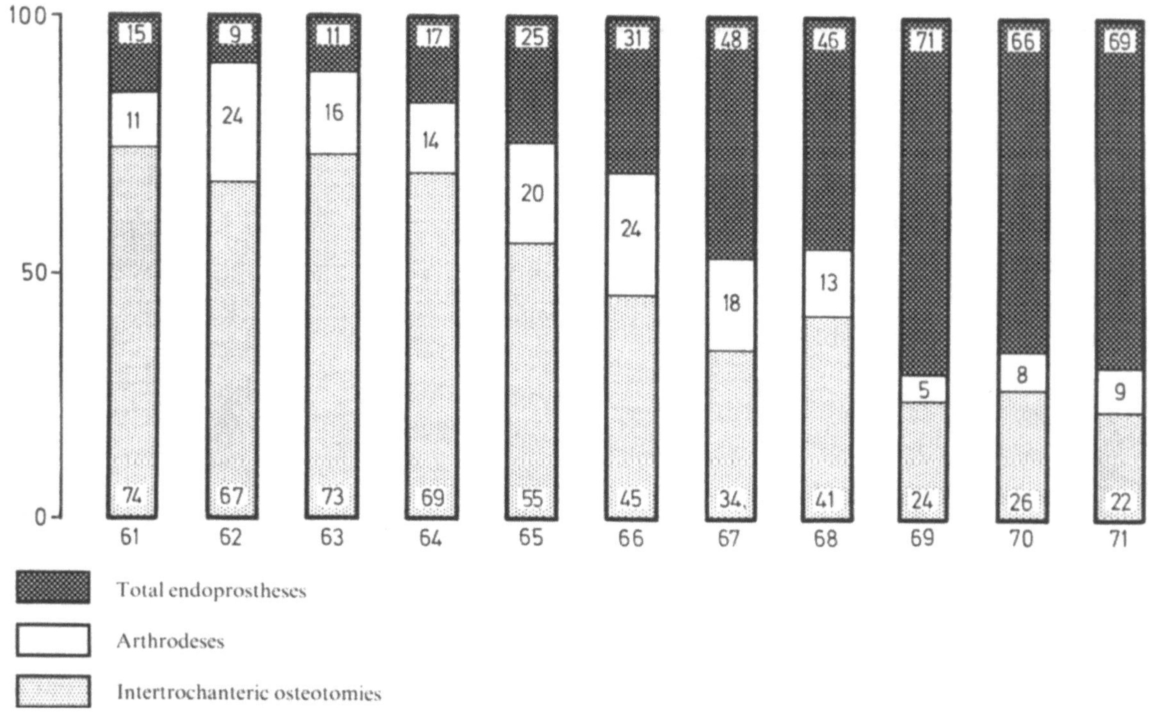

Fig. 69. *Surgical treatment of hip arthrosis from 1961 to 1971; classified by year and type of operation*

case which is suitable. The indication for TP is being examined somewhat more critically and this has resulted in increased applicability of HA. Thus in 1971, 34 HA were performed.

2 Diagnoses Leading to Hip Arthrodesis

Hip arthrosis remains the most frequent indication for HA (80.9%). This group includes idiopathic arthrosis and arthroses secondary to hip dysplasia, Perthes' disease and slipped epiphysis. Arthrosis secondary to rheumatoid arthritis was included in this group since monoarthritic rheumatoid arthritis or polyarthritic cases with relatively insignificant changes in the other joints do not present special problems as far as HA is concerned. Of the HA operations 19.1% were performed for other painful hip conditions.

In recent years, an increasing number of HA operations have been carried out following severe post-traumatic changes in the hip joint. The increase in severe highway accidents frequently involving young persons is clearly of significance here. Particularly important are hip changes following fracture of the acetabular roof and pelvis, or necrosis of the head of the femur (NHF) secondary to fractures of the femoral neck.

The cases of infective arthritis comprise a third group. Tuberculosis (Tb) of the hip is now less common and the cases in our series were almost all old inactive Tb infections, frequently

Table 2. Etiology (583 HA)

	No. of cases	%
Arthrosis and rheumatoid arthritis	391	67
Hip dysplasia	81	13.9
Post-traumatic	73	12.5
Infection		
Nontuberculitic	19	1.7
Tuberculitic	10	3.3
Idiopathic necrosis of the femoral head	8	1.4
Pathological fracture (secondary to tumor)	1	0.2

with fibrotic ankylosis resulting in hip deformity. The nontuberculitic hip joint infections comprise haematogenous arthritis in children, post-traumatic arthritis and iatrogenic arthritis. This group has recently gained in importance since it now includes infected loose hip protheses.

The last small group comprises the idiopathic femoral head necroses (Table 2).

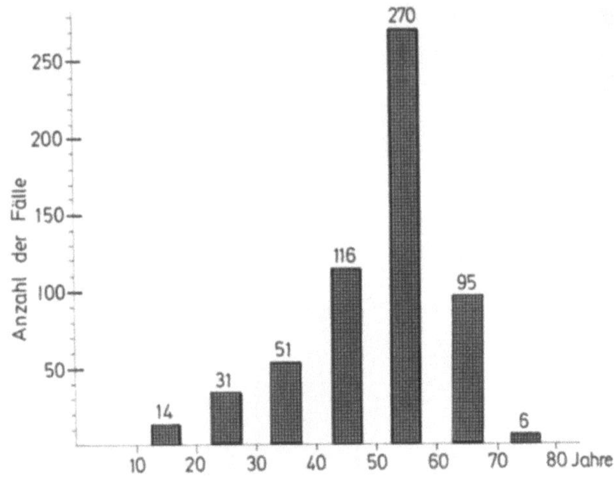

Fig. 70. *Age distribution of the 583 HA*

3 General Considerations

3.1 Age

The majority of patients were 40–55 years old at the time of operation. The mean age in our HA series was 51.4 years (Fig. 70, Table 3).

Our youngest patient (operated subsequent to resection of the head of the femur and Tb of the hip) was aged 11 years and our oldest patient was aged 77 years.

HA is rarely indicated before cessation of growth, e.g., following extensive destruction of the hip joint by Tb or nontuberculitic infection or in cases of fibrous ankylosis and deformity of the hip following unsuccessful operative treatment of a dislocation where no other surgical reconstruction is possible. The procedure may also be indicated following post-traumatic necrosis and disintegration of the femoral head.

In our opinion, the optimum age for HA lies between 20 and 50 years if the hips are in such a poor condition that there is no question of performing an IO. It is at this age that the patients are best capable of adapting to the new situation. Furthermore, they are too young for a TP. With certain exceptions (ankylosing spondylitis or extremely severe bilateral destruction of the hip joint secondary to arthrosis or rheumatoid arthritis) we only perform the latter operation in patients over 60 years of age.

The upper age limit for HA is generally given as 60 years. In our series however this limit was exceeded in 101 cases (17.3%). The reasons were:

a) In the first 5 years of our series, TP was still in its infancy and the more generally known IO and HA operations were more frequently performed.
b) TP is contraindicated during or following hip infection. HA is then the procedure of choice.
c) We consider the biological age of the patient to be much more important than the chronological age and for this reason the operation was performed in suitable patients who were over 60 years of age.
d) The new stable internal fixation procedures which allow early mobilisation of the patient without cast fixation have changed the outlook for HA.

Table 3. Age distribution of 583 HA

Age	No. of patients	%
10–20	14	2.4
20–30	31	5.3
30–40	51	8.7
40–50	116	19.9
50–60	270	46.3
60–70	95	16.3
70–80	6	1.0

3.2 General Condition of Patient

HA is still one of the most stressing hip operations. It frequently involves relatively severe blood loss which is a severe strain on the patient's physiology despite modern anaesthesia and intensive care. For this reason, HA is only performed in patients whose general condition is good and who have undergone thorough preoperative clinical examination. Thanks to improvements in technique and the fact that prolonged immobilisation is no longer necessary, the indication for HA may be extended and the procedure may also be carried out in older patients.

Table 4. Body weight and back complaints (206 patients with back complaints)

Ideal weight (kg)	63	118	*174 = 84.5%*
Over ideal weight by:			
Up to 5 kg	20		
6 – 10 kg	35		
11 – 15 kg	14	*32 = 15.5%*	
16 – 20 kg	7		
21 – 25 kg	5		
26 – 30 kg	4		
Over 30 kg	2		
Under ideal weight by:			
Up to 5 kg	19	*56*	
6 – 10 kg	24		
11 – 15 kg	11		
16 – 20 kg	2		

3.3 Somatic Type

HA patients are generally at a disadvantage if they are too large or markedly overweight. As regards obesity, we used to be very selective in our choice of patients; only 15% of the patients operated upon were overweight.

We did not consider the height of the patients to be so important; 15% of the patients were over 185 cm (Fig. 71).

Follow-up of our patients has shown that no particular disadvantages resulted in the 15% of patients who were overweight. On the other hand, obesity seems to be particularly detrimental to the success of TP.

Furthermore we could find no correlation between occurrence or worsening of back complaints and overweight. The proportion of overweight patients lies between 15% and 20% both in the total series as well as in the subgroup of patients who experienced occurrence or worsening of back complaints (Table 4).

Only 15.5% of overweight patients in the group had preexisting back complaints (Table 5).

Comparison of body height in the full series with that in the subgroup of patients in whom back complaints had occurred or become worse shows that 15 (15%) patients were over 185 cms. It follows that the height

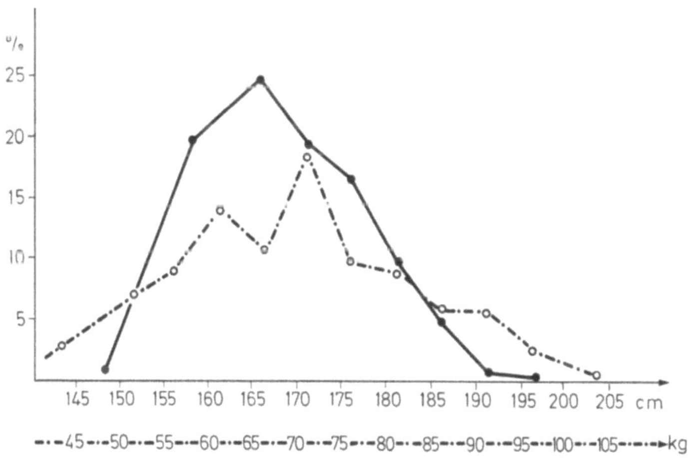

Fig. 71. *Height and weight of our HA patients*

Table 5. Body weight distribution among the 49 patients in whom back complaints arose or worsened following arthrodesis

Ideal weight (kg)	13	
Under ideal weight by:		
Up to 5 kg	3	
6–10 kg	5	39 = 80%
Over ideal weight by:		
Up to 5 kg	11	
6–10 kg	7	
11–15 kg	5	
16–20 kg	1	10 = 20%
21–25 kg	3	
26–30 kg	1	

of the patients is also of no particular significance.

3.4 Sex

HA operations were carried out on 326 men and 257 women. The problems which arise following HA differ markedly according to the sex of the patient and this should be noted by the doctor and taken into account when informing the patient. Problems associated with sexual intercourse following HA occur with significantly greater frequency in women (22%) than in men (11%) (Table 6).

Table 6. HA and sexual intercourse

		Difficulty with sexual intercourse
583 patients	326 men	36 (11%)
	257 women	66 (22%)

Closer questioning of the men (11%) who complained of this problem revealed that the HA is blamed for any reduction in potency, but there is certainly no causal connection. In our opinion the interference with sexual intercourse experienced by the women should not be underestimated, but is frequently exaggerated by both doctor and patient. It is important that the patient be carefully informed about this problem before the operation.

The HA may also render childbirth more difficult if there is simultaneous limitation of movement of the opposite hip or if the pelvic inlet is narrowed by excessive medial displacement following the PO which complements HA.

We tend to be cautious in performing HA if the patient wishes to have further children. Furthermore, marked medial displacement of the distal pelvic component following PO should be avoided if possible. A moderate or large degree of medial displacement may be expected to reduce the transverse diameter of the pelvic inlet by 2–4 cm and the oblique diameter by 1–2 cm. In the middle of the pelvis the narrowing still amounts to 50% of the above values. No narrowing may be observed at the minimum pelvic diameter or at the pelvic outlet. CECH et al. have investigated this problem in female patients over 20 years of age in whom a CHIARI osteotomy was carried out. It was found that narrowing of the true pelvis by the amounts given above leads to obstruction of delivery and makes Caesarean section necessary.

3.5 State of Joints Adjacent to the Arthrodesis

Every HA must be preceded by careful examination of the LS, the SIJ, the ipsilateral knee and ankle joints and the contralateral hip joint.

Arthrodesis of the hip produces widespread changes in the integrated dynamics of the locomotor system and the centres of movement adjacent to the arthrodesis must be fully capable of adapting to the changes imposed upon them.

3.5.1 Lumbar Spine and Sacroiliac Joint

A freely mobile lower vertebral column is a most important factor in successful HA. It

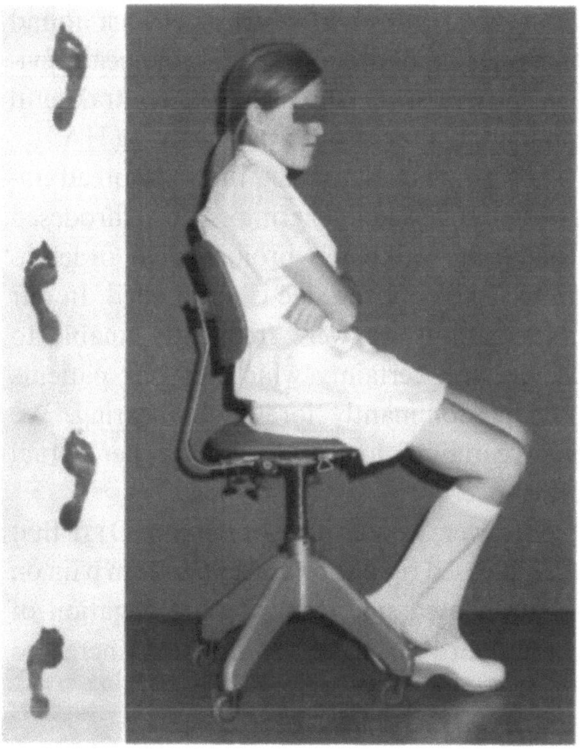

Fig. 72a. *Gait and sitting following HA*. N. I., ♀, aged 20 years, No. 118240

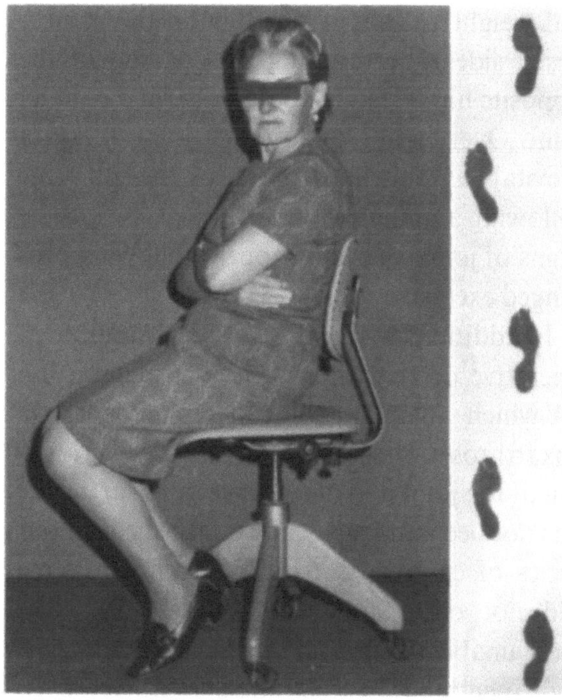

Fig. 72b. *Gait and sitting following HA*. B. J., ♀, aged 46 years, No. 150431

allows the patient to walk with a gait of normal appearance and to sit with little hindrance (Figs. 72a, 72b). The presence of spinal changes such as spondyloarthrosis, degenerative disc disease or vertebral deformity mitigates against HA. HA is still permitted in the presence of spondyloarthrosis of the LS if it does not bring about significant changes in the axis of the leg. Such changes would result in overloading of the LS which is no longer capable of adapting to the stresses imposed upon it. We have frequently seen improvement of back complaints in cases where the HA has resulted in correction of leg malposition (and of pelvic tilt).

3.5.2 Ipsilateral Knee Joint

HA almost always causes displacement of, and increase of, the loads on the ipsilateral knee joint. The surgeon should aim to leave the preoperative axis of leg loading unchanged if the latter is more or less normal. Conditions such as varus knee and particularly valgus knee, incipient gonarthrosis or femoropatellar arthrosis which hardly cause trouble will be detrimentally affected by the increased load. Arthrodesis of the hip will then almost certainly be followed by increased problems in the knee joint. In such cases, the HA may be carried out if one is prepared for subsequent axial correction (usually supracondylar femoral osteotomy) in the event of a significant worsening of the knee condition. Such corrective osteotomies are, however, relatively simple, usually well tolerated by the patient and very worthwhile procedures (pp. 89–92).

3.5.3 Contralateral Hip Joint

An intact and freely mobile contralateral hip joint is a prerequisite to a successful HA. In the first 2–3 postoperative months only partial weight bearing is possible on the arthrodesed side. The resulting overloading of the opposite hip certainly does not harm the intact joint. Overloading of an intact joint does not inevitably result in arthrosis of the hip (*vide* following amputation: FONTAINE, FASCYNSKI). Signs of joint wear only appear following prolonged excessive stress.

In addition, we have never seen rapid postoperative deterioration of a contralateral hip in which there was incipient preoperative coxarthrosis. The correlation between overloading of the joint and occurrence of coxarthrosis has not been unequivocally established. In our series of cases, arthroses due to overloading did not occur following faultless HA. We were unable to confirm the "delayed bilaterality" mentioned by HACKENBROCH. SEEWALD and DEBRUNNER were also of the opinion that increased stress is not detrimental to a normal, resilient hip joint. This opinion was confirmed by their investigations:

Sixty patients with unilateral ankylosis of the hip were examined, after an average period of 30 years, for the presence of coxarthrosis in the contralateral hip joint. An arthrosis frequency of 10% was established and this was primarily ascribed to biological causes and secondarily to mechanical causes.

Questioning of our 146 patients with bilateral coxarthrosis revealed subjective worsening on the nonoperated side in five cases and subjective improvement in a further five cases (Table 7).

Table 7. Effect of HA on the nonoperated side in 146 cases of bilateral arthrosis of the hip

Improvement following operation	5
Worsening following operation	5

In one case we were able to observe significant radiographic progression of the arthrosis. It would be reasonable to expect progression of a preexisting contralateral coxarthrosis and the progression which actually occurs following arthrodesis corresponds to the known behaviour of arthroses in general. HÖGER found only one case of pronounced radiologically evident progressive arthrosis in the contralateral hip joint in a series of 65 patients with HA.

According to FÜRMEIER, the widespread impression that weight bearing on an arthrodesed leg during walking is prolonged in order to protect the opposite side is unfounded. In our investigations we were frequently unable to decide with certainty which leg our patients used predominantly for weight bearing. We were certainly unable to find a percentual difference.

However, we share the opinion of OTTE that the increased rigidity and freedom from pain on the ankylosed side results in prolongation of the weight-bearing phase and thus increased stress on that side.

3.6 Occupation

Prior to every hip operation the surgeon should discuss and carefully enquire about the occupation of the patient, the stresses imposed upon the hip in the course of that occupation and the degree of occupational disability caused by the hip problem. Whilst we would tend to recommend a hip prosthesis for patients in sedentary occupations, HA is the operation of choice for labourers, agricultural workers and other manual workers who work mainly in a standing position. The latter patients must be able to continue full weight bearing on the hip joint without risk of failure. If a patient has already got used to his stiff hip, an improvement in mobility may not always result in the overall improvement expected. Frequently marked adjustment is necessary and sometimes the patient has to change his occupation (64 of 583 patients; 10.9%). Careful discussion of the latter possibility shortens the time required by the patient to readjust.

3.7 Social Circumstances

Careful enquiry should be made about the patient's social circumstances. The reintegration of the patient at his place of work and elsewhere should be carefully discussed and, if necessary, the social security authorities should be consulted. Sometimes racial or religious factors are important, e.g., HA should be avoided in Japanese since the latter are used to eating seated on the floor in a cross-leg position. This would be impossible following HA (KATAYAMA et al.).

The appropriateness of HA should be very carefully considered in patients who usually work in a sitting position and who are unable to change their occupation or in older persons who generally spend more time sitting. Here the following factors are particularly important:

a) Home circumstances (e.g., stairs, toilet, sitting bath)
b) Family circumstances, e.g., does the patient live alone? Is help available (pulling on stockings, tying shoes)?
c) Driving (if the automobile has a short distance between seat and pedals)
d) Sexual intercourse

Successful reintegration following HA can only be expected if careful enquiries are made about the above circumstances.

3.8 Sport

The decision to undergo HA is very difficult for patients who are or were active in sports. However, experience has shown that it is precisely these athletically active patients who adapt most rapidly and fully to the new circumstances. Very frequently the patients were active in sports before their operation despite marked limitation of movement and a painful limp. In the majority of cases this sporting activity persists following operation. Several of our HA patients still practise the following sports: walking (mountain walks of 6–8 h duration are not infrequent), skiing, cross-country skiing, tennis, sailing and even horse riding. Practising a sport in moderation can only be of advantage to the patient. The contact with the other participants in outdoor surroundings promotes accelerated readjustment to an almost normal way of life. Patients who are about to undergo an HA should be shown photographs of postoperative patients who practise sport. They offer courage and hope and favour a positive attitude to the operation (Fig. 73).

3.9 Psychological Factors

At first, the idea of a joint arthrodesis is always rejected or, at best, reluctantly accepted by the patient. Already the words "joint stiffening" are associated with loss, uselessness and disability. Unfortunately this negative attitude on the part of the patient is frequently reinforced by that of the doctor. As every orthopaedic surgeon knows, this frame of mind is unjustified. One has only to think of the results of ankle joint arthrodesis in a case of severe arthrosis. The abolition of pain and correction of deformity allows a gait of almost normal appearance.

The doctor-patient relationship is an extremely important factor in HA. It is the duty of the doctor to inform the patient fully, mentioning the disadvantages as well as the advantages. The mental conditioning of the patient should be taken to the point where the operation is not just accepted by him but positively desired. The postoperative cooperation of the patient is the key to success.

The doctor should introduce the patient to others who have undergone the operation. It is best to introduce women to women and men to men. In this manner the patients may discuss their problems without the direct influence of the doctor. Thus, they can get a clear picture

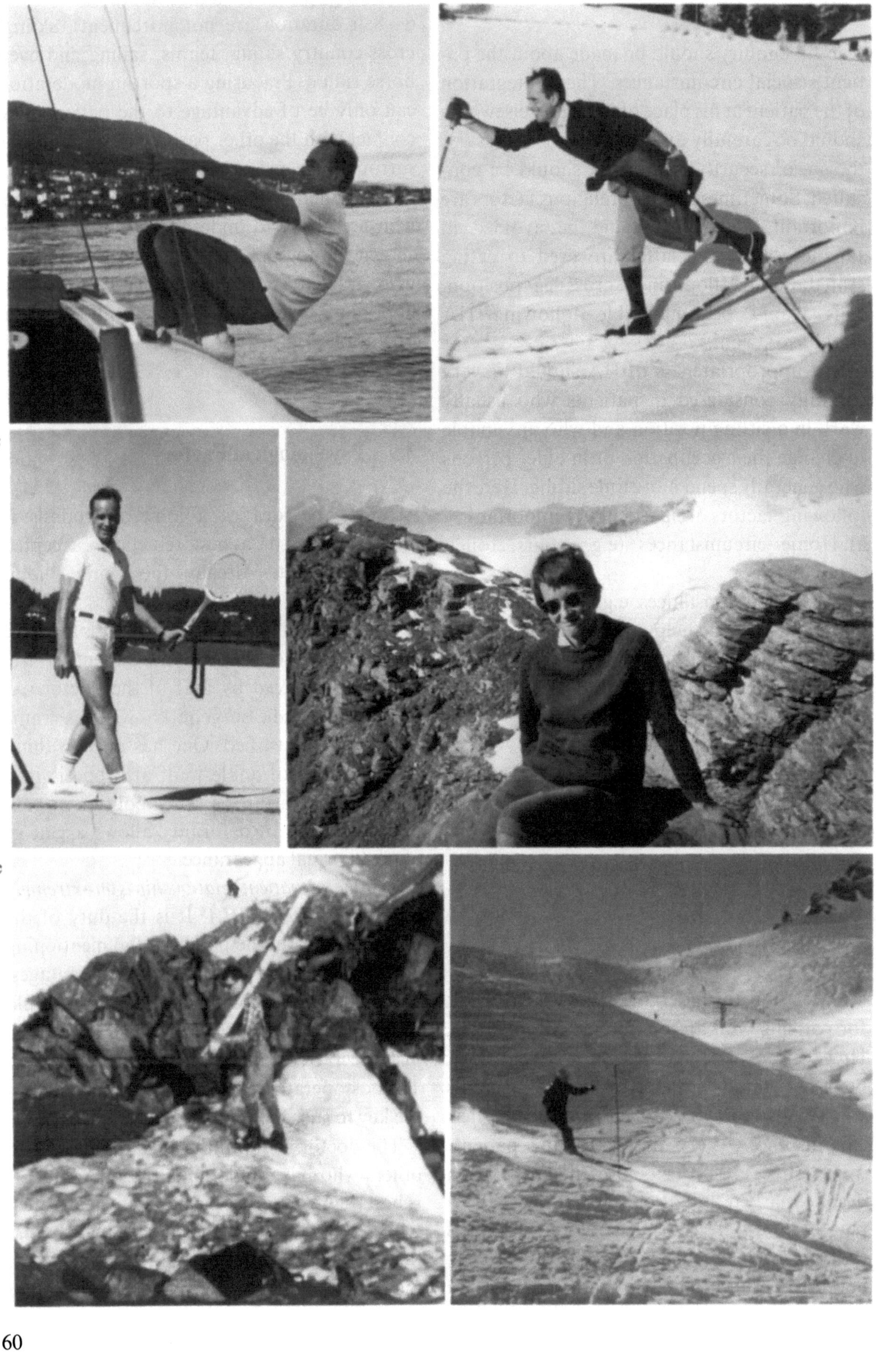

a b c d e f

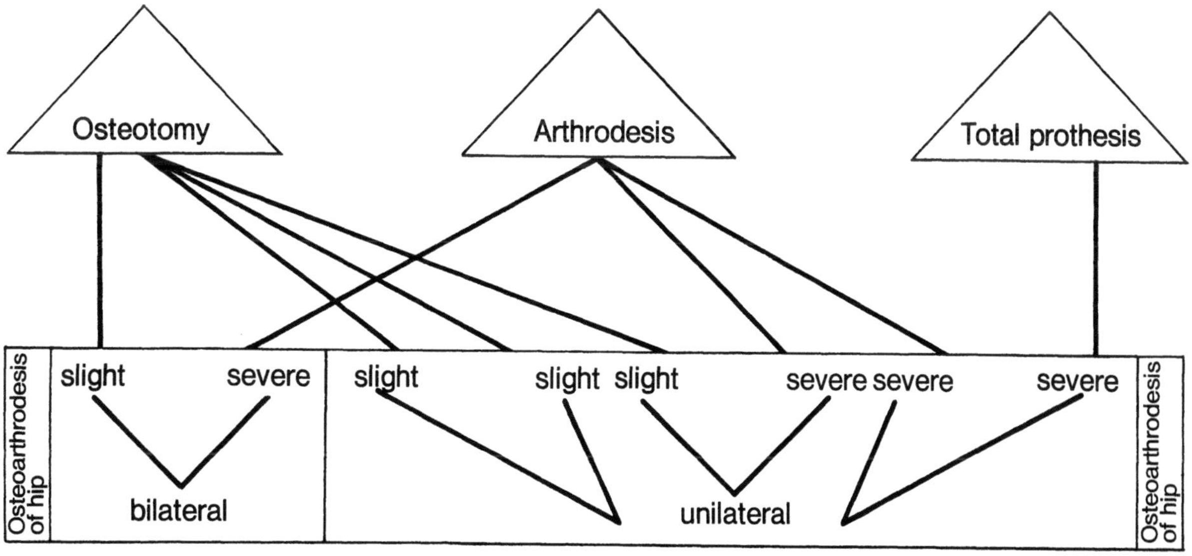

Fig. 74. *Indication for IO, HA and TP in young patients*

of the advantages to be expected from the operation.

Other solutions must be found for psychologically sensitive patients who become obsessed with thoughts of disfigurement or prolonged disability or for psychopaths or patients with depressive tendencies. Dynamic active and mentally adaptable patients with a positive attitude to life fulfill the prerequisites for HA.

Figs. 73a – f. *HA patients indulging in sport*

a – c) Two years following HA with cobra-head plate (see also Fig. 185): sailing, cross-country skiing, tennis (A. J.-Cl., ♂, aged 39 years, No. 105248).

d) Two years following Type I HA: walking, mountain climbing (seen here climbing the Wildstrubel, 3244 metres above sea level) (S. L., ♀, aged 37 years, No. 71355).

e and f) Ten months following Type II HA: skiing on the trail and in deep snow (A. L., ♂, aged 27 years, No. 103583)

4 Contraindications to Hip Arthrodesis

We differentiate between relative and absolute contraindications.

4.1 Relative Contraindications

- Poor general condition or reduced expectation of life
- Very young and very old patients
- Marked obesity
- Negative psychological attitude
- Reduced mobility of the lumbar spine (concave back, partially fixed lumbar lordosis) or reduced mobility of the contralateral hip and of the knee joint
  Varus knee or exaggerated degree of valgus knee (additional corrective osteotomy necessary)
- Severe destruction of the contralateral hip (particularly in young patients)
- Active infection

4.2 Absolute Contraindications

- Stiff ipsilateral knee
- Stiff contralateral hip
- Severe degenerative LS changes

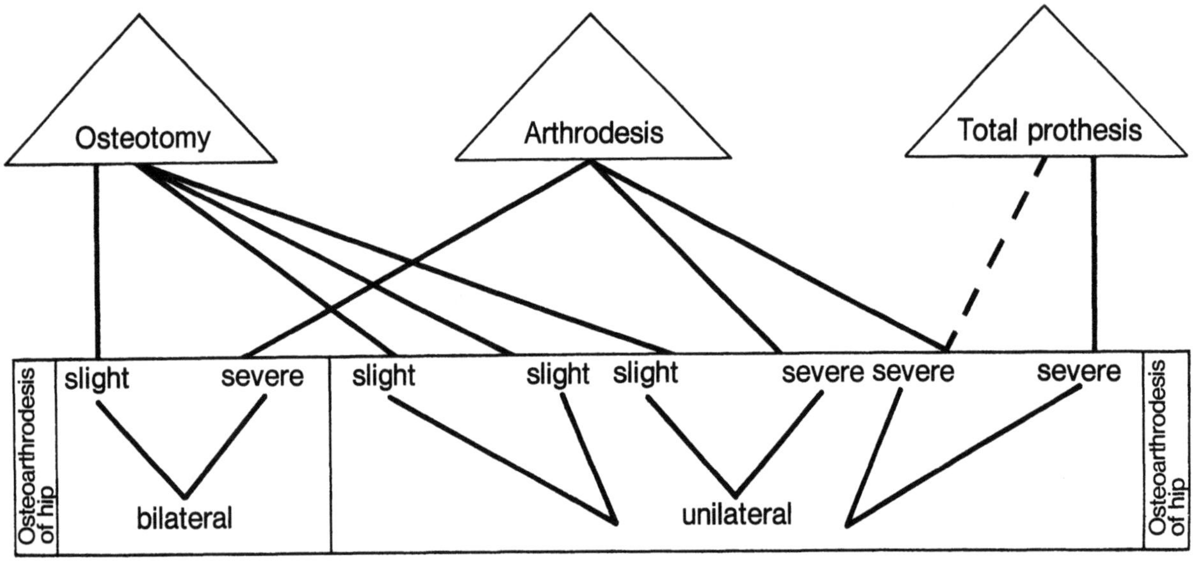

Fig. 75. *Indication for IO, HA and TP in middle-aged patients*

5 Choice of Operation

The three following figures illustrate our policy on the choice of IO, HA or TP in arthrosis of the hip. The factors considered are age, unilaterality or bilaterality and severity of the changes in the hip joint (Figs. 74–76).

In young patients we prefer IO (particularly where the degenerative dangers are slight) or HA (particularly in severe arthrosis of the hip). We are cautious in our approach to TP and will remain so until better solutions have been found to the problems associated with implant material and prosthesis fixation. The surgeon's options are not restricted on failure of an IO (WEBER) whereas at present the complications which are occurring with increasing frequency following TP leave one with few therapeutic alternatives (Fig. 74).

The considerations are similar in middle-aged patients. Only in exceptional cases do we perform bilateral TP in persons with bilateral severe coxarthrosis (Fig. 75).

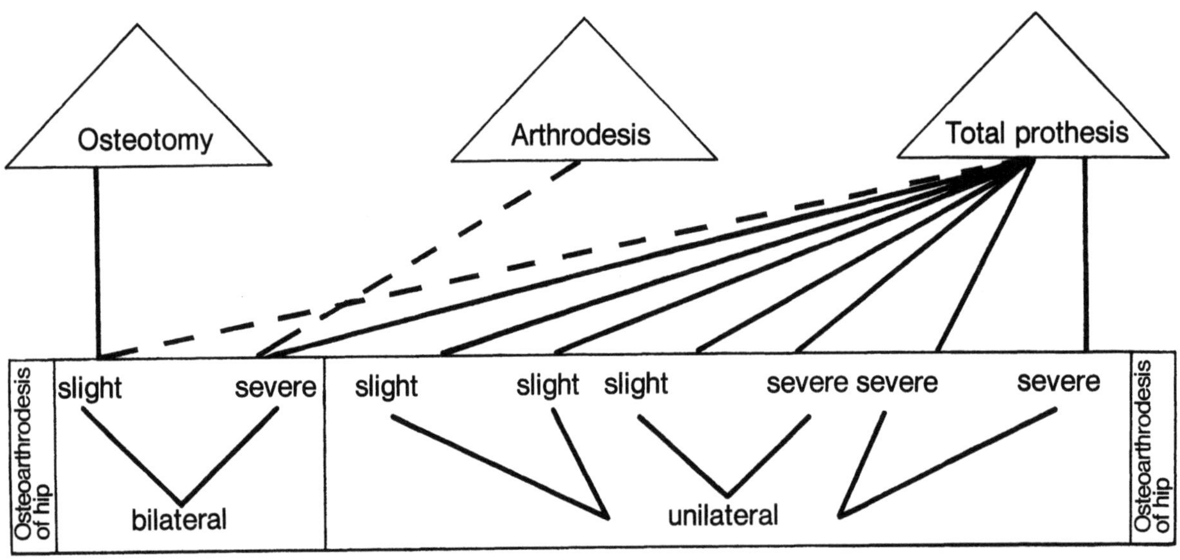

Fig. 76. *Indication for IO, HA and TP in elderly patients*

Subsequent to the development of prosthetic replacement we came to prefer this procedure in older patients. Now we only seldom perform an IO, perhaps wrongly. HA remains the exception but is still performed where the circumstances are ideal (Fig. 76).

6 Summary

The range of indications for HA has narrowed since the introduction of prosthetic replacement. In certain cases, however, HA has remained without substitute. If offers the clear advantages of definitive relief of pain together with total rigidity and ability to bear weight.

The chances of a successful HA have in creased as a result of improved technique and better understanding of the factors which determine whether or not the operation is indicated in a particular case. Both duration of hospital stay and of postoperative treatment have been significantly reduced by the use of rigid internal fixation with double plates or with the cobra-head plate. Such techniques allow one to dispense with prolonged postoperative cast fixation. In addition, weight and height are no longer so important. The early postoperative mobilisation of patients (an average of 7–10 days) has fundamentally reduced the danger to the neighbouring joints. For this reason, advanced age is no longer on its own an absolute contraindication to HA.

If strict attention is paid to the choice of patients and care is taken with their psychological conditioning, HA is the safest of the three main hip joint procedures and, in addition, the final result is permanent.

V. Operative Technique

1 Introduction

Basic changes have been made in our operative technique over the years 1961–1971. The earlier arthrodesis methods have been largely replaced by rigid internal fixation. The latter allows early mobilisation, functional postoperative treatment with no necessity for cast fixation, short duration of hospital stay and rapid rehabilitation both at work and elsewhere. The operation is still a severe stress for the patient, particularly if combined with PO, and also places great demands on the surgeon and anaesthesiologist. The operation can only be successfully carried out by a surgeon with considerable experience in hip surgery, a thorough grasp of hip biomechanics and an understanding of the principles of internal fixation. An HA which is incorrectly performed with rigid internal fixation has more serious consequences than earlier operations in the event of incorrect positioning of the hip; the latter mistake can only be corrected by reoperation. The methods available today allow a suitable arthrodesis to be performed in every case. In addition they have all withstood the test of time. The individual techniques are now discussed with their specific indications.

2 Preoperative Work-up

The patient should be thoroughly investigated preoperatively. Careful medical, radiological and orthopaedic examinations are obligatory.

2.1 Medical Examination

Apart from the routine tests (blood sedimentation rate, blood film, urinalysis) patients over 40 years of age should have an electrocardiogram and estimation of the serum electrolytes.

2.2 Radiological Examination

This includes:

- a/p and lateral thoracic films
- Lumbar vertebral films (both axes) and, if necessary, functional films in maximum inclination and reclination
- Plain film of the pelvis and, if necessary, functional views with the hips in maximum abduction and adduction
- Special views may be indicated in cases of post-traumatic disease of the hip joint (posterior dislocation of the hip, fracture of the acetabular roof with bone gap, etc.) and infection (sequester?).
- If there are problems in the neighbouring joints, particularly on the ipsilateral side, corresponding additional views may be necessary.

2.3 Orthopedic Investigation

This includes:

- Orthopedic history; previous operations or infections; occurrence, duration, localization and character of the complaints as well as the extent to which they are influenced by standing, sitting, lying and weight bearing; aids and therapy (cane, crutches, analgesics)
- Physical build, weight, height, occupation
- Gait, type of limp (Trendelenburg, Duchenne; limps caused by pain; leg shortening and joint stiffening)
- Examination of the back: posture, mobility, particularly that of the lumbar spine (finger-toe distance)
- True and apparent leg lengths; pelvic tilt
- Range of motion in the hips, knee joints and ankle joints
- Examination of the musculature and simple neurological examination
- Assessment of psychological state, family and social circumstances, activity in occupation and private life

3 Preparation for Operation

Since this is the same for all our HA operations, this topic is dealt with at this point.

3.1 Anesthesia

HA is always carried out under general anesthesia with endotracheal intubation. There is frequently considerable blood loss and four blood units should therefore be cross-matched.

3.2 Positioning of the Patient

We use the same lateral approach for all types of arthrodesis and the patient is therefore placed supine on a standard operating table. A traction table may be useful in special cases (high congenital dislocation or post-traumatic dislocation with a high femoral head) but is not absolutely necessary (Fig. 77).

3.3 Draping

The lower leg and foot are sterile wrapped and freely movable. Transparent self-adhesive plastic drapes are used to cover the whole upper leg to just above the knee as well as the hip which is to be operated and both iliac crests. The rest is draped with towels. Both malleoli should be palpable in order to allow checking of apparent leg length during the operation (Fig. 78).

4 Operative Technique

Thorough asepsis and gentle operative technique are essential to any internal fixation. Asepsis starts with the preparation of the patient for surgery and finishes with wound healing. Gentle "anatomical" operative technique largely prevents soft tissue necrosis and thus reduces the danger of infection to a minimum.

Orthopedic operations on the skeleton and particularly procedures which involve implantation of large foreign bodies require extensive prophylactic measures against infection. The danger of infection is dependent on the degree of asepsis and the powers of resistance of the patient. Apart from the universally valid rules of asepsis in orthopaedic surgery (disinfection of the hands, cotton gloves worn over surgical rubber gloves) the quality of the operating room plays an important part. Orthopedic surgery and particularly internal fixation procedures should not be carried out in the same room as abdominal surgery. Sterile operating

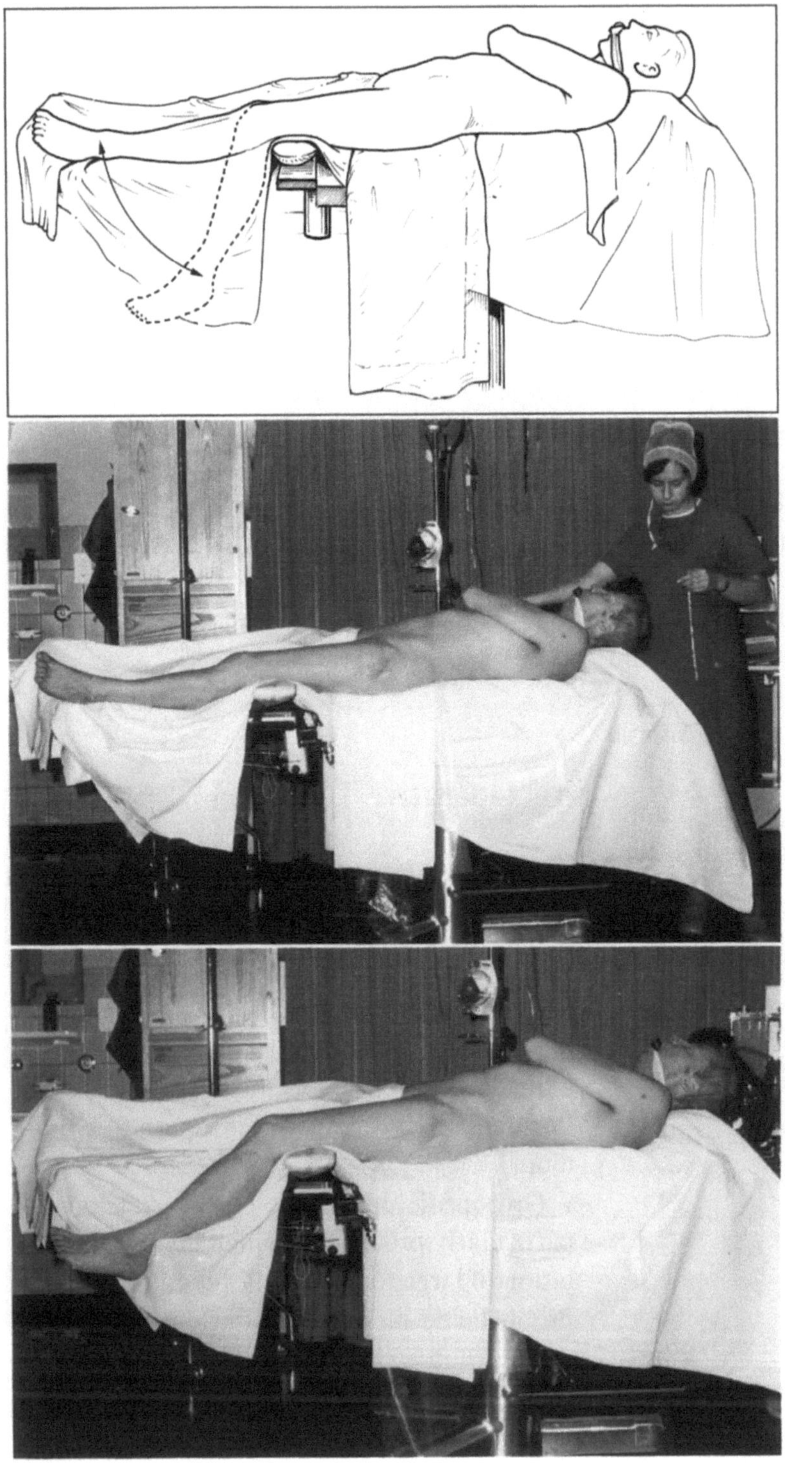

a

b

c

Fig. 77. *Positioning of the patient.*

a) Diagram. Patient lies supine on normal operating table. The well-padded board which is slid under the distal thigh allows free movement of the lower leg on the side being operated on.

b) and c) As above (photographs)

a b c

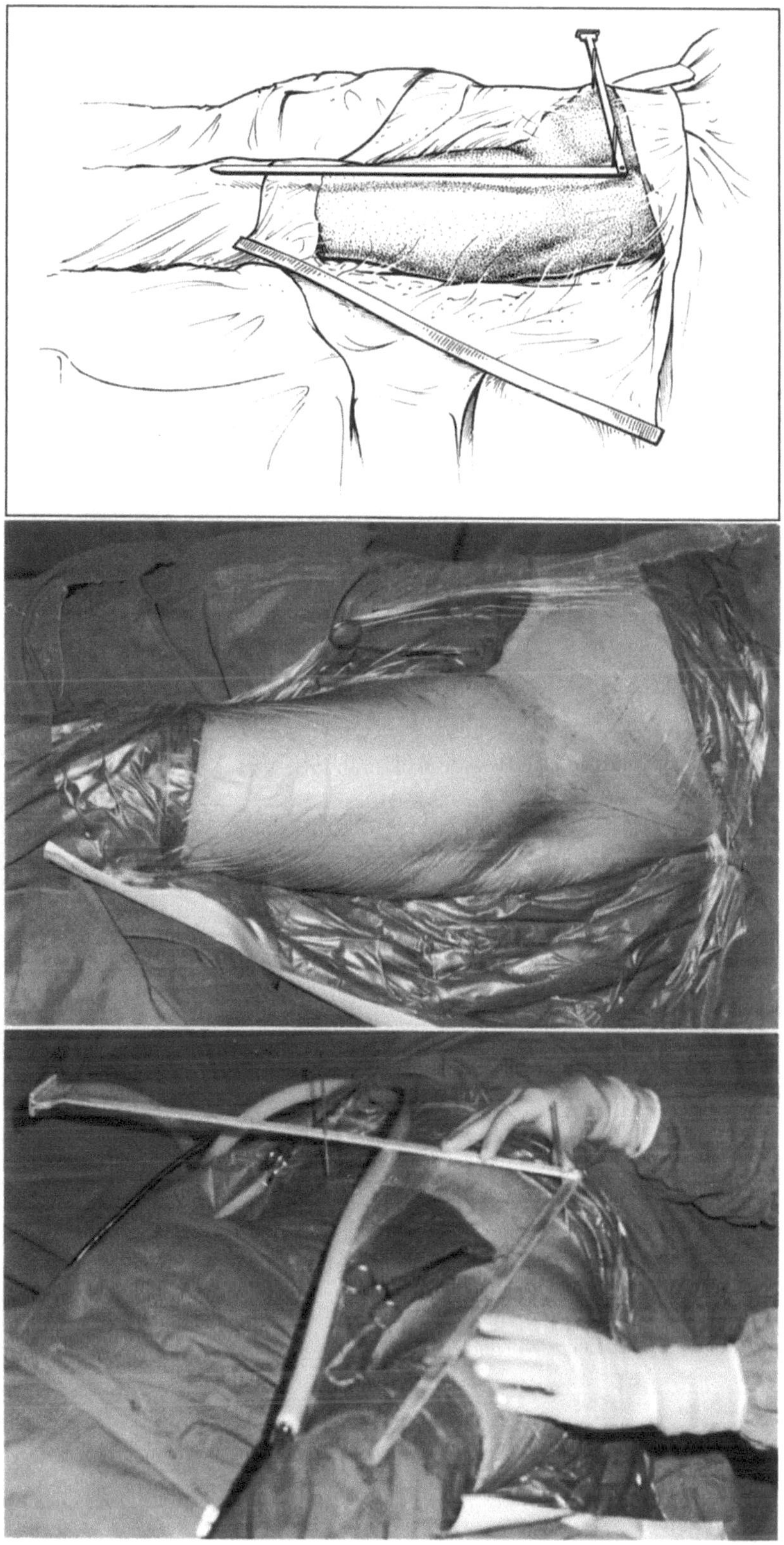

Fig. 78. *Draping patient.*

a) Diagram. K-wires have been driven into both anterior superior iliac spines (reference points for determining leg position using the special device).

b) and c) As above (photographs). The transparent self-adhesive plastic film allows precise determination of leg position. The lower leg and foot on the side being operated on are draped in such a way that they are freely movable

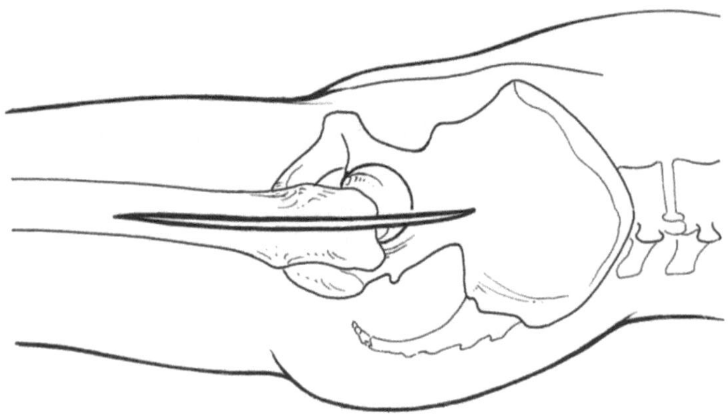

Fig. 79. *Skin incision.* Strictly lateral approach from the femoral diaphysis to a point 8 – 10 cm above the tip of the greater trochanter

boxes offer the best environment and reduce the chances of contamination of the wound by bacteria from the surrounding air (WEBER et al.).

In certain cases we increase the resistance of our patients by active immunisation with a polyvalent staphylococcal antigen (LIECHTI et al.). Until now we have mainly used this prophylactic immunisation in TP cases (bringing about a reduction in hip joint infection rate following TP from 6.8% to 2%) but it should also be applied systematically to any extensive orthopaedic procedure (particularly IO and HA).

4.1 Usual Operative Approach

We use basically the same approach for all our HA types. It is a strictly lateral approach from the femoral diaphysis to a point above the tip of the trochanter. The length of the incision is dependent upon the type of HA and is longest (25 – 30 cm) in Type IV arthrodeses (cobra-head plate arthrodeses) (Fig. 79).

In arthrodesis Types II – IV we proceed as follows:

Lateral skin incision (25 – 30 cm) along the femoral diaphysis to a point 8 cm cranial to the tip of the greater trochanter. The fascia lata is

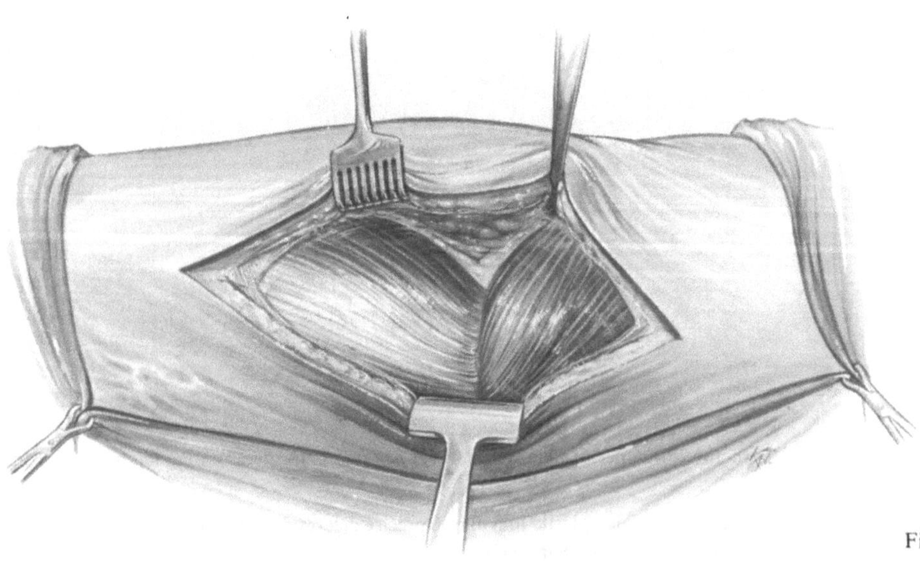

Fig. 80. *Splitting the fascia lata*

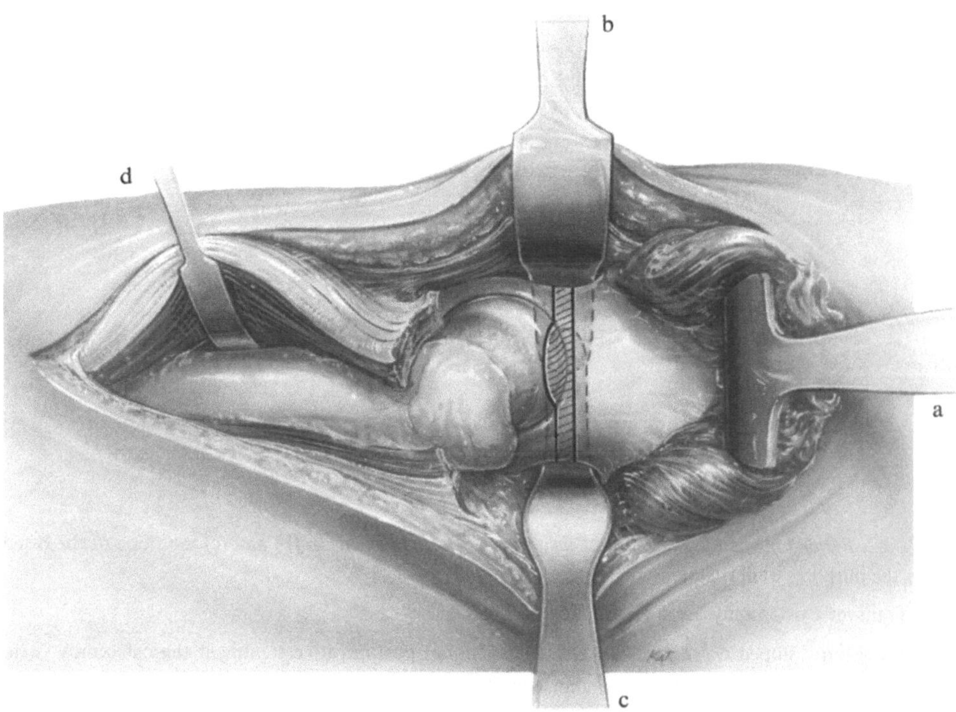

Fig. 81. *Positions of the Hohmann retractors*. Broad Hohmann retractor in the ala iliaca (*a*). Broad blunt Hohmann retractor over the iliopectineal eminence (*b*). Blunt Hohman retractor in the sciatic notch (*c*). Hohmann retractor over the femoral diaphysis (*d*) The interrupted lines show the contours of the blunt Hohmann retractors. The disc of bone which is to be removed is cross-hatched

split (Fig. 80). The joint capsule is exposed between M. tensor fascia lata and M. glutaeus medius. A retractor is placed between the joint capsule and the gluteal muscles, immediately medial to the tip of the trochanter. M. gluteus minimus and M. gluteus medius are divided from the greater trochanter and are freed along the joint capsule in a cranial direction up to the acetabular roof using scissors and osteotome. The pelvitrochanteric muscles can also be separated from the greater trochanter by slicing off a small disc of bone with its muscular attachment using the osteotome. M. vastus lateralis is opened proximally. It is freed along the linea aspera and is separated from the femur in an anteroposterior direction following display and ligature of the perforating vessels.

Three Hohmann retractors are now inserted (Fig. 81). The tip of the first broad retractor is driven into the ala iliaca 6–8 cm cranial to the acetabular rim; it retracts the pelvitrochanteric musculature in a cranial direction and exposes the roof of the acetabulum. The second broader, blunt retractor is slid over the ileopectineal eminence between the pelvis and M. iliacus and protects the pelvic contents. The final retractor is blunt but narrow and is inserted into the greater sciatic notch. It meets the broad retractor so that the whole pelvis is surrounded at this point, thus protecting nerves and vessels.

A further Hohmann retractor holds the M. vastus fibularis away from the femur in a ventral direction.

The freshened greater trochanter and the cranial surface of the femoral neck are sliced off with the oscillating saw and retained. The trochanteric fragment can later be inserted as a graft between the lateral aspect of the acetabular roof, the freshened neck of the femur and the plate.

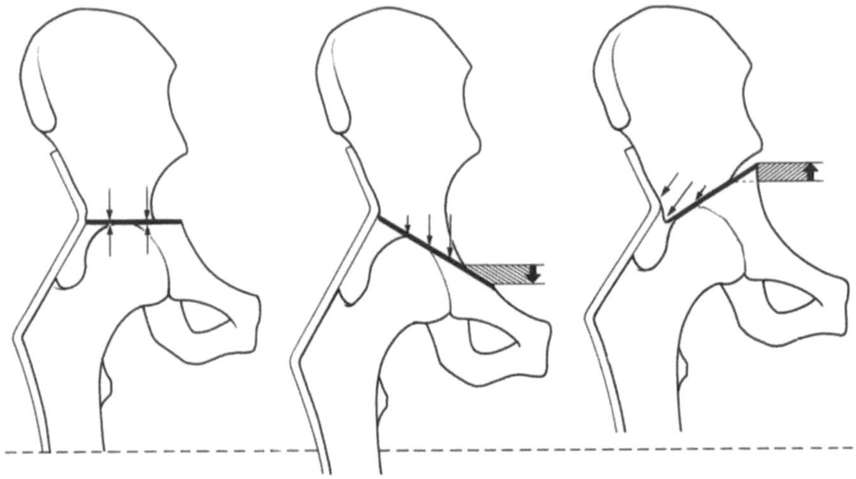

Fig. 82. *PO and medial displacement of the distal pelvic component.* In (b) and (c) the slope of the osteotomy has been exaggerated for the purposes of illustration.

a) Transverse osteotomy. Even distribution of forces.

b) Osteotomy sloped downwards. 1. During functional postoperative treatment the osteotomy is, for all intents and purposes, compressed vertically, allowing maximum stability. 2. Load particularly medial. 3. Small increase in length if medial displacement pronounced.

c) Osteotomy sloping upwards. 1. Shear forces act on the osteotomy. 2. Bone contact area diminished. 3. Increased load on the plate. 4. Pronounced medial displacement results in slight shortening of the leg

4.2 Pelvic Osteotomy

The joint capsule is resected cranially, ventrally up to the middle of the femoral neck and in a dorsal direction. The cranial segment of the femoral head is resected with the oscillating saw or with a broad thin osteotome. This makes the acetabular roof visible from the hip joint. The acetabular roof is osteotomised approximately 1 cm higher up, precisely in the transverse plane of the body. The osteotomy should run transversely or slightly sloped downwards (Figs. 82a–82c). A complete disc should be resected stepwise from the pelvis until the internal cortex is visible. The two blunt Hohmann retractors offer full protection during this procedure. The stepwise removal of the disc of bone down to the internal cortex is fully visible and completely safe. A distractor is now inserted (Fig. 83) and the internal cortex is sliced through stepwise with a long narrow osteotome, thus completing the PO.

Medial displacement of the femoral head under the iliac bone is usually necessary in order to improve contact between the raw cancellous surfaces of the acetabular roof and the femoral head. The medial displacement is easily encouraged using a suitable vanadium lever (known to us as the tire lever) (Fig. 84). Rotation of the distal pelvic fragment at the symphysis occurs and in some cases this results in full dislocation of the symphysis. However, the latter does not give rise to complaints and is only noticeable as a radiological curiosity. Rosen recommends cutting the symphysis in order to facilitate medial displacement. We have never done this but we are of the opinion that it could be useful if a particularly large degree of medial displacement were necessary.

Following medial displacement, the leg is placed in the position finally intended. The raw surfaces of the acetabular roof and femoral head should lie precisely parallel to each other. If this is not the case, a further resection of a

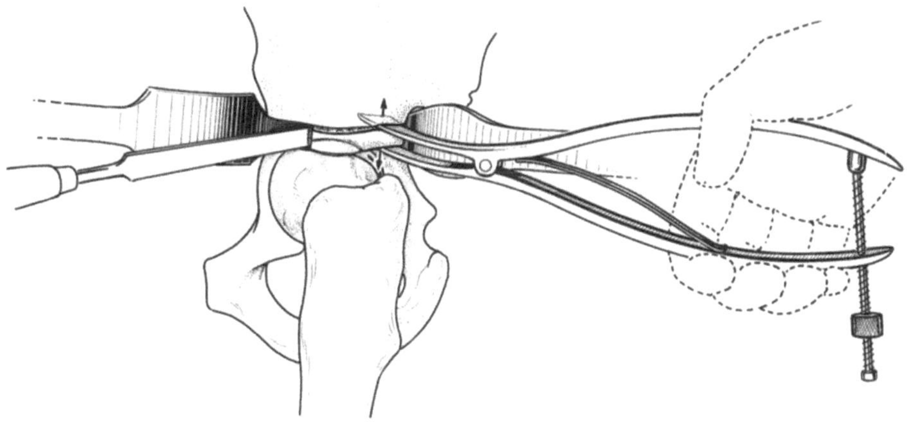

Fig. 83. *PO*. Following removal of the bone disc, use of the distraction clamp allows the internal cortex to be cut through under direct vision without danger to surrounding anatomical structures

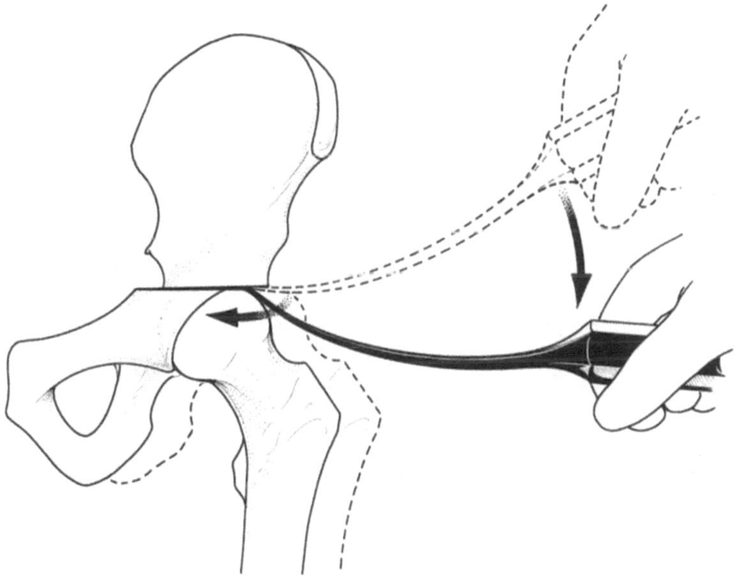

Fig. 84. *Medial displacement following osteotomy*. Medial displacement is simplified by the leverage provided by the vanadium "tire lever"

small amount of the femoral head may be carefully performed. It is preferable that the osteotomy surfaces be concave rather than convex in order that the contact points be at the periphery and not at the centre (Fig. 85). This concavity increases stability and usually makes the additional bone graft unnecessary. The lateral acetabular roof is now trimmed so as to prevent it projecting laterally and to render it flat. This allows the implant (straight plates or cobra-head plates) to fit snugly against the bone.

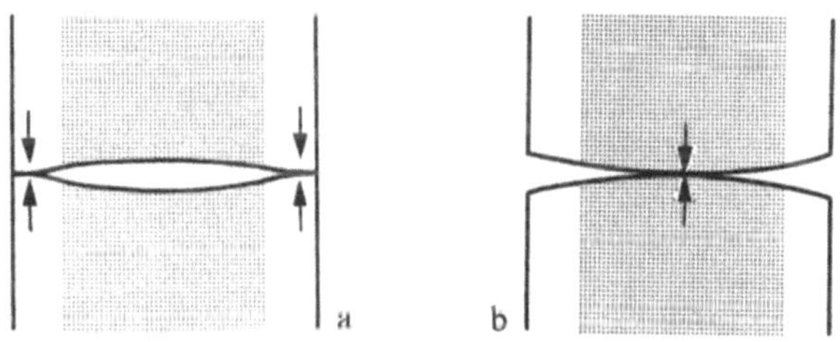

Fig. 85. *Diagrammatic representation of the osteotomy*.

a) Concave osteotomy surfaces. Good contact between the cortices results in improved stability.

b) Convex osteotomy surfaces. Disadvantageous (slight peripheral gaping with separation of the cortices)

4.3 Intertrochanteric Osteotomy

This was usually carried out as part of the Type I HA. Now it is particularly carried out in atypical hip arthrodeses. The advantages are:

- In certain cases, an increase in leg length is possible.
- The final leg position may be adjusted postoperatively ("Flexible arthrodesis").
- Because the long femoral lever arm no longer acts directly on the proximal femur, the stress on the internal fixation is markedly reduced. This is useful where only a minimal degree of internal fixation is possible, e.g., in the presence of infection.
- If possible, M. vastus lateralis is not freed. It is simply split longitudinally and the IO field is exposed with two small Hohmann retractors.

Extensive elevation of the periosteum should also be avoided. A *transverse* osteotomy is made with the oscillating saw precisely between the Hohmann retractors. This allows

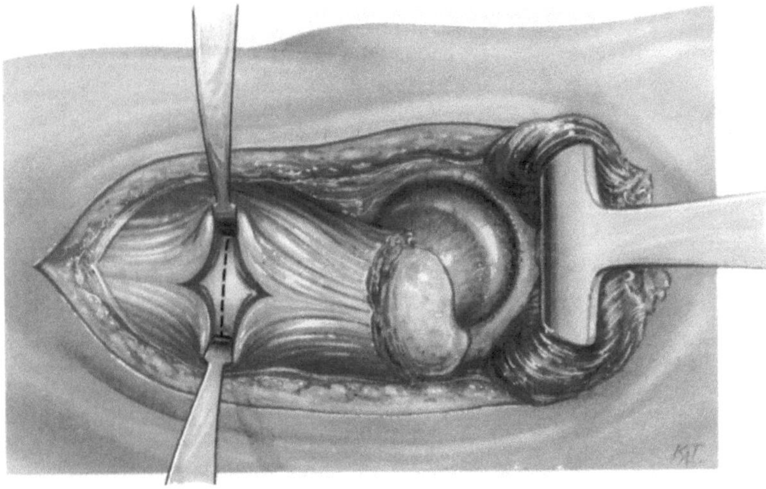

Fig. 86. *Intertrochanteric or subtrochanteric osteotomy.* The vastus lateralis muscle is split but not freed from the bone. Transverse osteotomy between the small Hohmann retractors

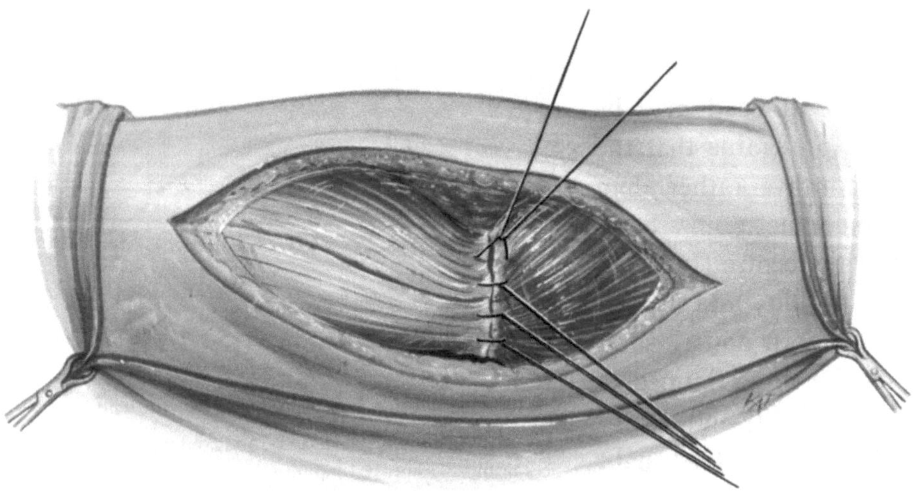

Fig. 87. *Wound closure.* The pelvitrochanteric muscles are sutured to the vastus lateralis muscle with single sutures

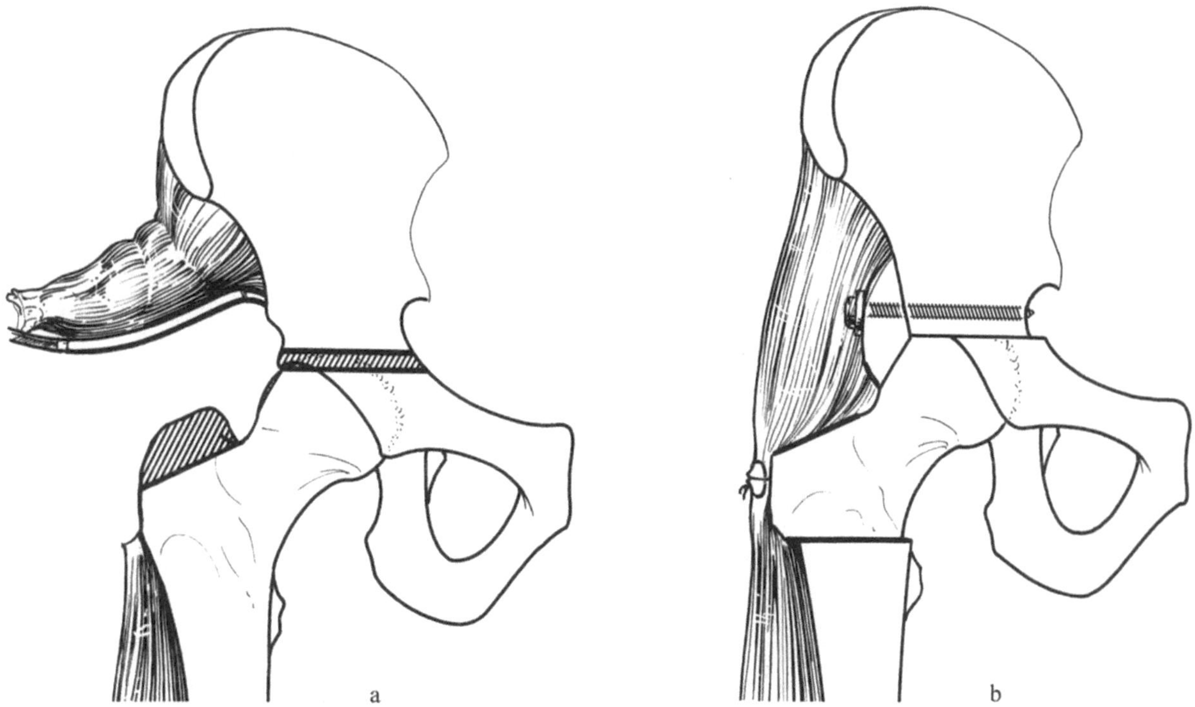

Fig. 88. *Type I Hip arthrodesis*. Freshening arthrodesis with IO. The greater trochanter is used as an iliofemoral graft and is fixed to the pelvis with a lag screw. The vastus lateralis muscle is not freed

the final leg position to be adjusted without disturbing the relationship between the femoral head and the iliac bone (Fig. 86).

If freeing of M. vastus lateralis and extensive periosteal elevation are avoided, the soft tissues form a cuff around the bone and the muscle lends a degree of stability to the IO. The resulting light pressure accelerates bone union.

If it unexpectedly becomes necessary to perform an IO following extensive freeing of the soft tissues at the level of the osteotomy, it is recommended that a thick K-wire (or a flexible Oberholzer nail) be inserted into the medullary cavity from the trochanter in order to increase the stability of the IO (Fig. 99c).

4.4 Wound Closure

Wound closure is the same following all methods (Fig. 87). The whole operative field is generously rinsed with Ringer solution. Two deep suction drains and two subcutaneous suction drains are left in place. Careful suture of the pelvitrochanteric musculature to M. vastus lateralis is very important. The latter is in turn sutured dorsally to the tendon of M. glutaeus maximus. The fascia lata and skin are closed in layers.

5 Operative Technique: Particular Features of the Different Arthrodesis Types

The HA Types I–IV and the atypical HA are discussed individually. In particular, the type of HA, the special indications and the postoperative management are explained in each case. The reader is referred to pp. 26–37 for technical details of the operations.

5.1 Type I Hip Arthrodesis

This is an arthrodesis with freshening of the bone surfaces and IO. The greater trochanter is used as an iliofemoral graft and is fixed with

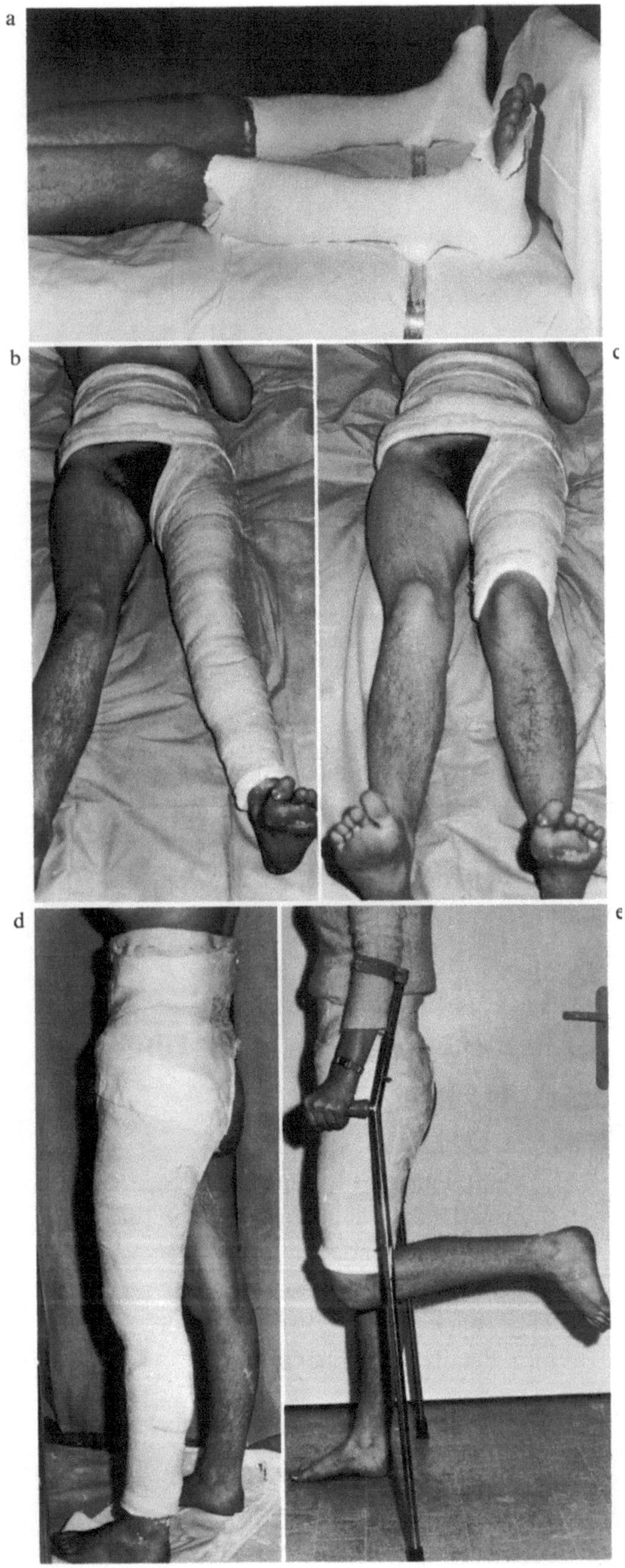

Fig. 89. *Postoperative cast fixation.*

a) Postoperative cast with slight abduction.

b and d) Two weeks after operation. Hip spica with patient lying (b) and standing (d).

c and e) Four weeks following operation. Short hip spica with patient lying (c) and standing (e)

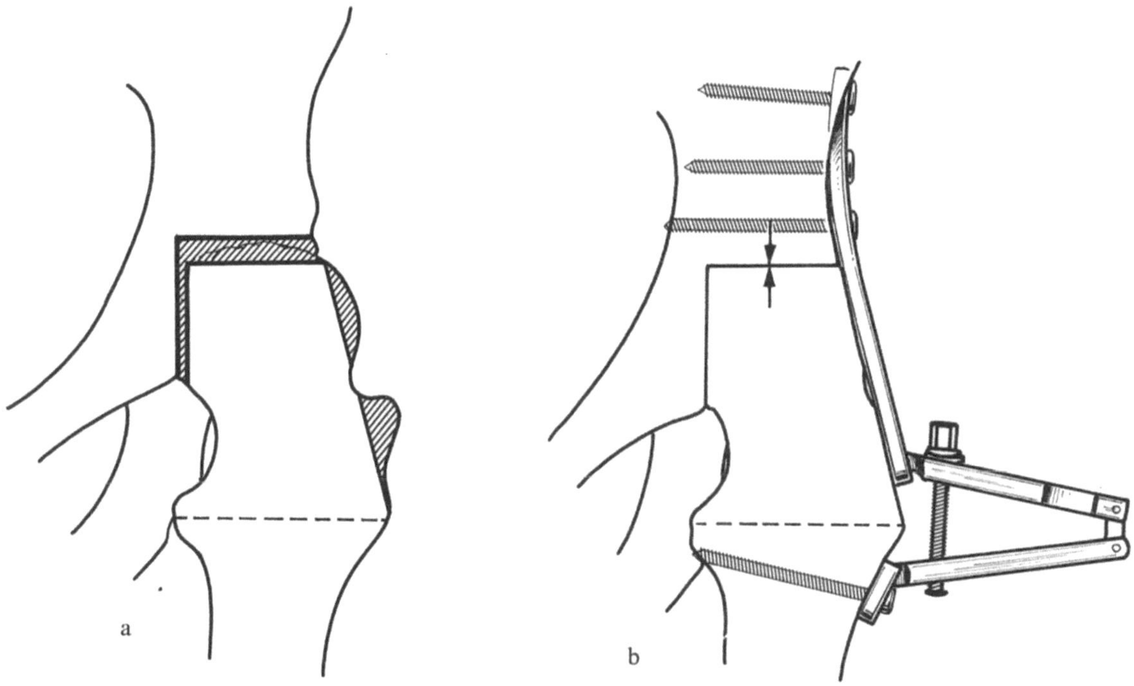

Fig. 90. *Type II HA without PO*. Following freshening of the joint surfaces and resection of the lateral femoral head and trochanter (a) a straight plate is fixed to the pelvis and tensioned with the special device (b). Subsequently IO is performed

a compression screw. This graft prevents dislocation of the femoral head and fixes the femoral neck in the required degree of valgus. The Type I may optionally be combined with PO.

Freeing of M. vastus lateralis is to be avoided in this type of arthrodesis (Fig. 88).

In our series of cases, 156 such procedures were carried out. However, in the last 5 years it has been replaced by the HA with stable internal fixation.

Postoperative management: Both lower legs are placed in a cast. The cast is joined by a bar with moderate symmetrical abduction. The patient is laid flat in bed (Fig. 89a).

At 2 weeks postoperatively, the patient is placed in a hip spica down to just above the ankle in general anaesthesia. The leg is abducted 10° more than required. The patient then gets up and walks with canes; heel-to-toe movement is allowed on the operated side (Figs. 89b and 89d). At 4 weeks postoperatively, the cast is shortened to just above the knee joint. Active and passive knee joint exercises commence (Figs. 89c and 89e). Discharge is 12 weeks following operation with removal of the cast and radiological control. If the HA and IO are united cast-free weight bearing is increased over a period of 6 weeks and then a further radiological check is carried out.

5.2 Type II Hip Arthrodesis

In this type, the joint components are fixed with a plate following decortication. In addition, an IO is carried out (Figs. 90, 91).

This HA can also be optionally combined with a PO. It was a transition to HA with rigid internal fixation. In our series, 20 such arthrodeses were performed.

This method is still particularly useful in the following indications:

- Increase in leg length (varus hip, idiopathic or posttraumatic NHF). Valgus correction causes lengthening of the proximal femur and following IO there is an increase in leg length.

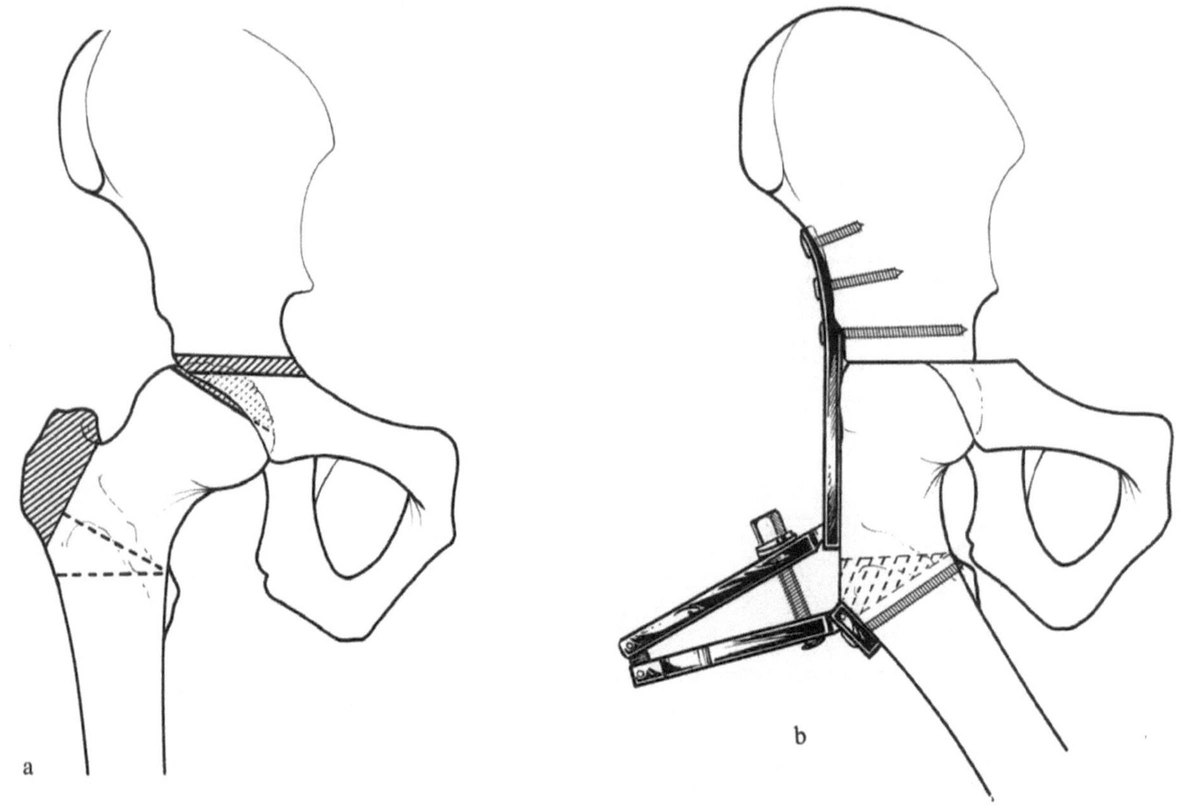

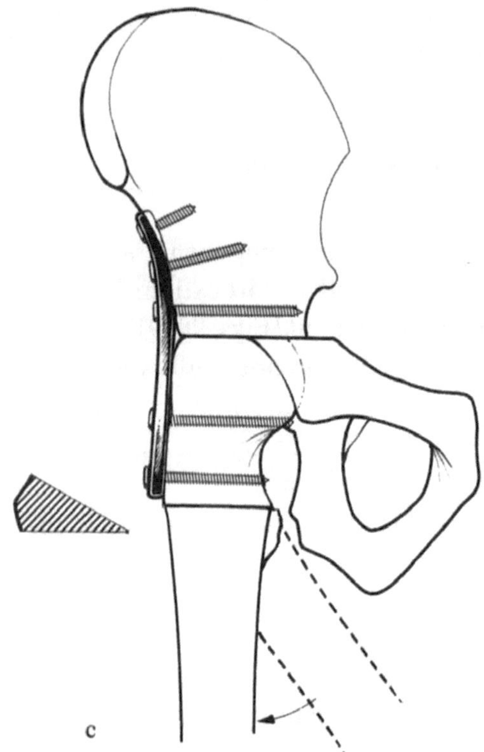

Fig. 91. *Type II HA to increase leg length.*

a) Resection of the trochanter, PO, resection of a small disc from the femoral head with the leg in adduction.

b) Adduction of the leg brings the femoral neck into valgus. The plate is applied and tensioned.

c) IO is performed with removal of a small lateral wedge to correct the adduction deformity

- If the plate is only to fulfill a buttress function (following reduction of a high congenital dislocation).
- In certain cases of GH, the method may be used to prevent redislocation of the greater trochanter which has been brought into the acetabulum.
- If an increase in length is intended, a PO is carried out as described but with the leg in adduction. The femoral neck is in valgus so that leg lengthening occurs following IO. Following PO, the greater trochanter is cut off and the lip of the acetabular roof is smoothed off somewhat in order to allow a better fit to the thick 6-hole plate. The plate is screwed to the ala iliaca with at least three screws and with the leg in abduction. The special jointed tensioning device already described is screwed into place distal to the plate and hooked into the plate. The freshened head of the femur is thus forced against the iliac surface of the PO. Compression internal fixation results. Following fixation of the plate with the last distal screw, transverse IO is carried out. The adduction deformity of the leg is corrected by removal of a small lateral wedge and, in this manner, the leg length is increased by 2 – 3 cm (Fig. 91).

Postoperative management: Same as for Type I. For this reason the arthrodesis Types I and II which require more prolonged cast fixation are more suitable for younger patients.

5.3 Type III Hip Arthrodesis

The double-plate arthrodesis with or without PO had already been recommended by MÜLLER in 1953 (Fig. 47). It was the first HA using stable internal fixation. In our series it was carried out in 108 patients. It allowed early mobilisation and was therefore indicated in older patients. This type of arthrodesis has been completely replaced by HA using the cobra-head plate but the end effect is identical. The procedure is only exceptionally indicated but may be valuable in the following situations:

a) In cases of PA subsequent to cobra-head plate arthrodesis
b) If cobra-head plate arthrodesis is impossible for technical reasons (e.g., severe changes in anatomy as a result of trauma, steeply angled ala iliaca) or if the fixation of the cobra-head plate in the bone immediately above the osteotomy is inadequate

Postoperative management: No cast; quadriceps exercises and immediate mobilisation of the knee joint. Patient gets up 10 days postoperatively. Walking with two canes for 3 months with gradual increase in weight bearing. Radiographic follow-up with full weight bearing when complete bone union has occurred.

5.4 Type IV Hip Arthrodesis

The HA developed by SCHNEIDER in Switzerland uses the cobra-head compression plate and is a refinement of MÜLLER's double-plate arthrodesis. It is almost always combined with PO; the degree of medial displacement depends on the anatomical relationship between femoral head and acetabulum. It has been the method of choice since 1967 (258 cases in our series) (Figs. 92, 93).

This arthrodesis has the following advantages:

a) Large area of cancellous bone contact
b) Stability
c) No postoperative cast fixation or immobilisation; early mobilisation and exercise are integral parts of the technique. For this reason there is no longer any worry about knee stiffness which used to be such a problem. Furthermore, early mobilisation benefits circulation and respiratory function and reduces the danger of decubitus, which is particularly important in older patients.
d) Short hospital stay (2 – 3 weeks).

A moderate to large degree of medial displacement following PO results in improved

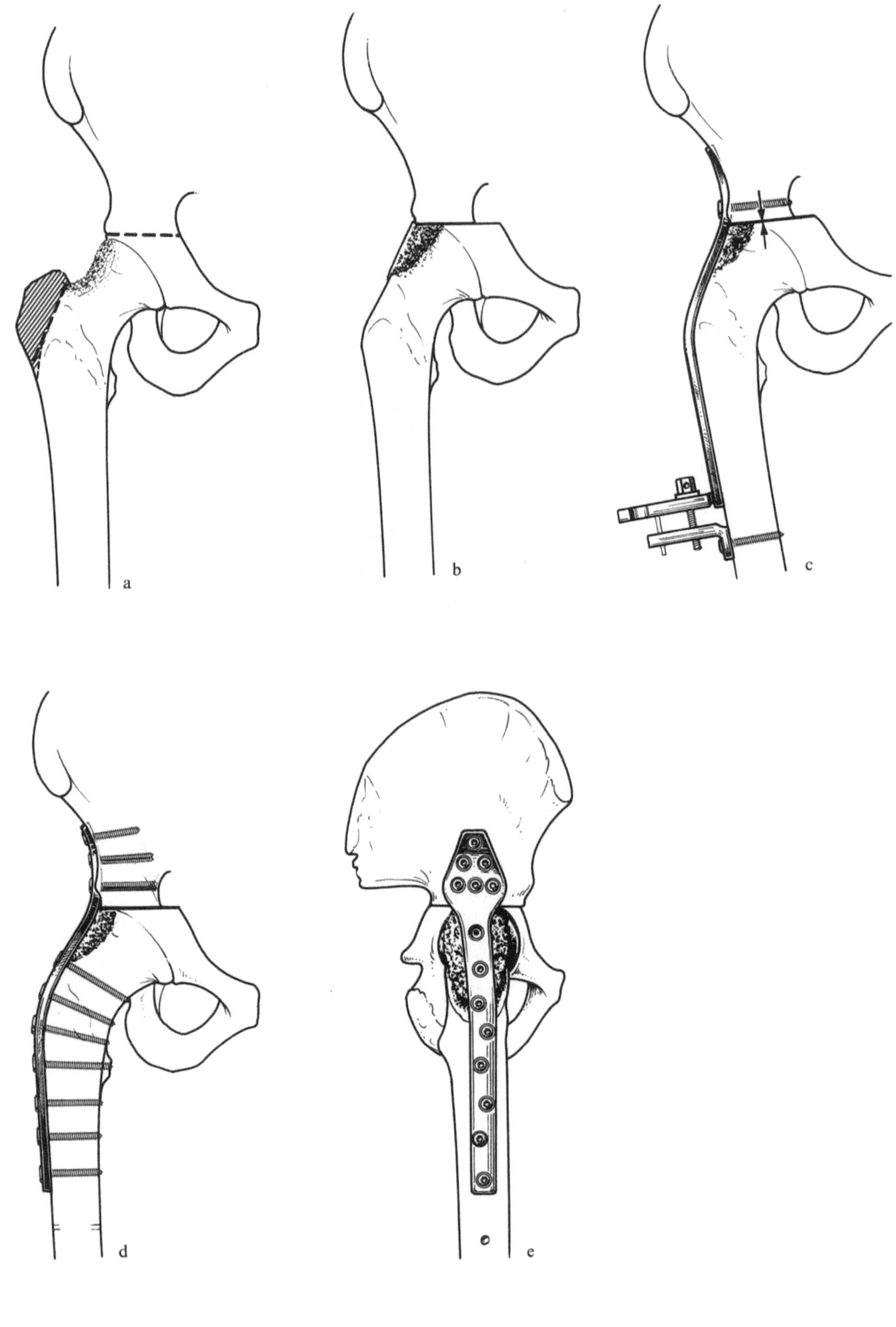
a
b
c
d
e

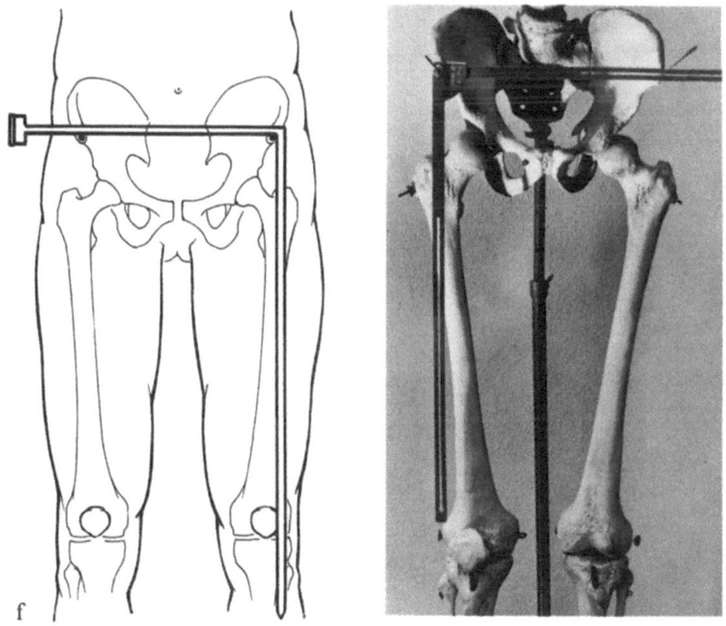

Fig. 92. *Type IV HA; operative technique (cobra-head plate arthrodesis).*

a) The greater trochanter is removed and the lateral aspect of the femoral neck is freshened. PO.

b) If there is considerable medial displacement of the femoral head, the freshened greater trochanter is inserted into the space between the femoral neck and the cobra-head plate.

c) The cobra-head plate is fitted to the bone, using the bending irons or plate press to contour the plate if necessary. The plate is temporarily fixed with a cortex screw through the middle hole of the head of the plate. The screw passes through the middle of the acetabular roof, 1 cm cranial to the PO. The plate is gently tensioned with the AO tensioning device.

d) Fixing the plate. First the proximal screw is driven into the acetabular roof. The freshened greater trochanter is inserted into the space between the freshened femoral neck and the plate. The plate is tensioned so as to impact the osteotomy surfaces. The leg position is again checked with the special apparatus; if the position is correct the line joining the iliac spines should subtend an angle of 90° to the line joining the iliac spine to the lateral femoral condyle. When positioned correctly (zero position or up to 5° of adduction), the lower arm of the positioning device should lie against the lateral border of the patella. All the screws are driven into the femoral diaphysis. Reduction in functional leg length 0 – 1 cm.

e) Position of the cobra-head plate seen from the side.

f) Correct application of the special positioning device for HA. The K-wires which have been driven into the anterior superior iliac spines are used as points of reference. If the leg is in the zero position with respect to abduction/adduction following fixation of the plate (i.e., at the end of the operation) the vertical arm of the positioning device should touch the lateral border of the patella. Before tensioning the plate the position is checked: rotation, flexion, adduction (10° – 15°). The ideal flexion position is obtained by placing a small towel roll under the leg. With the correct degree of adduction the functional length of the operated leg is 4 – 5 cm less than the opposite side.

g) Application of the special positioning device, demonstrated on the skeleton

a
b
c
d
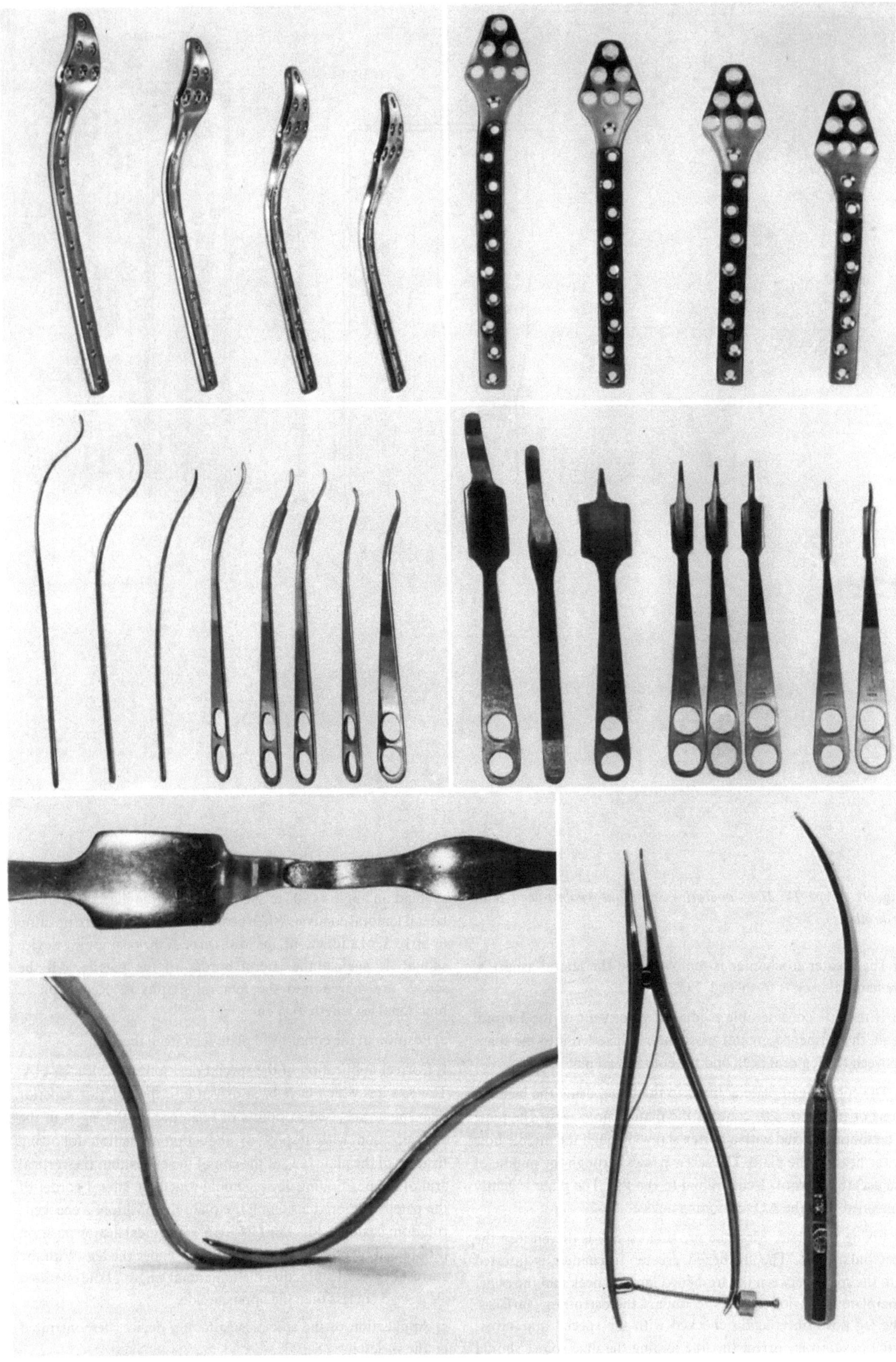

e

f

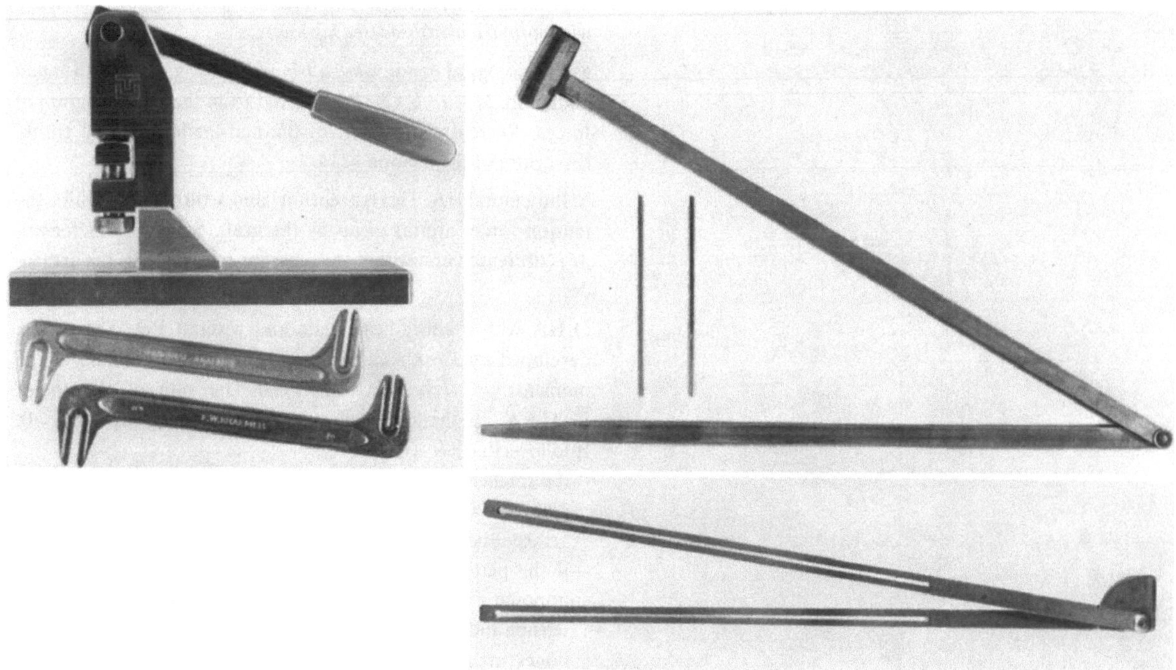

g

Fig. 93. *Important instruments for cobra-head plate arthrodesis.*

a) Long cobra-head plates seen from the front and side.

b) Hohmann retractors: blunt ribbed retractor; broad retractor, known as the "spade-Hohmann"; various broad sharp retractors.

c) The two blunt Hohmann retractors (seen from the side and front) are juxtaposed in this manner so as to allow the PO to be safely performed.

d) Right: so-called "tire lever", made of vanadium. Left: distraction clamp.

e) Plate-bending instruments. Above: bending press. Below: bending irons.

f) Aiming device and K-wires.

g) Müller's improved version of the instrument (grooves for the K-wires and built-in protractor)

distribution of the forces acting on the skeleton of the leg since the leverage is reduced (Figs. 94–97).

It must be emphasised once more that this operation imposes a greater stress on the patient and that the operative technique is sufficiently complex to require a practised hand.

Postoperative management: The leg is laid in a foam rubber splint. Immediate quadriceps exercises and mobilisation of the knee joint, bed rest for 5 days followed by walking with two crutches; the foot is placed on the ground without weight bearing. Gradual increase in load with full weight bearing at the end of 3 months. The radiological follow-up at 3 months almost always shows full primary bone union. Fibrous ankylosis is extremely rare (Fig. 113).

5.5 Atypical Hip Arthrodeses

Almost all HA operations can be carried out using the cobra-head plate or one of the other techniques mentioned. However, the following techniques are available in exceptional cases, e.g., in infected hips or in GH; following removal of a TP; in cases of high congenital dislocation; following certain fracture dislocations; in almost completely ankylosed hips with angular deformity.

5.5.1 Hip Arthrodesis in the Presence of Infection

Classically, in cases of hip infection the infection itself was first treated and the arthrodesis was carried out at a later stage. Our

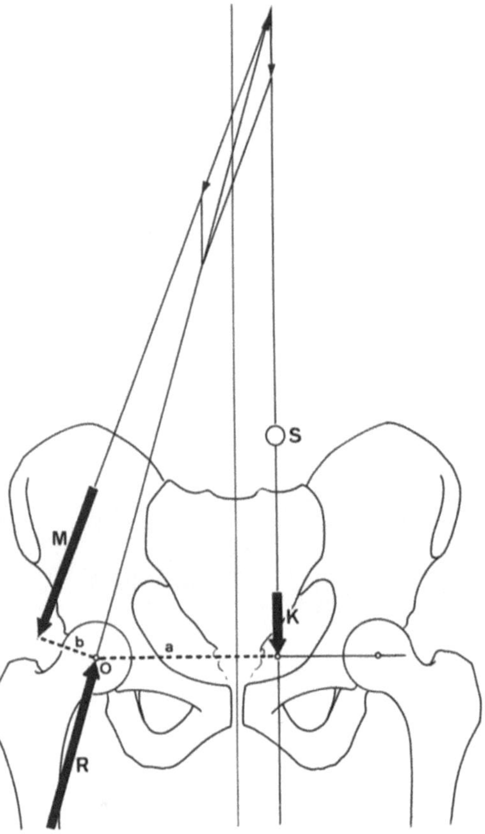

a

Fig. 94. *Analysis of the forces which act when standing on one leg with normal and arthrodesed hip joints.*

a) Physiological conditions: $a/b=3/1$ (see Fig. 19). With intact abductors $M\times a=b\times K$. R is derived from the parallelogram of forces. S=centre of weight of the non-loaded leg and trunk. O=centre of the femoral head.

b) Iliofemoral HA. This is a tension band arthrodesis in which the tension forces are taken up by the graft. Since b is increased, $\vec{M}$ is decreased and with it the pressure acting across the arthrodesis.

c) HA with a cobra-head plate and without PO. The torque developed by $\vec{K}=\vec{K}\times a$. For O at equilibrium: the sum of the moments $=\ O\rightarrow a\times\vec{K}+\vec{M}\times b=0$ The sum of the forces $=O\rightarrow\vec{K}+\vec{M}$ the forces acting in the arthrodesis gap $(\uparrow\uparrow\uparrow)=0$. It follows that:

—the smaller $\vec{K}\times a$, the smaller becomes M (the tension on the plate) and the smaller becomes the pressure across the arthrodesis gap.

—if the plate is removed then 1) the tension forces must be opposed by restoration of abductor activity or 2) additional tension and compression forces are generated in the arthrodesed bones (in the abductor arthrodesis system precise detection and measurement of these forces is hardly possible; it is only possible to make semiquantitative estimates).

d) HA with cobra-head plate, PO and medial displacement of the distal pelvic component. Reduction in the magnitude of a lessens the torque acting about the point O. This in turn proportionately reduces all the tension and compression forces acting on the arthrodesis. By medial displacement, the lever (a) over which K is distributed is shortened and this causes increased stress, particularly on the lateral femur

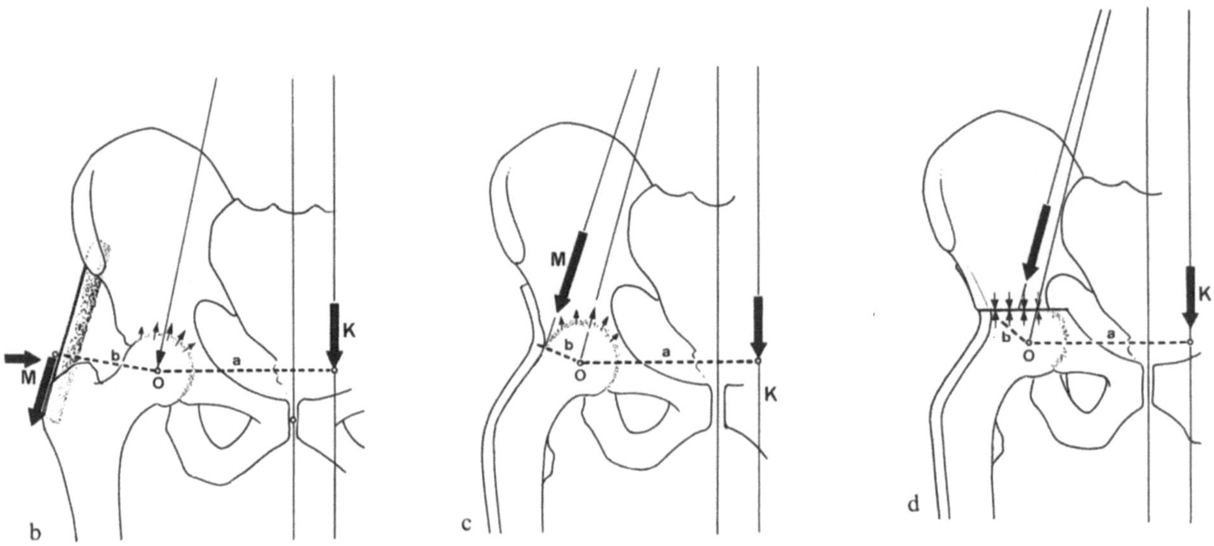

b c d

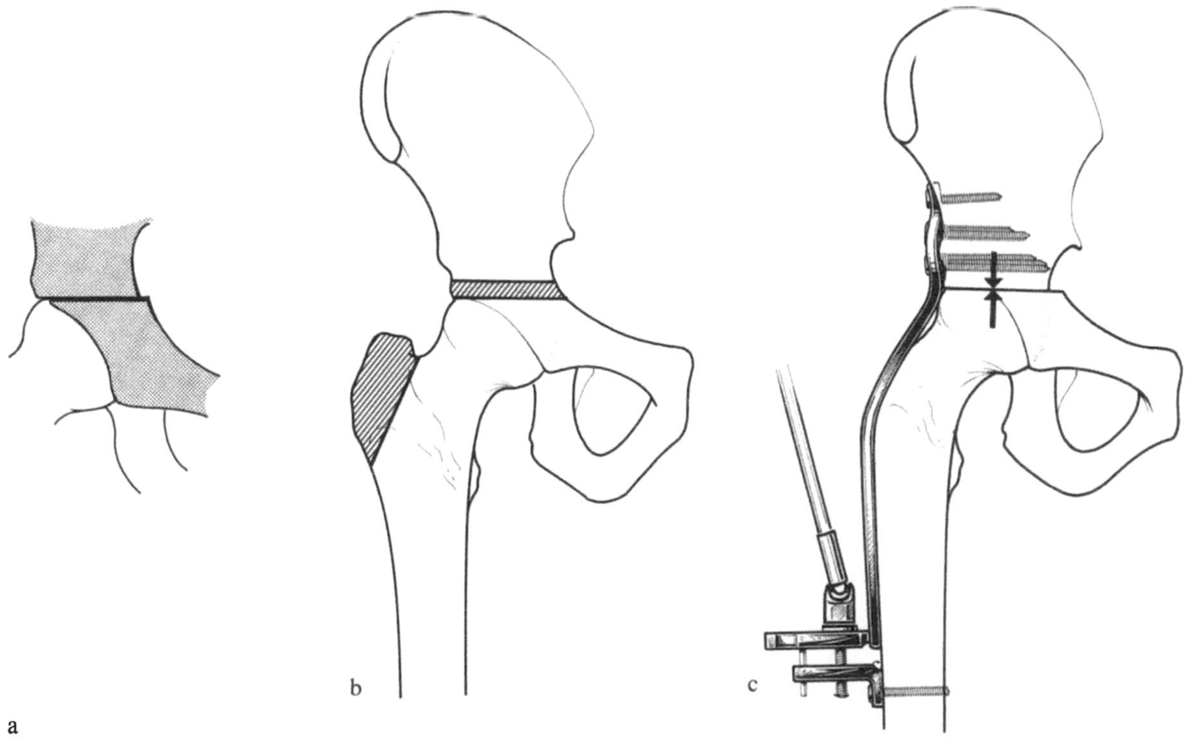

Figs. 95 – 97. *Medial displacement of the femoral head following PO*

Fig. 95. *Small medial displacement*

a) Diagrammatic representation of the medıal displacement.

b) A small medial displacement suffices if the femoral head lies completely within the acetabulum.

c) Large surfaces of contact. The plate touches the bone at all points

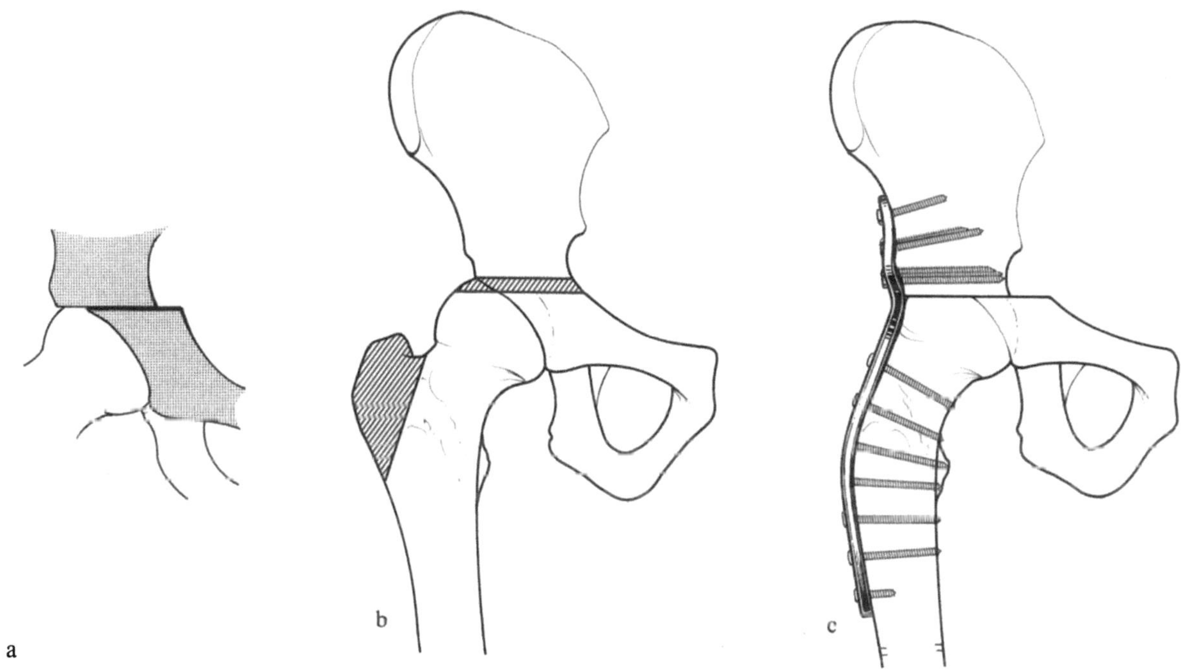

Fig. 96. *Moderate medial displacement*

a) Dıagrammatic representation of the displacement.

b) If subluxation of the femoral head has occurred greater medial dısplacement is necessary in order to bring the head well under the proximal pelvis.

c) The plate has been bent to fit the bone closely at all points

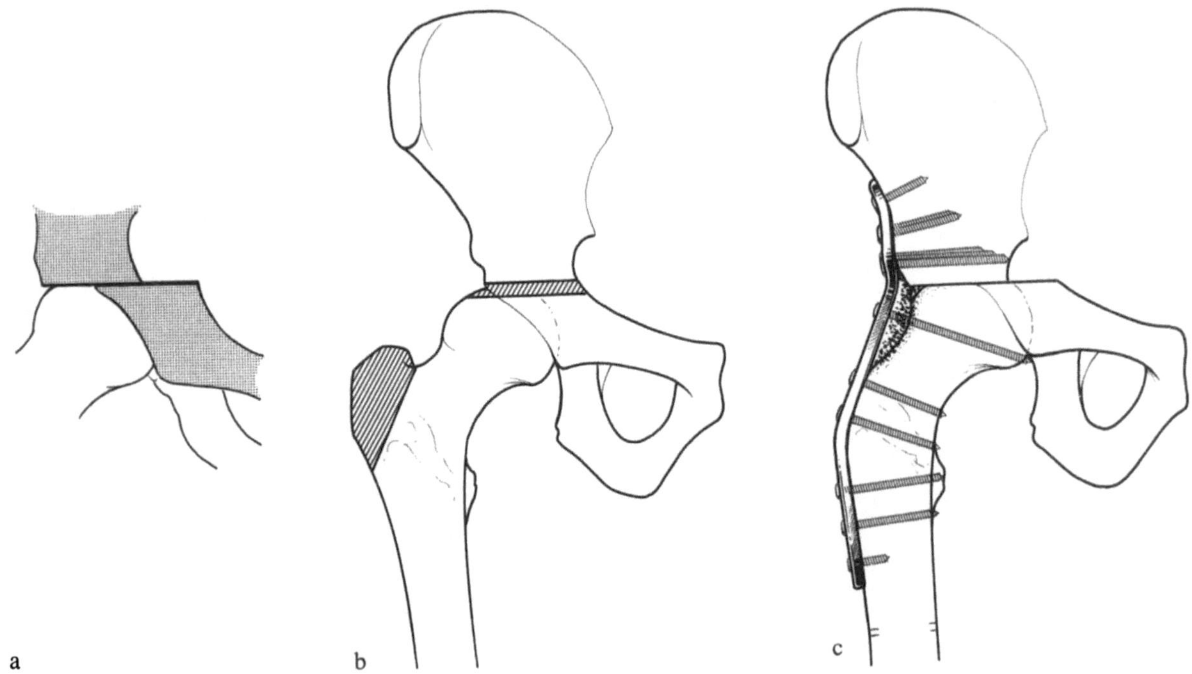

Fig. 97. *Large medial displacement*

a) Diagrammatic representation of the displacement.

b) Subluxation of the femoral head. PO and resection of the trochanter.

c) If the plate does not fit perfectly against the bone the cavity between the femoral neck and the plate may be filled with the freshened trochanteric bone

approach is as follows. The acute active infection is treated by sequesterotomy, drainage and administration of antibiotics. This seldom results in healing; the acute infection simply becomes quiescent.

In the presence of the quiescent infection we now combine evacuation of the infection with simultaneous stabilisation by arthrodesis of the hip. This is similar to the treatment of infected PA. Extensive internal fixation (e.g., with a cobra-head plate) is contraindicated and for this reason we perform minimal internal fixation using compression screws.

Technique: Restricted lateral approach; débridement, removal of sequester and cartilage; internal fixation with two cancellous compression screws. The first passes immediately under the innominate tubercle through the femoral neck and femoral head into the pelvis. The second passes level with the innominate tubercle and at right angles to the femoral axis into the pubic ramus. With this technique, freeing of M. vastus lateralis is never necessary (M. vastus lateralis is simply split at the level of the lesser trochanter where the IO is performed). Good wound drainage is important.

Postoperative management: Plaster boot for 3 weeks followed by hip spica for 4–6 weeks and then a short hip spica for a further 6 weeks; administration of appropriate antibiotics. The drains are left in place until secretion ceases. Radiological follow-up at 3 months.

5.5.2 Arthrodesis of Girdlestone Hips or Similar Conditions

This procedure is always troublesome because of the disadvantageous biomechanical circumstances, the reduction in bone vitality and the

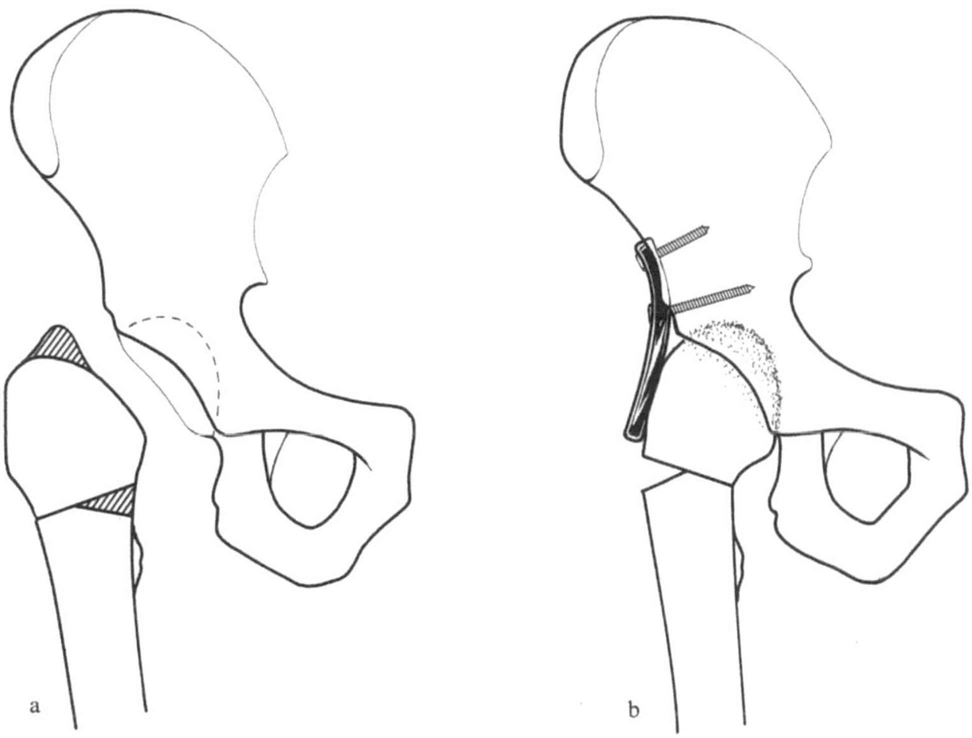

Fig. 98. *Arthrodesis of a Girdlestone hip*

a) The greater trochanter is freshened and the acetabulum is slightly deepened.

b) A straight plate which is only fixed to the pelvis is used to buttress the end of the femur. The abduction deformity is corrected by subtrochanteric osteotomy

possibility that a quiescent infection may be present.

Technique: Restricted lateral approach. The musculature is detached from the greater trochanter and the latter is freshened to form a conical knob of cancellous bone. The acetabular cartilage is removed, particularly around the acetabular roof. The cancellous bone is hollowed out somewhat in the direction of the iliac bone. With the leg in abduction, the greater trochanter is fitted into the acetabulum.

If there is inadequate cancellous bone, particularly following removal of prostheses and bone cement, a cancellous bone plasty with material removed from the iliac crest is indicated.

In order to hold the proximal end of the femur in place in the acetabulum, a straight buttress plate is fixed on to the pelvis with screws. Screws inserted into the femur would prevent subsequent impaction of the greater trochanter in the pelvis. A subtrochanteric osteotomy may be performed immediately or at a later date if correction of abduction deformity is necessary. If the latter procedure is to be performed at a later date, the leg is left in abduction following placement of the greater trochanter in the acetabulum and a suitable hip spica is immediately applied. The corrective subtrochanteric osteotomy is carried out after 6 weeks bed rest (Fig. 98).

If *infection* is suspected, the *osteotomy* is performed but not using the same lateral approach. *A second separate direct ventral approach is taken.*

Postoperative management: If the subtrochanteric osteotomy was carried out at the same time as the arthrodesis, the postoperative management is the same as in Types I and II.

In the other case, the short hip spica is retained for 6 weeks until the subtrochanteric

Fig. 99. *Arthrodesis of a high dislocated femoral head*

a) Before operation.

b) The head is brought into the true acetabulum and a plate is fixed to the pelvis to prevent further dislocation. If the plate is also to be fixed to the proximal femur it is first tensioned with a special tensioning device.

c) The proximal femur is fixed to the pelvis with the plate. A flexible Oberholzer nail prevents displacement at the level of the subtrochanteric osteotomy

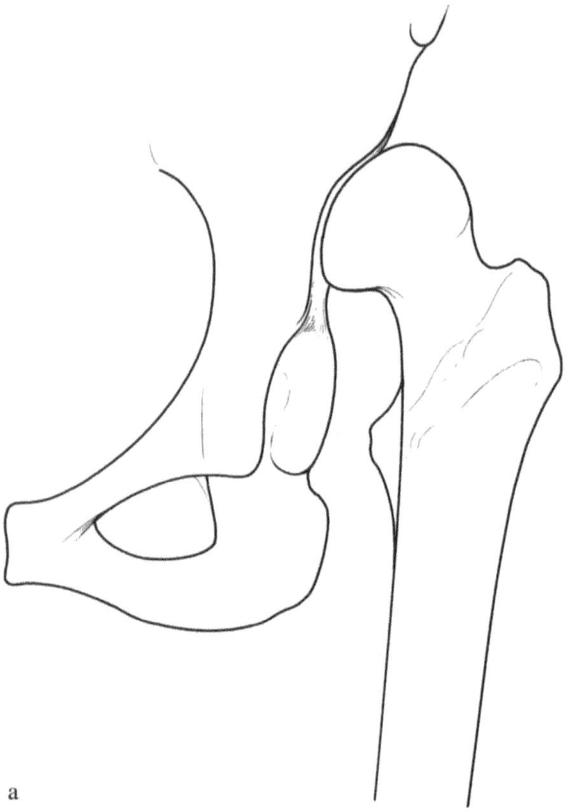

a

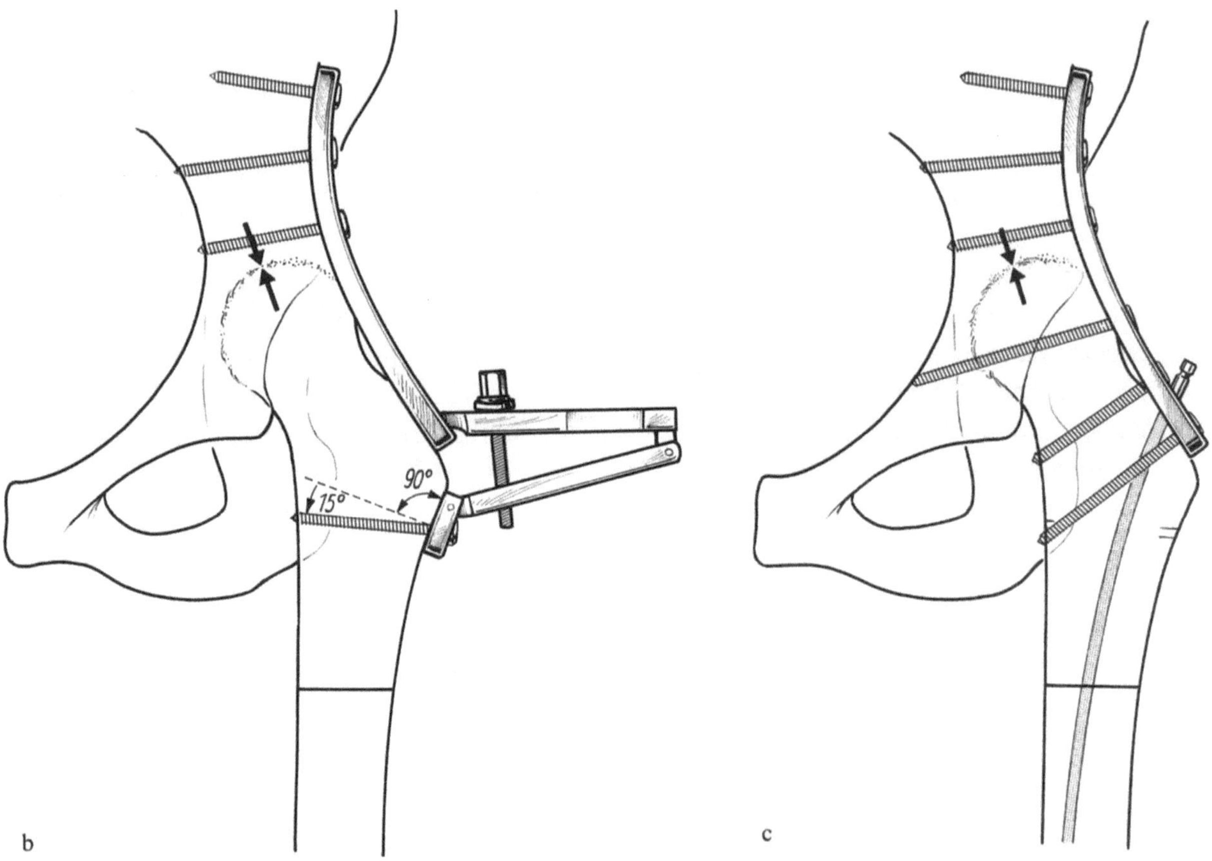

b

c

osteotomy is performed. The leg is then brought into the functional position, i.e., adducted, and a new hip spica is applied. The patient can get up after 6 – 8 days. At 4 weeks following osteotomy, the cast is shortened to just above the knee. The cast is removed 16 weeks following the arthrodesis.

5.5.3 Arthrodesis of a High Dislocated Femoral Head

In these special cases two problems predominate:

a) The head of the femur must be returned to its original position.
b) Redislocation must be prevented.

Technique: Two steps are usually necessary:

a) Supracondylar traction with Steinmann pins for an average of 10 days prior to the planned HA. This greatly eases reduction and the muscle tone is almost completely adjusted to its normal postoperative level. The latter reduces postoperative complaints. In certain cases, reduction is also rendered easier by adductorotomy.
b) As in the GH arthrodesis, a plate is used which is only fixed to the pelvis in order to prevent redislocation of the head of the femur. Alternatively the proximal end of the femur is fixed to the pelvis with the plate (Fig. 99).

Postoperative management: As in Type I.

5.5.4 Hip Arthrodesis in Cases of Incomplete Painful Ankylosis of the Hip (Intertrochanteric Valgus Osteotomy)

This HA is a rarity. It should be considered if almost total ankylosis of the hip is accompanied by malposition. Valgus correction causes pressure to be exerted on areas where ankylosis is absent or incomplete and thus promotes rapid bone union. The IO makes simultaneous correction of any malposition possible.

This technique may also be used to bring about arthrodesis in patients who are opposed to primary arthrodesis despite the fact that there is no useful motion left in the hip joint. HA would be the best operation for such patients and this procedure allows one to carry it out by performing an IO.

We have been pleased with the results of this procedure. Following complete ankylosis, the patients were always satisfied by the abolition of pain.

Technique: The technique is that of a normal IO. Lateral approach to the hip with partial freeing of M. Vastus lateralis; exposure of the intertrochanteric area; IO with the oscillating saw, bearing in mind the desired angular correction. The plate is driven in. With the aid of the compression device which is fixed with a screw, the osteotomy surfaces are compressed and the plate is fixed with screws. Anatomic wound closure leaving in place two deep suction drains and two superficial suction drains (Figs. 100, 101).

Postoperative management: Quadriceps exercises; 4 days bed rest followed by walking with canes; gradual loading to full weight bearing within 2 months. Precise instructions for physiotherapy: only functional treatment of the knee joint (and not the hip joint) necessary. Radiological follow-up at 3 months usually shows the IO to be united with complete ankylosis of the hip joint.

6 Corrective Osteotomies

Malposition following HA and ankyloses is not rare. Whilst the leg position may be corrected postoperatively following Type I and Type II arthrodeses or subsequent to atypical HA combined with IO, adjustment is no longer possible following Type III and Type IV arthrodeses. This may be the reason why we have found malposition to occur most frequently following cobra-head plate arthrodesis.

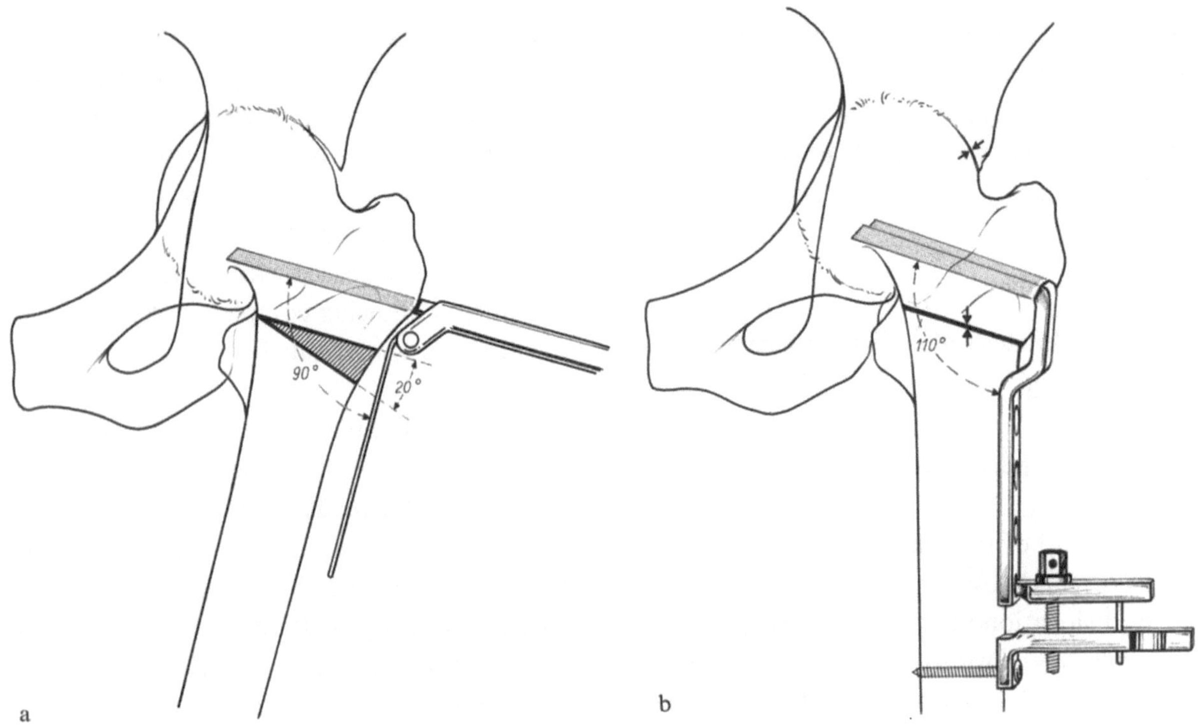

a b

Fig. 100. *HA by intertrochanteric valgus osteotomy.*

a) Valgus osteotomy, in this case with correction of 20° (wedge with lateral base).

b) Compression of the osteotomy followed by fixation of the plate with screws

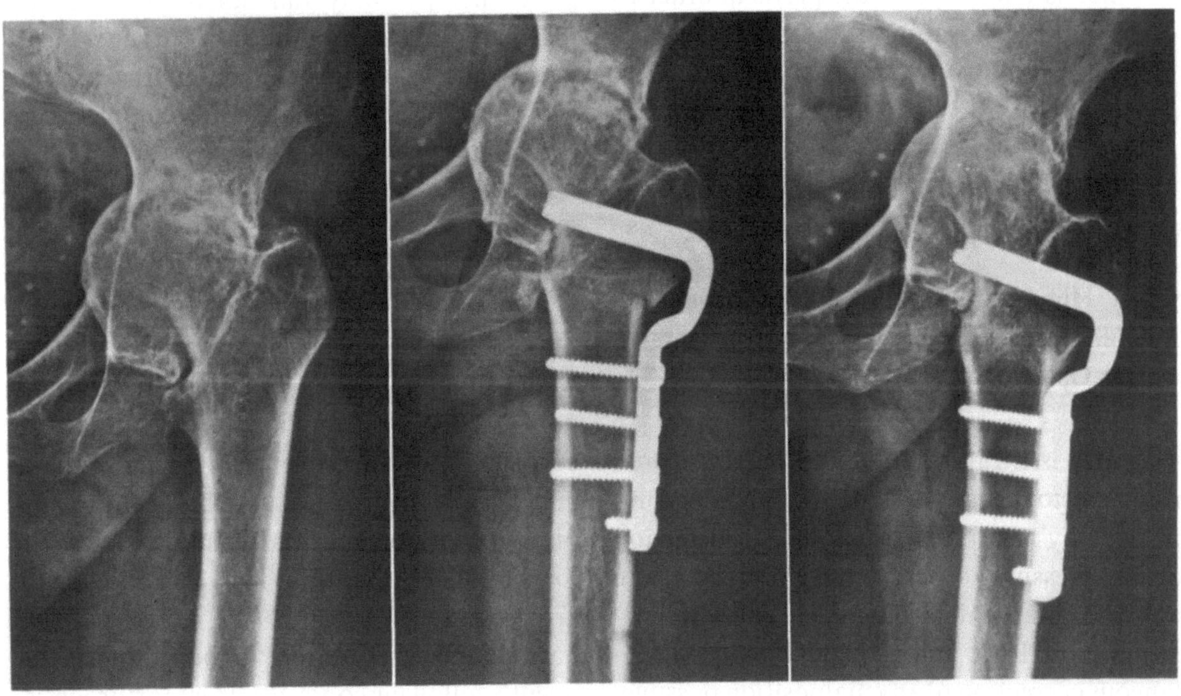

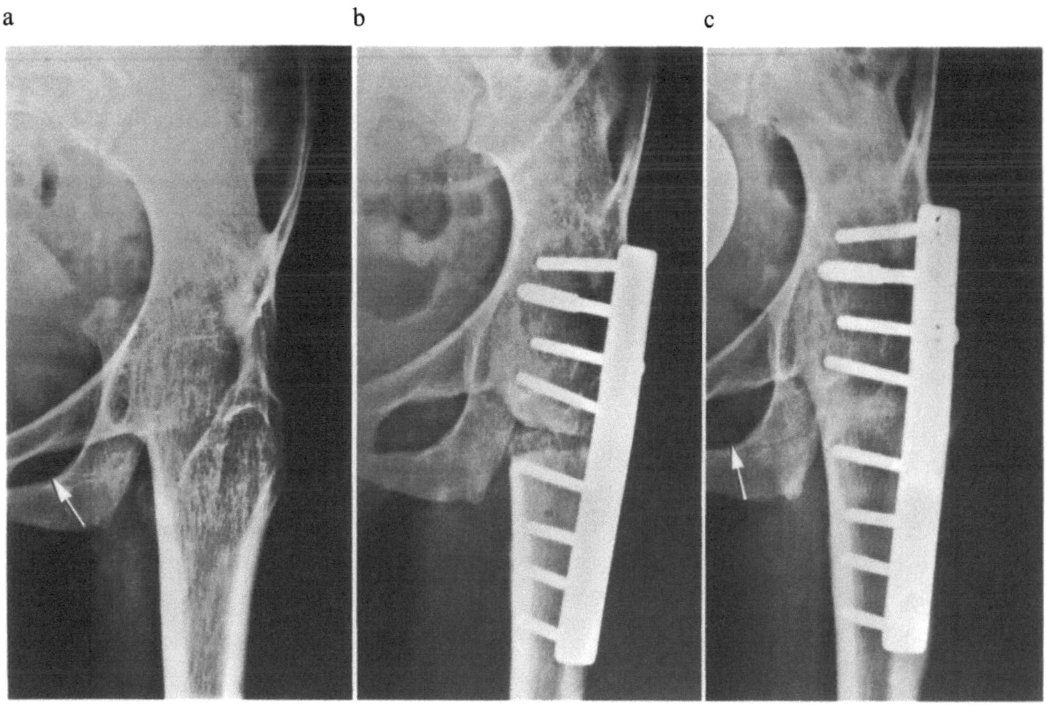

Fig. 102. *Correction of flexion deformity by intertrochanteric osteotomy*. (Hip ankylosis secondary to nontuberculitic juvenile hip infection). A. A., ♂, aged 28 years, No. 109885.

a) Three years following hip ankylosis. Flexion deformity can be deduced from the "narrow" obturator foramen.

b) Immediately following operation.

c) Three months later. Normal position with "broad" obturator foramen. Full bone union

Fortunately, malposition which gives rise to problems following HA may easily and reliably be corrected by osteotomy followed by rigid internal fixation (wedge osteotomy and compression plate fixation).

If knee problems occur following HA a valgus or varus knee may be corrected by supracondylar femoral osteotomy.

←

Fig. 101. *HA by intertrochanteric valgus osteotomy*. W. A., ♀, aged 78 years, No. 145692.

a) Painful partial ankylosis with adduction deformity and corresponding leg shortening of 3 cm.

b) Three months after valgus IO (20°) with 100° AO angled blade plate.

c) Eleven months following IO. The osteotomy has united. Hip fully ankylosed in ideal position. No difference in leg length. Patient complaint-free

6.1 Intertrochanteric Corrective Osteotomy

The most frequent deformities are adduction or external rotation. However, they frequently fail to bother the patient appreciably and correction is therefore not carried out. On the other hand, abduction or internal rotation and flexion deformities in particular cause considerable disability.

In such cases corrective osteotomy is always indicated. The desired correction is easily carried out by wedge osteotomy followed by stabilisation by compression plate fixation. Other advantages of this procedure are the immediate mobilisation, reduced period of bed rest and short hospital stay (2 weeks) (Fig. 102).

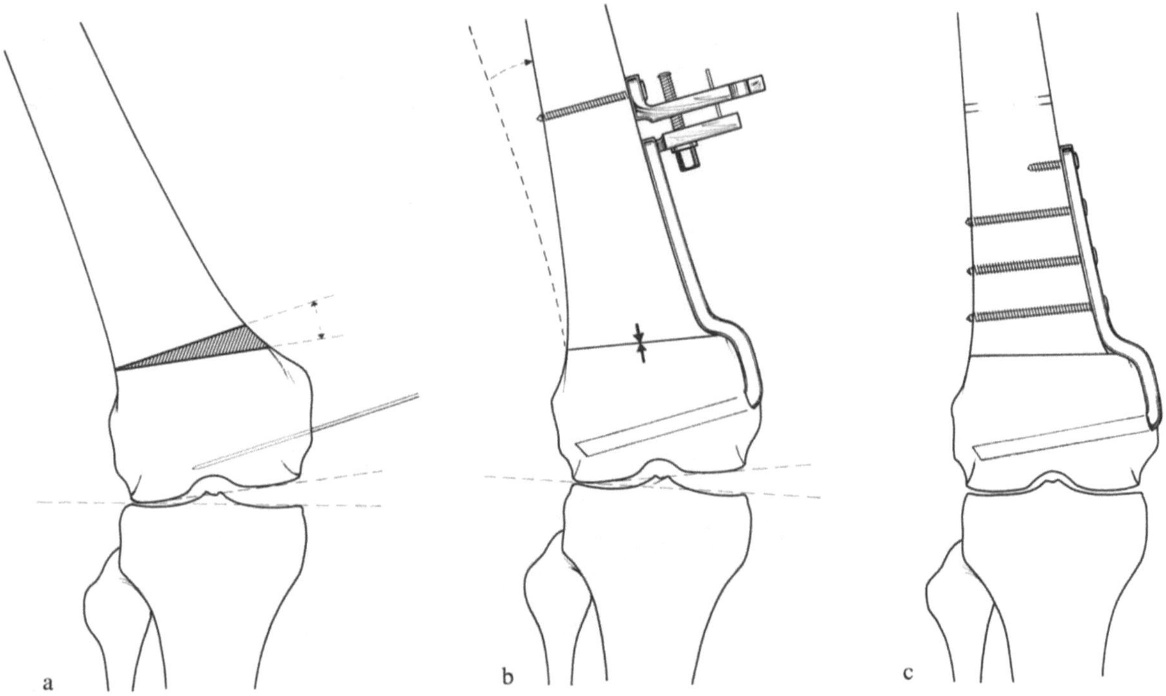

Fig. 103. *Correction of valgus knee by supracondylar osteotomy.*

a) Intended direction of blade is marked with a K-wire. The plate seating device is driven in and varus osteotomy is performed with removal of a medial wedge.

b) The plate seating device is replaced by the blade of the 90° angled plate. If necessary, the plate is fixed distally with a cortex screw or cancellous screw and it is then tensioned so as to compress the osteotomy.

c) Screw fixation of the plate and removal of the plate tensioner. Postoperative management: leg in right angled splint; quadriceps exercises on first postoperative day; patient gets up on fourth day

6.2 Supracondylar Corrective Osteotomy

If the leg is in valgus or varus and knee complaints arise as a result of the overloading of the fibular or tibial side of the joint, a supracondylar corrective osteotomy will bring benefit. The technical procedure is described in the AO manual.

6.2.1 Correction in Cases of Valgus Deformity

This deformity usually results if the hip is arthrodesed in abduction since the latter malposition is only partly compensated for by pelvic tilt. Knee pain results. The patient walks on the arthrodesed abducted leg and with each step weight bearing leads to increased valgus stress on the knee joint. Thus, one should not attempt to compensate for leg shortening by carrying out a hip arthrodesis in abduction. On the other hand, adduction arthrodesis of the hip is recommended if the knee is preoperatively in valgus (Figs. 103, 104).

Fig. 104. *Supracondylar corrective osteotomy for arthrosis of a valgus knee and ankylosis of the hip.* R. A., ♀, aged 60 years, No. 125163.

a) Before operation. Advanced arthrosis of the knee with narrowing of the lateral joint space.

b and c) Immediately following corrective osteotomy (right angle plate; 20° varus correction).

d and e) 4 years later. Widening of the joint space. Flexion/extension 65s – 0s. Patient complaint-free

a b c

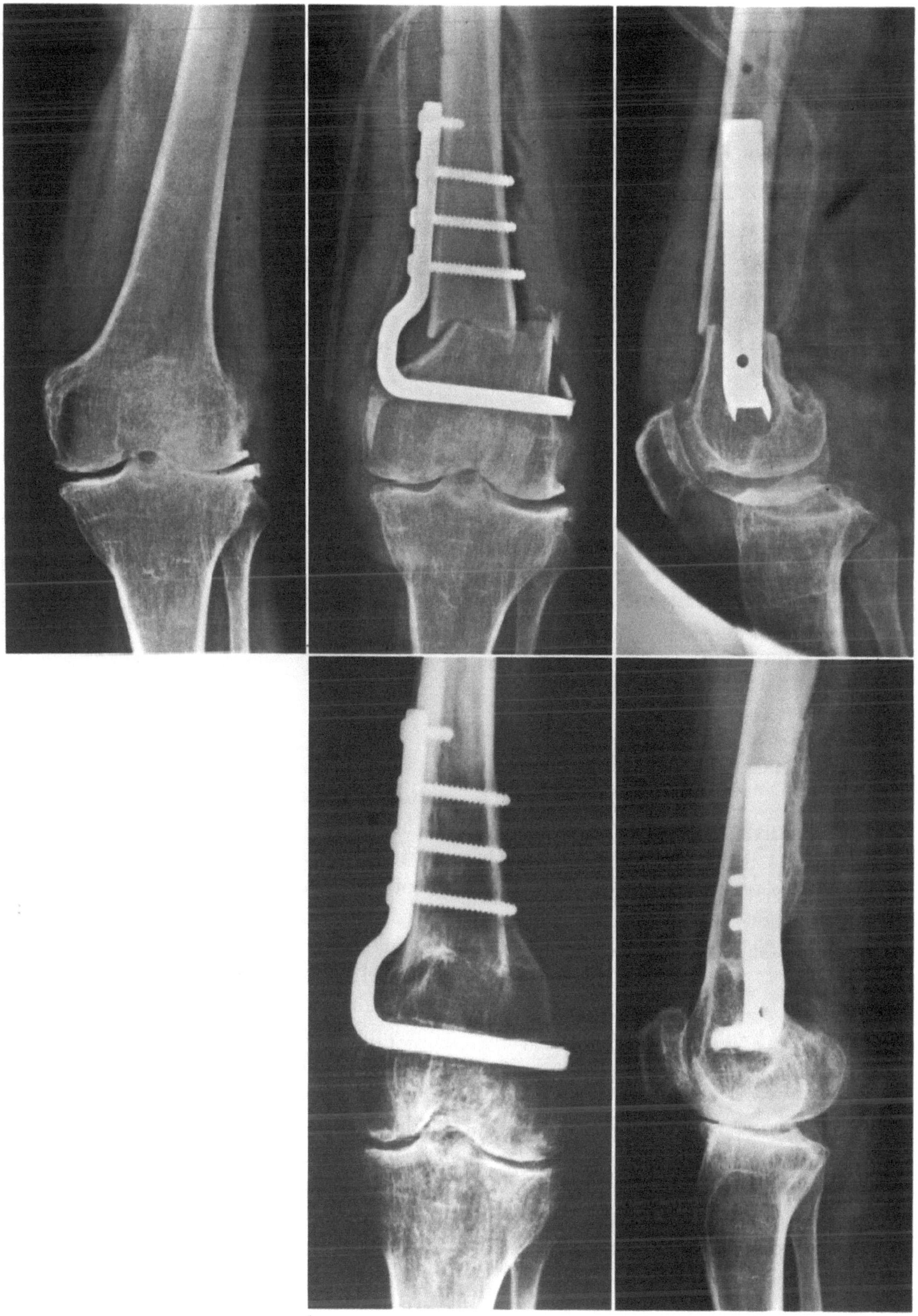

d e

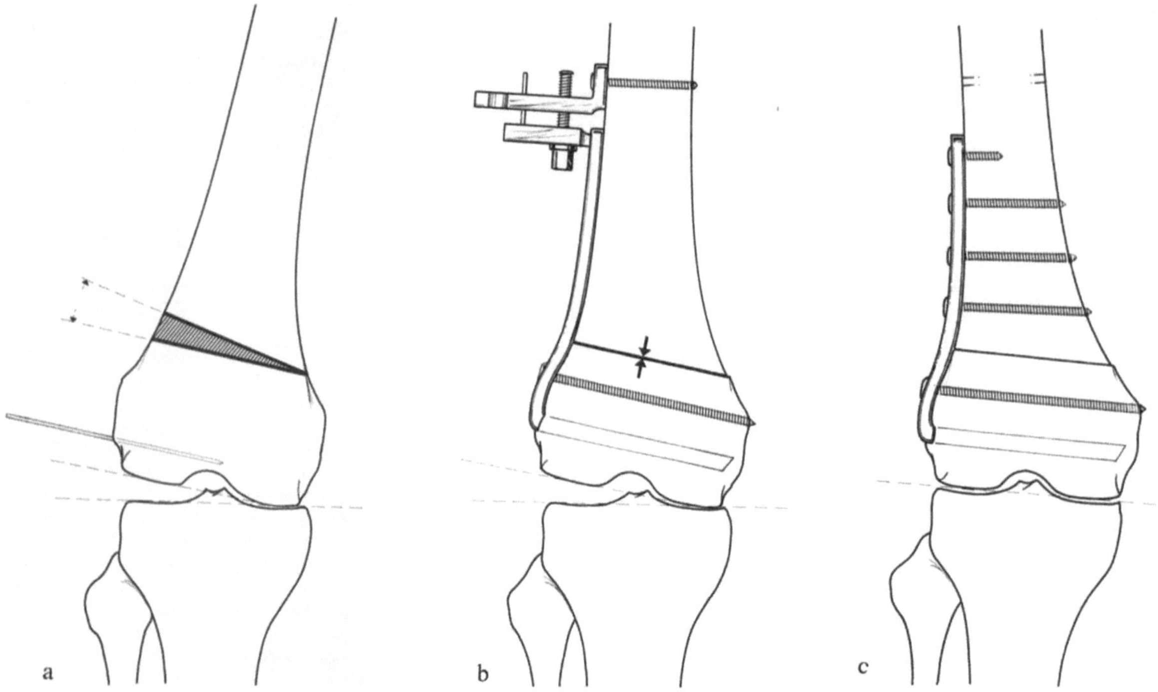

Fig. 105. *Correction of a varus knee by supracondylar valgus osteotomy*

a) A K-wire is driven into the femoral condyle parallel to the intended osteotomy. The lateral wedge is marked.

b) Tensioning of the plate.

c) Screw fixation of the plate. Postoperative management same as varus osteotomy

6.2.2 Correction in Cases of Varus Deformity

No case of varus deformity had to be operated on in our series. Such cases could be corrected by supracondylar osteotomy (Figs. 105, 106). Varus knee is, however, corrected by osteotomy of the head of the tibia.

7 Summary

HA is always a difficult operation. Careful preoperative work-up and adequate knowledge of the different operative techniques are essential. Whenever possible in older or elderly patients a HA should be performed which offers maximum rigidity, immediate mobilisation and a minimal period of bed rest without cast fixation. Only young healthy patients should be subjected to the ordeal of HA with prolonged postoperative treatment (cast for 3 months).

The cobra-head plate arthrodesis is preferable in the majority of cases. However, by using the other techniques special problems may be solved such as: later adjustment of leg position; leg lengthening; ankylosis in cases of hip infection, GH or similar conditions; high dislocation of the femoral head (post-traumatic or congenital dislocation); incomplete and painful ankylosis. Thanks to the availability of a variety of operations, account may be taken of the general condition of the patient, his primary disease and local circumstances in the hip.

Again, the multiplicity of available operations allows choice of the optimum technique for the individual case.

Malposition may be easily corrected by osteotomy (intertrochanteric or supracondylar) followed by rigid internal fixation.

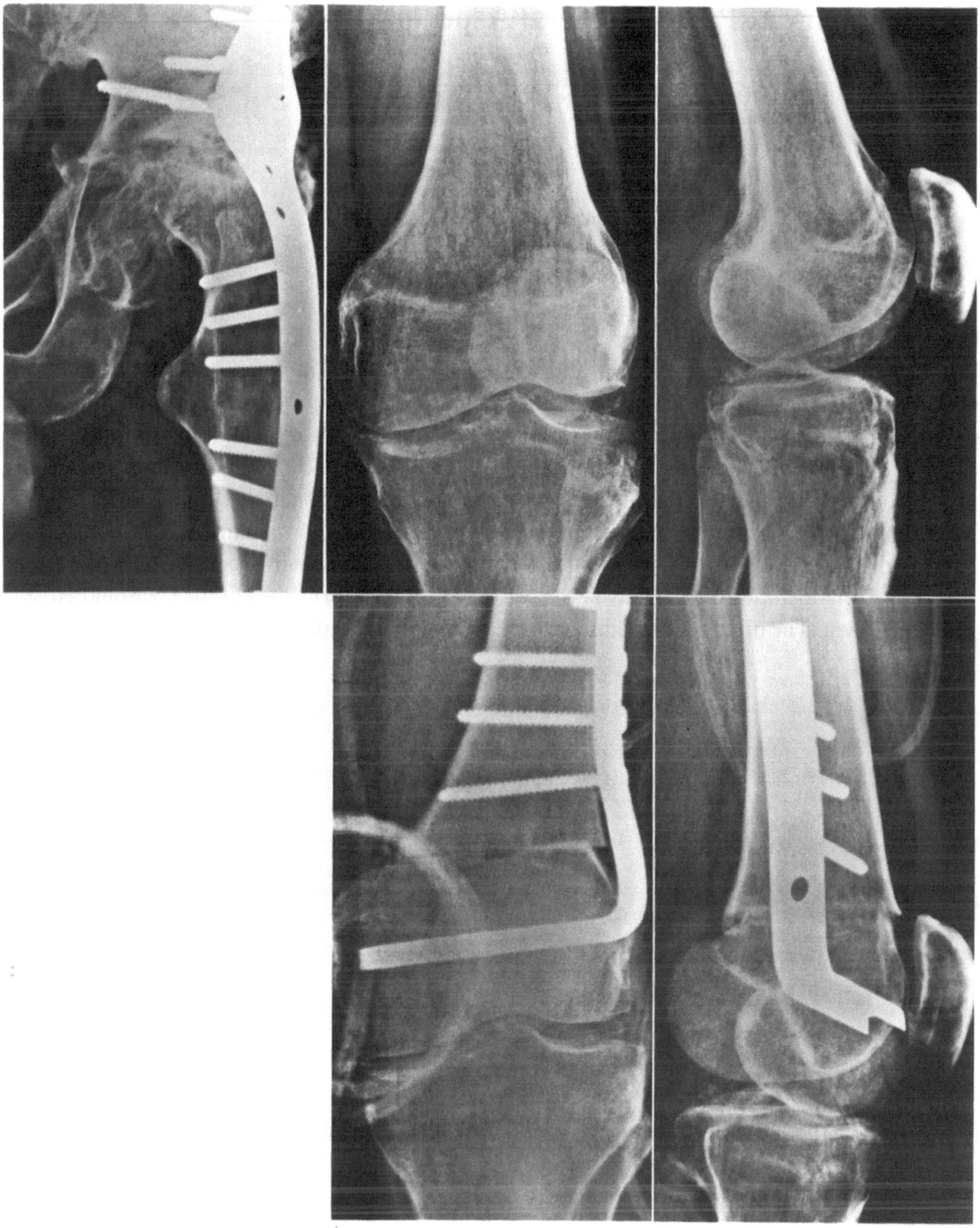

Fig. 106. *Supracondylar valgus osteotomy for arthrosis of a varus knee with arthrodesed hip*. H. U., ♂, aged 59 years, No. 97511.

a) Advanced bone union 8 months following HA.

b and c) Before operation. Narrowing of the medial joint space.

c and d) Immediately following corrective osteotomy

VI. Summary of Part I (General Aspects)

The structural principles of the hip and leg skeleton enunciated by PAUWELS, the static and dynamic changes induced by HA and the influence of arthrodesis on the neighbouring joints have been discussed. Logical conlusions were drawn with respect to indications and contraindications for HA and guide lines for the choice of operation (IO, HA, TP) have been laid down. The different procedures have been described in detail and the stress distribution resulting from certain operations has been analysed using a laboratory model.

Prior to Part II, the most important results are once again concisely summarised:

a) Of the extra-articular, para-articular and intra-articular arthrodeses, only the latter type was performed at the Cantonal Hospital in St. Gall. Rigid internal fixation was a

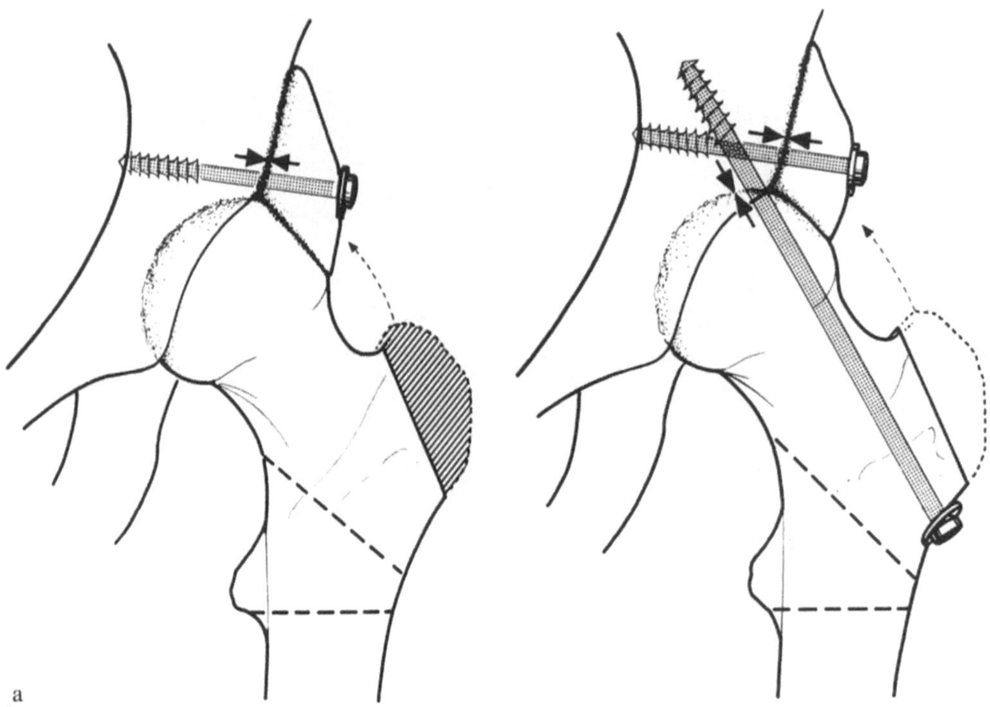

a

Fig. 107. *Summary of the various types of HA*

a) Type I c) Type III

b) Type II d) Type IV

e) HA with minimal internal fixation (infection)

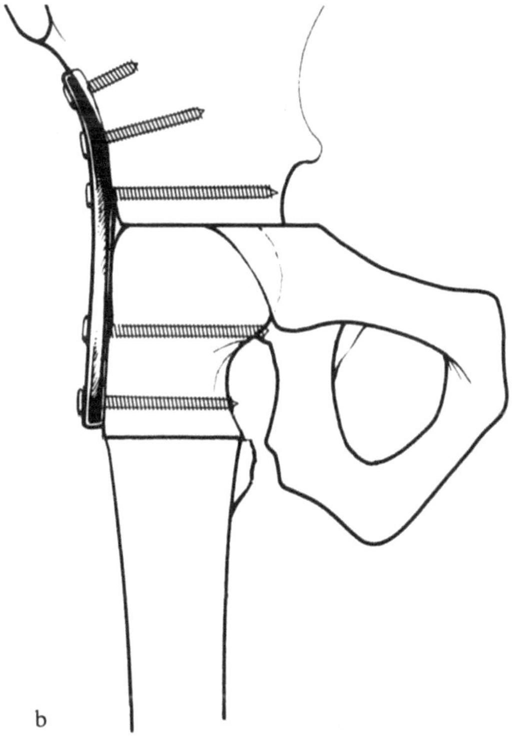

b

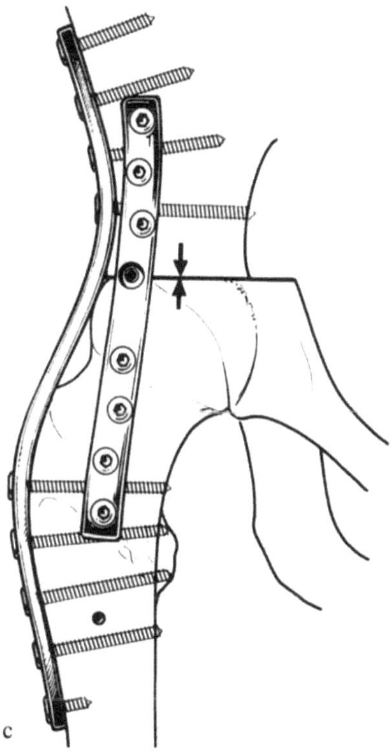

c

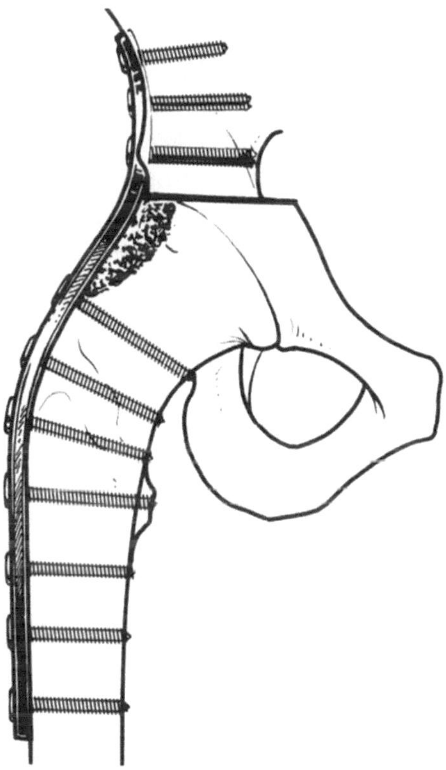

d

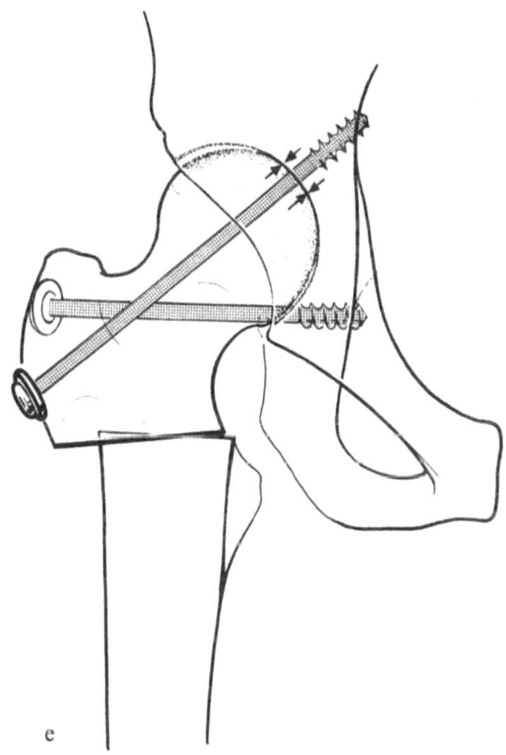

e

basic advance in the history of HA. Since its introduction we have been able to dispense with postoperative cast fixation in the majority of cases and the patient can be mobilised at an early stage. The latter simplifies nursing, shortens the hospital stay and reduces the duration of postoperative treatment. In addition, younger patients may be expected to resume work 2–4 months following the operation.

b) The decision to perform HA should only be made following careful medical examination (operability, psychological state, examination of the neighbouring joints, i.e., hips, knee, SIS, LS) and careful questioning of the patient (occupation, social circumstances). The patient should be fully informed.

Absolute contraindications: Stiff ipsilateral knee; stiff contralateral hip; severe lumbar spinal changes.

Relative contraindications: Poor general condition; age; weight; psychological state and attitude to life; reduced range of motion in the neighbouring joints; severe degrees of varus or valgus knee; active infection.

c) Deformities or differences in leg length cause inadequate or excessive stress on the neighbouring joint. They may cause degenerative changes in the latter with resulting subjective problems. They should therefore be corrected or compensated for.

Examination of our follow-up data together with consideration of the biomechanical principles suggest the following angulation to be ideal for a hip arthrodesis: flexion 15° – 20°; abduction/adduction in the zero position or in slight adduction (up to 5°); rotation in the zero position or slight external rotation.

An optimum distribution of tension forces following PO results if the osteotomy is performed transversely (neither upwards nor downwards) with moderate medial displacement of the distal pelvic component. Excessive medial displacement should always be avoided if possible in the presence of valgus knee since the valgus is accentuated by the reduction in length of the lever arm and medial displacement of the line of weight bearing.

d) HA is a difficult operation and always represents a severe stress for the patient. Careful preoperative work-up and adequate knowledge of the techniques and operative possibilities available are essential. Since 1966 we usually perform HA using the cobra-head plate. Nevertheless, in the following illustrations we have summarised the most common arthrodesis types, some of which are no longer or only rarely used. (Fig. 107)

Part II Specific Problems and Case Material

I. Evaluation of Case Material

1 Methods

Prerequisite to an objective and critical examination of the results of the HA operations carried out in our clinic from 1961–1971 were:

- Extensive study of the case histories and radiographs
- Completion of an extensive questionnaire by all our postoperative patients
- Personal examination of the majority of patients (more than 300), particularly those who were dissatisfied or only partially satisfied with the final results of HA or in whom adequate clinical and radiological evidence of complete bone union had not been obtained. Particularly worthy of mention is the readiness of patients to cooperate in the study. In more than 80% of the cases, the 41 questions were very extensively and accurately answered. Only 58 questionnaires (11.9%) were not returned. In addition, the patients readily attended the clinic for follow-up examinations. Only one patient, an anxious individual whose HA had probably ended in PA, failed to attend for follow-up despite repeated requests (Table 8).

Table 8. Questionnaire sent to patients

No. of patients	510	
No. deceased	24	4.7%
Questionnaire		
Answered by patient	403 (82.9%)	88.1%
Answered by third party	25 (5.1%)	
Questionnaire not answered	58	11.9%

The data obtained from questionnaire, case history, radiographs and clinical examination were stored on punched cards (Fig. 108).

2 Characteristics of Case Material

2.1 Sex

257 females, 326 males

2.2 Age

The majority of our patients were between 40 and 55 years of age at the time of operation. The mean age was 51.4 years, the youngest patient was 11 years old and the oldest patient was 77 years old. There was no significant difference in the mean ages of the patients subgrouped according to arthrodesis type (Table 9).

Table 9. Mean age of the patients

Type of arthrodesis	Age (years)
Freshening	46.1
Nailing	46.5
CHARNLEY	55.5
Type I	53.5
Type II	43.2
Type III	49.6
Type IV	52.4
Type V	41.4
Mean age	51.4

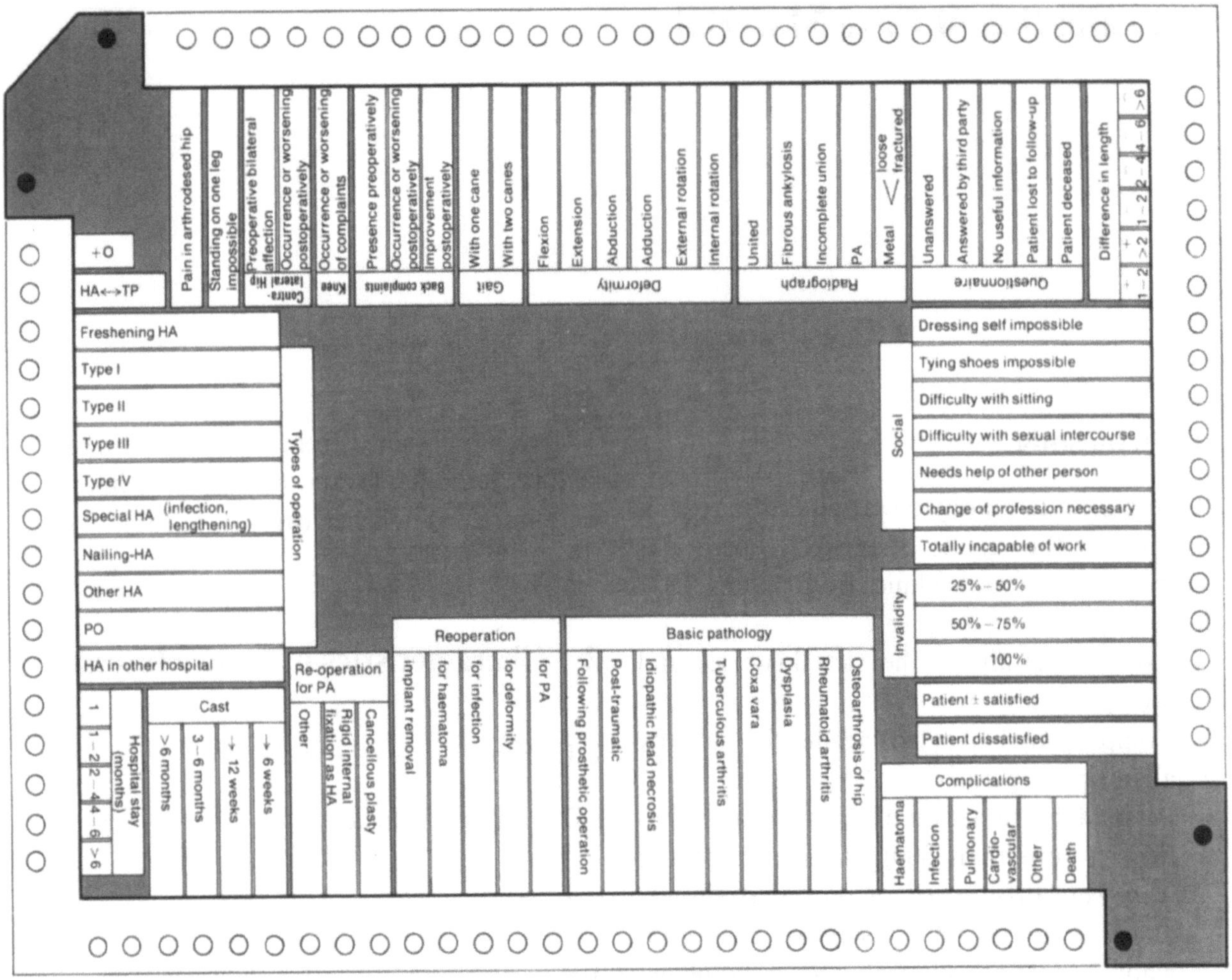

Fig. 108 Punch card for processing case data. Ninety parameters can be stored in this simple manner

2.3 Etiology

See Table 2. Half of our patients had unilateral hip disease. In the others, both hips were affected at the time of HA and bilateral arthrosis of the hip was clinically and radiologically confirmed in 146 patients.

3 Types of Operation

We performed 583 HA in 513 patients (Fig. 109). A single arthrodesis was carried out in 449 patients, two arthrodeses in 59 patients, three arthrodeses in four patients and four attempts at arthrodesis in one patient (Table 11).

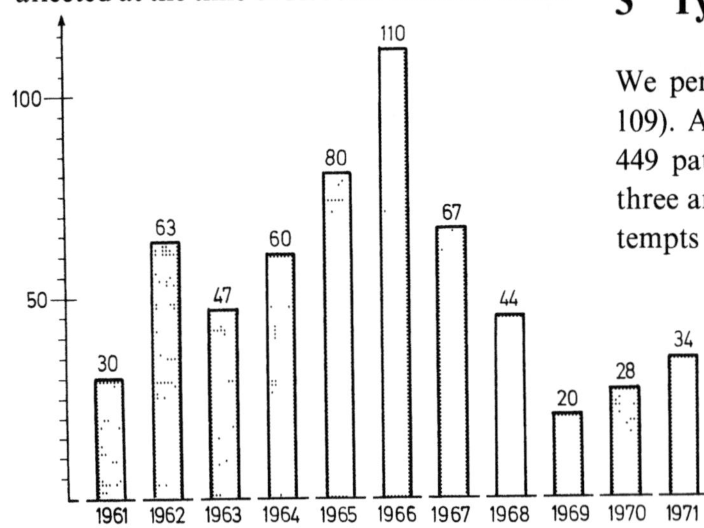

Fig. 109. Arthrodeses and rearthrodeses from 1961 to 1971

Table 10. Types of HA (1961 – 1971)

Year	Freshen-ing	Nailing	CHARNLEY	Type I	Type II	Type III	Type IV	Atypical	Total
1961	5	1	1	18	–	5	–	–	30
1962	2	–	–	50	2	9	–	–	63
1963	1	–	–	38	–	8	–	–	47
1964	3	1	1	20	4	31	–	–	60
1965	7	–	–	22	1	22	28	–	80
1966	6	–	–	5	7	8	82	2	110
1967	4	–	–	2	3	13	45	–	67
1968	1	–	–	–	2	3	38	–	44
1969	–	–	–	–	–	4	15	1	20
1970	1	–	–	–	–	3	23	1	28
1971	2	–	–	1	1	2	27	1	34
Total	32	2	2	156	20	108	258	5	583

The number of HA rose in 1965 and 1966, partly because of the successful introduction of the cobra-head plate technique. The number then decreased from 1967 – 1969 and subsequently increased again.

The development of the operative technique in our clinic from 1961 – 1971 is shown in Fig. 110. Three groups stand out: Type I ("freshening" arthrodesis with IO and compression screw fixation of the greater trochanter as an iliofemoral graft), particularly from 1961 – 1965; the Type III arthrodesis (double-plate arthrodesis) may be regarded as a transition phase prior to use of the cobra-head plate (Type IV) which was used from 1965 onwards. The cobra-head plate arthrodesis is also numerically the most frequent type (258 cases) followed by Types I, III and II in that order (Table 10).

Table 11. Cases from 1961 – 1971; 449 HA, 134 re-arthrodeses

Arthrodeses	Patients	%	Arthrodeses and re-arthrodeses
1 operation	449	87.5	449
2 operations	59	11.5	118
3 operations	4	0.8	12
4 operations	1	0.2	4
Total	513	100.0	583

Table 12. Duration of hospital stay

Arthrodesis type	Died during or after op.	Months				
		up to 1	1 – 2	2 – 4	4 – 6	more than 6
Freshening	–	2	14	10	5	1
Nailing	–	–	1	–	–	–
CHARNLEY	–	–	1	1	–	–
Type I	–	2	115	36	2	1
Type II	–	3	12	5	–	–
Type III	1	32	64	11	–	–
Type IV	2	157	93	4	2	–
Atypical	–	2	–	3	–	–

3.1 Postoperative Course

3.1.1 Duration of Hospital Stay

HA with rigid internal fixation has allowed a considerable shortening of the hospital stay. The Type I and Type II HA, which almost always involve postoperative cast fixation, required an average of 6 – 9 weeks while cobra-head plate arthrodesis requires only 4 – 5 weeks. Recently we have taken to discharging the patients 15 – 20 days following a Type IV HA (5 – 7 days bed rest followed by 2 – 3 days walking with a walking frame and then two crutches) (Table 12).

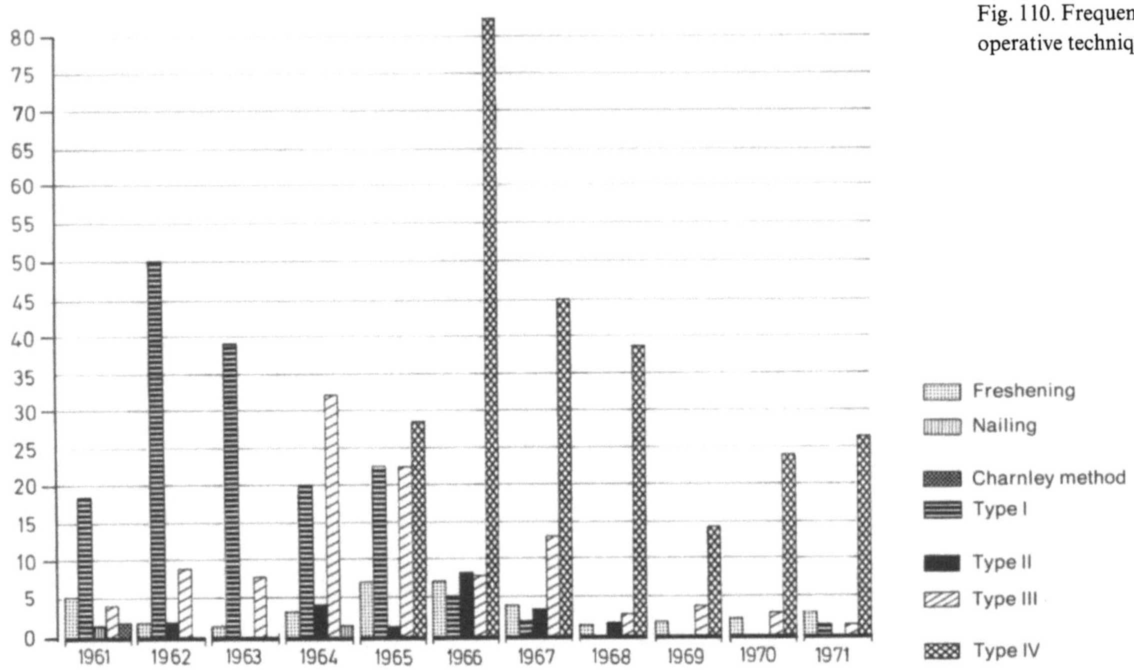

Fig. 110. Frequency of operative techniques

3.1.2 Postoperative Cast Fixation

Introduction of HA with rigid internal fixation has allowed us to dispense almost totally with this troublesome postoperative precaution. Cast fixation for 3–4 months was the rule in HA of Types I and II. It was also used as a precaution in half of the double plate arthrodesis cases. Conversely, only one of our 258 Type IV HA required a cast for $4^1/_2$ months because of delayed bone union (Table 13).

The length of hospital stay and postoperative cast fixation is dependent on the type of arthrodesis (Fig. 111).

The brevity of the hospital stay and the chances of dispensing with a cast are proportional to the rigidity of the internal fixation which complements the arthrodesis.

3.2 Intraoperative and Postoperative Complications

We differentiate between *systemic complications*, *local complications* and *localised operative failures*.

Table 13. Arthrodeses and cast fixation

Arthrodesis type	Up to 6 weeks	Up to 12 weeks	3–6 months	Over 6 months	Total	%
Freshening	–	17	14	1	32	100
Nailing	–	–	1	1	2	100
CHARNLEY	–	2	–	–	2	100
Type I	1	115	35	5	156	100
Type II	–	10	4	–	14	70
Type III	–	32	15	–	47	44
Type IV	–	–	1	–	1	0
Atypical	–	2	3	–	5	100
Total	1	178	73	7	259	44.6

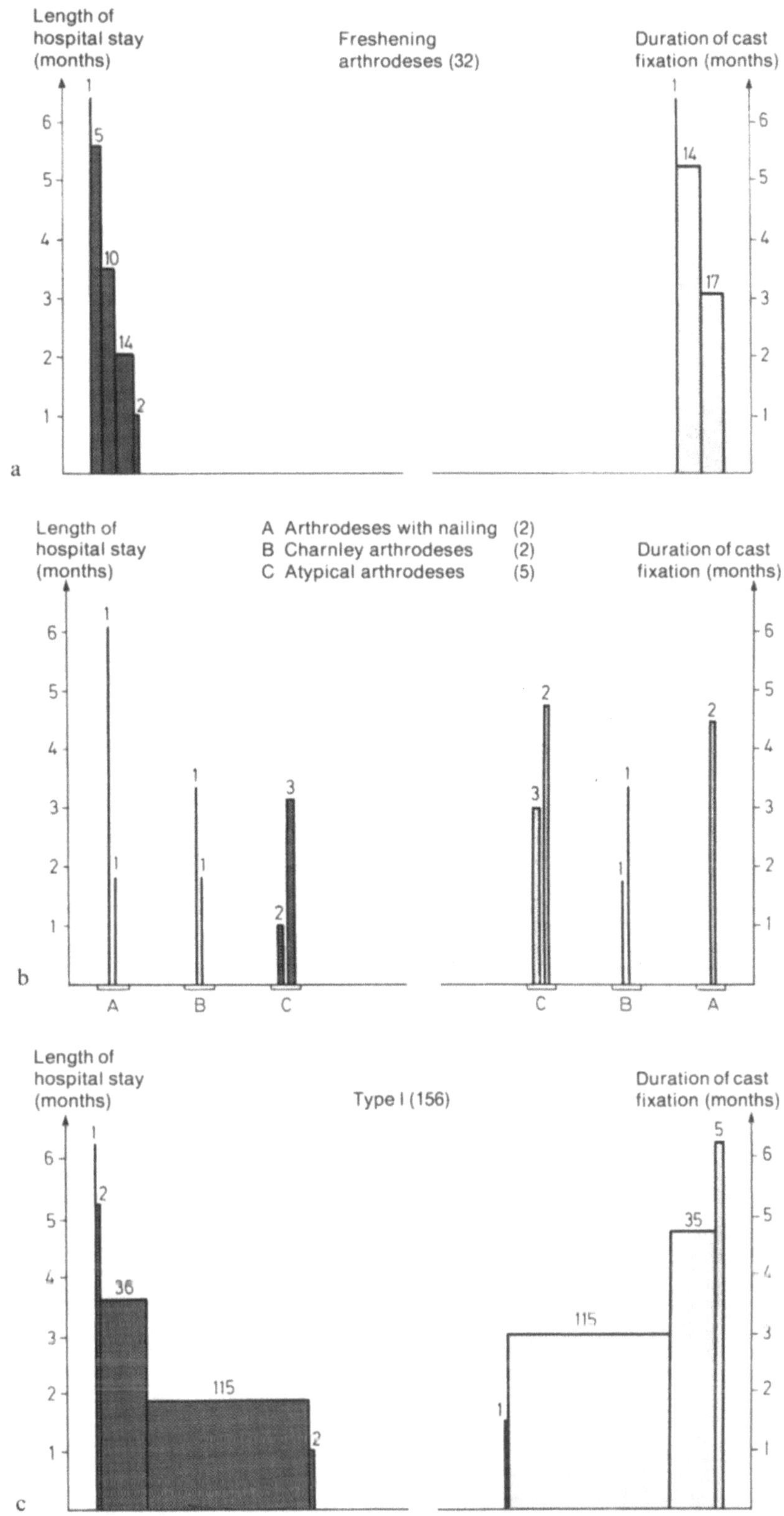

Fig. 111. *Length of hospital stay, duration of cast fixation and type of hip arthrodesis*

a) Freshening arthrodeses

b) Charnley arthrodeses, arthrodeses with nailing and atypical arthrodeses

c) Type I

d) Type II

e) Type III

f) Type IV; cast fixation in only one case; length of hospital stay between 3 – 5 weeks

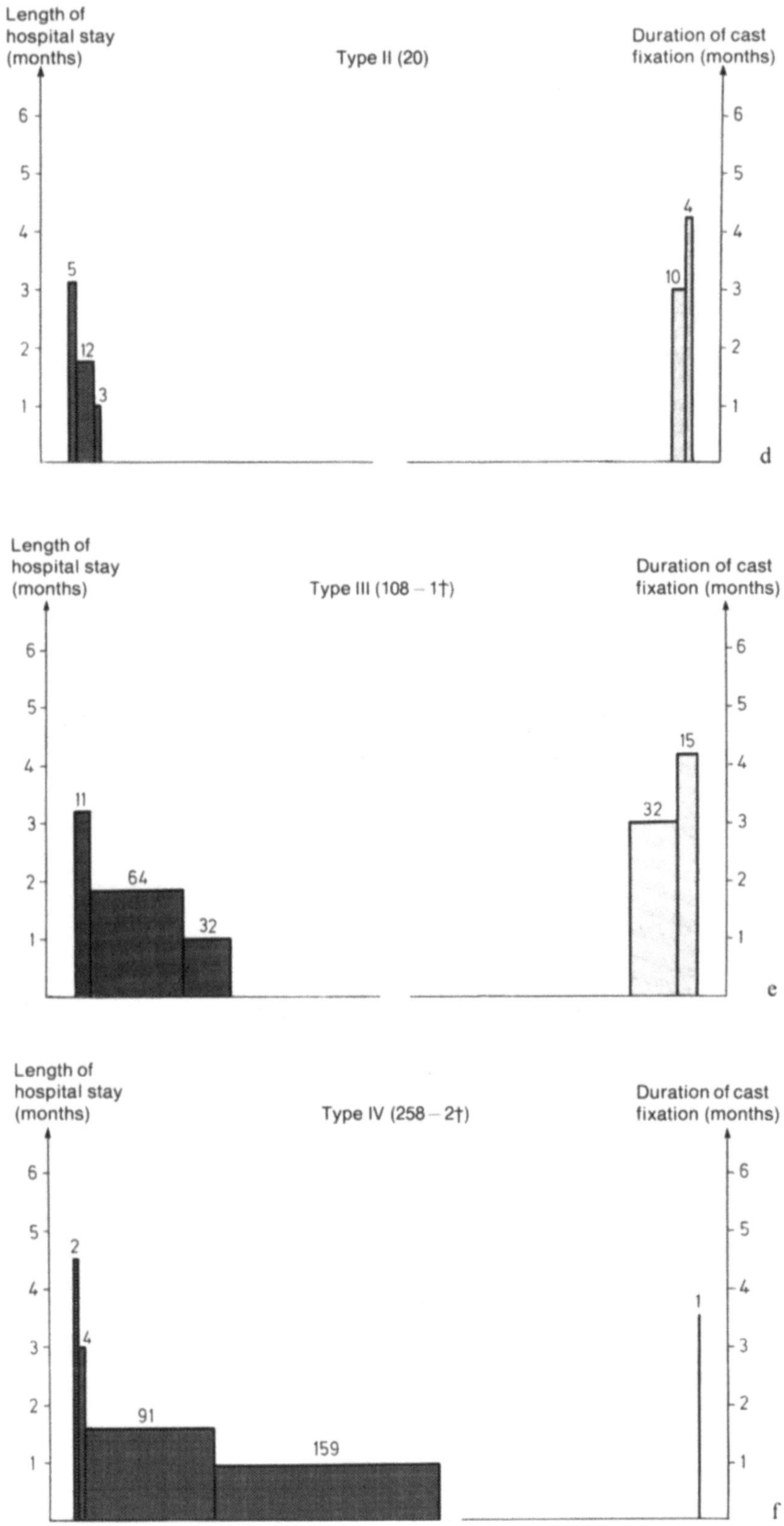

Fig. 111 d – f Legend see page 103

Table 14. Causes of death

1. Anesthetic incident (air embolus)
2. Diffuse intraoperative bleeding (clotting defect, hypofibrinogenemia, acute fibrinolysis leading to shock and cardiac arrest)
3. Vomiting with massive inhalation of vomit (12 h after operation)

3.2.1 General Complications

Three deaths (0.5%) occurred in our 583 HA. The causes of death are mentioned in Table 14. In addition we observed:

- Pulmonary complications in 11 patients (1.9%); these comprise 10 pulmonary emboli and one case of pneumonia.
- Cardiovascular complications in seven patients (1.2%) of which six were cases of thrombophlebitis and one of angina pectoris.
- Abdominal complications in three patients (0.5%), comprising one stress ulcer, one paralytic subileus and one case of cholecystitis.

The systemic and local complications are summarised in Table 15. There seems to be no direct connection between complications and ages of the patients (Table 16).

3.2.2 Local Complications

Hematoma occurred postoperatively in 29 patients (5%) and an infection in 24 patients (4.1%). It must be emphasised once more that occurrence of a hematoma is an indication for immediate revision of the wound with evacuation of the hematoma. Of our total of 24 infections, 11 occurred following wound hematoma (Table 17).

3.2.3 Localised Operative Failures

The majority of these cases were pseudarthroses followed in frequency by malposition and also, to a certain extent, excessive differences in leg length. Damage to nerves is mentioned as an intraoperative complication (Table 18).

Table 15. Systemic and local complications following HA (classified by arthrodesis type)

Complication	Freshening	Nailing	CHARNLEY	Type I	Type II	Type III	Type IV	Atypical
Death	–	–	–	–	–	1	2	–
Embolus	–	–	–	4	–	4	2	–
Pneumonia	–	–	–	1	–	–	9	–
Thrombophlebitis	3	–	–	3	–	2	9	–
Hematoma	1	–	–	8	1	4	15	–
Infection	3	–	–	5	–	6	9	1
Other	3	1	–	9	1	8	14	–

Table 16. Complications related to age of the patients

Complications (87)		Age of the patients											
		15–20	20–25	25–30	30–35	35–40	40–45	45–50	50–55	55–60	60–65	65–70	70–75
Death	(3)	–	–	–	–	–	2	–	1	–	–	–	–
Pulmonary	(11)	–	–	–	–	–	1	–	4	4	2	–	–
Vascular	(17)	–	–	–	–	–	1	2	5	4	4	–	1
Abdominal	(3)	–	–	–	–	–	–	–	1	1	1	–	–
Hematoma	(29)	–	–	–	–	1	4	5	5	6	5	3	–
Infection	(24)	1	2	–	1	–	5	–	4	4	6	1	–

Table 17. Hematomas and infections following HA

Arthrodesis type	Hematoma	Infection following hematoma	Other infections
Freshening	1	1	2
Nailing	–	–	–
CHARNLEY	–	–	–
Type I	8	3	2
Type II	1	–	–
Type III	4	2	4
Type IV	15	5	4
Atypical	–	–	1
Total	29	24	
%	5	4.1	

Table 18. Complications of 583 HA in St. Gall from 1961 – 1971

Pseudarthroses	84 (14.5%)
Deformities	80 (13.8%)
Fatigue fractures	7 (1.2%)
Nerve damage	12 (2%)

a) Pseudarthrosis

In our series, 84 PA (14.5%) occurred together with 14 cases (2.4%) in which complete bone union was radiologically absent at follow-up of a patient who was clinically well (full weight bearing possible, freedom from pain) (Figs. 112, 113).

Two fibrous ankyloses (0.3%) occurred which did not give rise to subjective complaints and following repeated arthrodeses only 14 PA (2.4%) remained. Of these 14 patients, four could not be followed up personally (domiciled abroad), one anxious patient failed to appear despite repeated requests and three had only slight subjective problems and were satisfied with the result. Reoperation was rejected by three patients and was impossible in a further three patients for medical reasons.

a b c

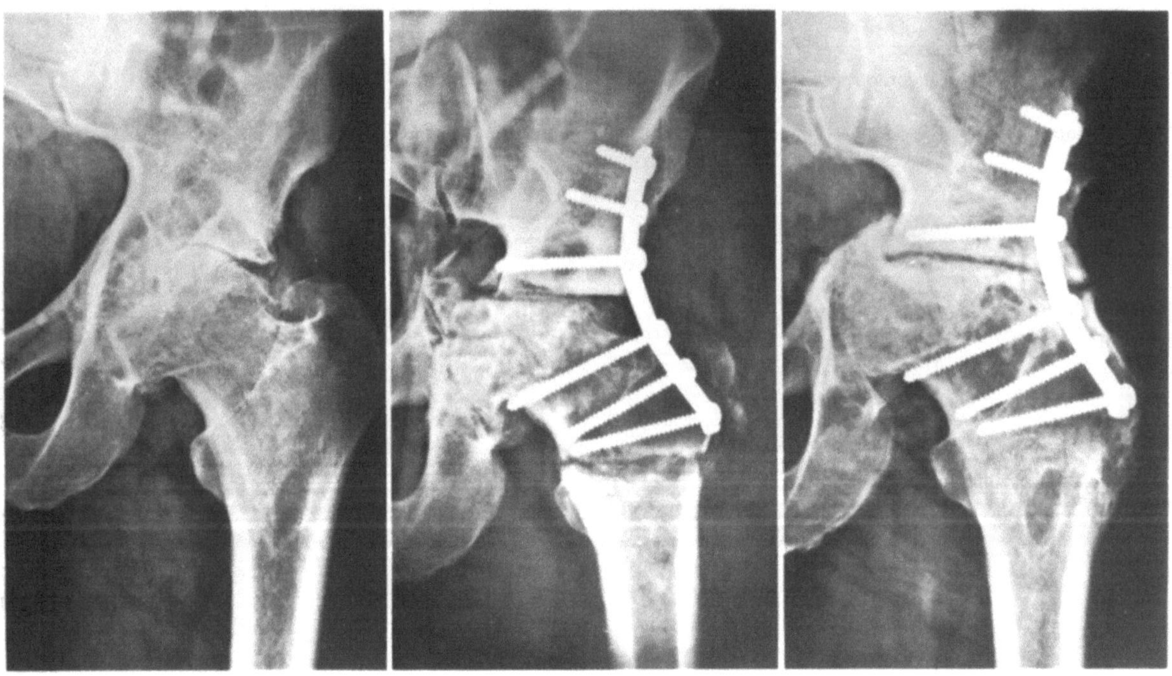

Fig. 112. *Fibrous ankylosis following HA*. H. A., ♂, aged 46 years, No. 99531

a) Severe arthrosis of the hip.

b) Immediately following Type II HA with PO.

c) Follow-up 6 years later. Fibrous ankylosis. Patient complaint-free

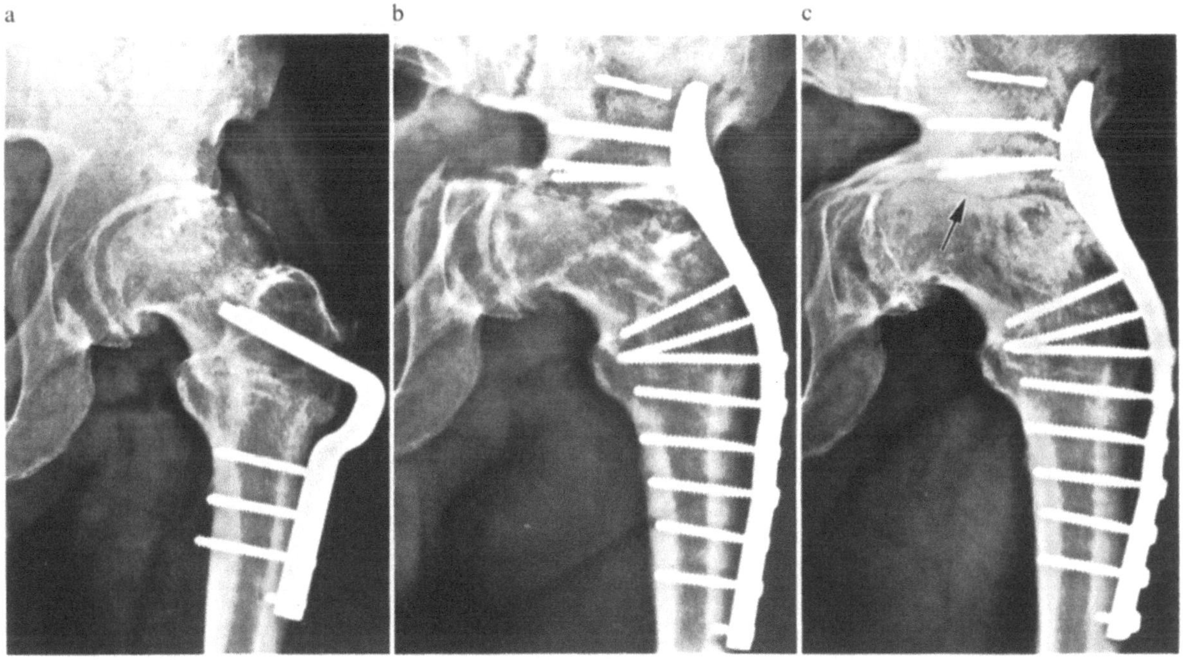

Fig. 113. *Fibrous ankylosis following cobra-head plate arthrodesis.* K. S., ♂, aged 49 years, No. 71895.

a) Painful partial ankylosis 2 years after IO.

b) One month after cobra-head plate arthrodesis with marked medial displacement following PO.

c) Four years later. Marked PA gap. No subjective problems whatsoever

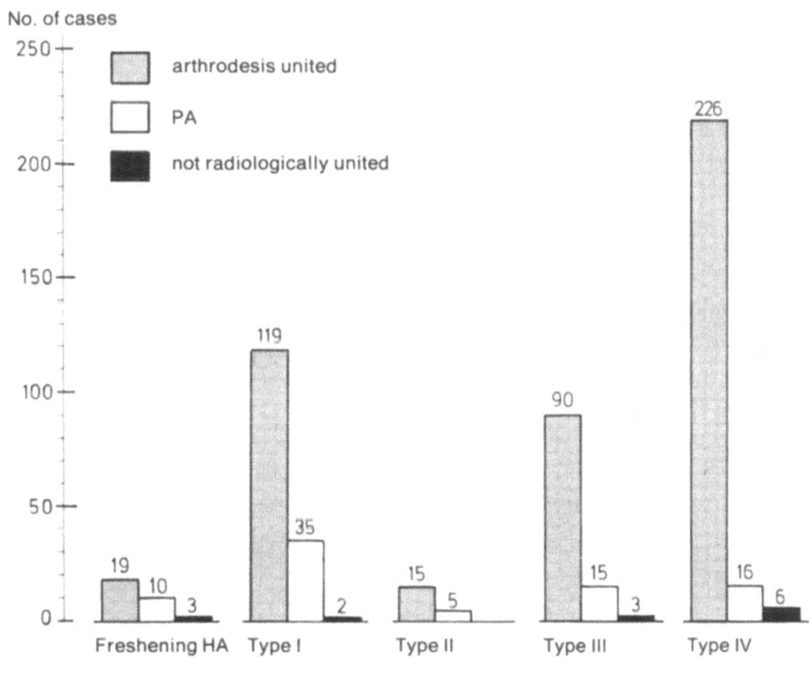

Fig. 114. *PA frequency following different types of arthrodesis.* Marked reduction in PA frequency following Type IV HA. (Rigid internal fixation.)

Table 19. Duration of postoperative cast fixation related to % PA frequency; classified by author and technique

Author	No. of cases	Duration of cast	PA (%)	HA method
WATSON-JONES (1956)	120	16 weeks	6	Nail + intra-articular graft
CHARNLEY (1956)	95	6 months	47	Own method
LINDSTRÖM (1956–1957)	41	∅	5	Smith-Petersen nail + intra-articular graft
McKEE (1957)	50	∅	6	Screw arthrodesis
DEBEYRE (1959)	100	8 weeks	42	CHARNLEY method
HUGGLER (1960)	59	8 weeks	12	CHARNLEY method
MORTENS u. JENSEN (1960)	39	16 weeks	22	CHARNLEY method
PIGGOT (1960)	91	12 weeks	26	CHARNLEY method
PADOVANI (1961)	308	12 months	16	Nail + intra-articular graft
AXER (1961)	19	∅	26	Own method
LIPSCOMB (1961)	371	?	22	Various methods
CHAPCHAL (1962)	91	16 weeks	3.3	Nail + intra-articular graft
GARDINER (1962)	53	∅	11.3	Smith-Petersen + graft
CINCCARELLI (1962)	79	?	29	2 intra-articular screws
MERLE D'AUBIGNÉ (1964)	114	8 weeks	24	Smith-Petersen + intra-articular graft
ONJI (1965)	20	∅	11.1	Küntscher nail
ADAMS (1966)	125	6 weeks	21	Nail + ischiofemoral graft
MORRIS (1966)	55	8 weeks	23.6	CHARNLEY method
LAM (1968)	57	∅	13	Nail + intra-articular graft
BECK (1969)	20	∅	5	Cobra-head plate arthrodesis
ALVIK (1969)	634	∅	6.6	Own method
DREYER and PINGEL (1969)	27	∅	11	Cobra-head plate arthrodesis
WIEDMER (1969)	48	∅ (– 3 months)	6.3	Cobra-head plate arthrodesis
GOESSENS (1970)	57	∅	5.3	Cobra-head plate arthrodesis
GÖRDES (1970)	54	2 1/2 months	24	Axer-Viernstein method
STEWART and COKER (1970)	109	4 months	30	Various methods
GÖRDES (1971)	64	∅	18.7	Cobra-head plate arthrodesis
CARTER (1971)	100	4 months	37	Various methods
AUTHOR'S SERIES (1973)	583	0–3 months	14.5%	Various methods
	of which			Cobra-head plate arthrodesis
	258	∅	6.2	Cobra-head plate arthrodesis

The number of PA has certainly been significantly reduced by the introduction of HA with rigid internal fixation (Fig. 114).

We have surveyed the literature with respect to bone union following HA and the results are summarised by author and technique in Table 19. Results of cobra-head plate arthrodesis published by various authors (GOESSENS, GOERDES, DREYER, WIEDMER) confirm our observations; PA only occurred in 6%–7% of cases.

b) Malposition

In 80 patients (13.8%) malposition occurred and in 21 of them a corrective osteotomy was necessary. The other patients experienced no significant problems as a result of the malposition and were satisfied with the result.

c) Difference in Leg Length

Shortening of up to 1 cm on the arthrodesed side is desired. Frequently, however, the degree of shortening is greater, particularly following arthrodeses for hip dysplasia, NHF or GH. In such cases, the difference in leg length must be corrected by raising the heel or by the use of orthopaedic shoes. Leg lengthening is rarer and is usually a consequence of abduction deformity on the arthrodesed side which leads to excessive weight bearing on the contralateral hip, particularly on standing. For this reason we

Table 20. Difference in leg length following arthrodesis

Type of arthrodesis	Leg lengthening		0	Leg shortening			
	1–2 cm	>2 cm		1–2 cm	2–4 cm	4–6 cm	>6 cm
Freshening	–	–	6	9	12	4	1
Nailing	–	–	–	1	1	–	–
CHARNLEY	–	–	–	1	1	–	–
Type I	3	–	14	69	52	14	4
Type II	2	–	1	9	6	1	1
Type III	1	–	19	46	30	7	5
Type IV	5	–	40	133	66	13	1
Atypical	–	–	–	1	3	1	–

prefer a shortening osteotomy with simultaneous correction of the malposition or we equalise the difference in leg length by raising the heel on the healthy side (Table 20).

d) Nerve Damage

Intraoperative damage to the sciatic nerve (only the fibular branch) occurred on nine occasions and damage to the lateral cutaneous nerve of the femur on three occasions (total of 2.0%). These were usually reversible; irreversible damage to the fibular branch only occurred in one case.

Table 21. Re-operations

Arthrodesis type	Pseudarthrosis	Deformity	Infection	Hematoma	Implant removal
Freshening	7	8	3	–	2
Nailing	1	–	–	–	–
CHARNLEY	1	–	–	–	–
Type I	29	4	4	–	7
Type II	4	1	–	–	3
Type III	3	6	5	–	7
Type IV	14	2	8	6	10
Atypical	1	–	1	–	1
Total	60	21	21	6	30
	138				

e) Fatigue Fractures

This late complication is frequently mentioned by a number of authors (ADAMS, MERLE D'AUBIGNÉ, MORRIS) but it only occurred in seven of our cases (1.28%). The operative treatment of these fatigue fractures using rigid internal fixation is not particularly difficult.

Reoperation was necessary in 108 cases in which PA, malposition, hematoma or infection occurred (Table 21).

All complications associated with our 583 HA operations are summarised in Table 22.

3.3 Sociomedical Problems

3.3.1 Postoperative Fitness for Work.

HA with rigid internal fixation has significantly accelerated the patients' return to work. Of the 258 patients with cobra-head plate arthrodeses (Table 23), 195 were at least 50% capable of work 1–6 months following operation; 64 patients (10.9%) had to change their job after HA. In 65% of cases there was a significant improvement in working capacity following HA; in 25% it was unchanged and in 10% it was worsened.

3.3.2 Disability

Our analysis is based on the degrees of disability assessed by the insurers (disability insurance,

Table 22. Summary of all complications following HA

Complications	Freshening	Nailing	CHARNLEY	Type I	Type II	Type III	Type IV	Atypical	Total	Percent
Death						1	2		3	0.5
Embolus				5		4	2		11	1.9
Thrombophlebitis	3			3		2	9		17	2.8
Hematoma	1			8	1	4	15		29	5.0
Infection	3			5		6	9	1	24	4.1
Stress ulcer							1			
Paralytic subileus				1						
Delirium tremens				1						
Angina pectoris							1			
Cholecystitis							1			
Decubitus ulcer				1						
Strep. wound infection							1			
Furunculosis (buttock)							1			
Parotitis							1			
Femoral art occlusion (→ amputation)						1				
Allergies										
a) To cast material				1						
b) To Mastix	1			1						
c) To Sintrom (anticoagulant)				1						
Postoperative fracture:										
a) Femoral neck		1					}			
b) Intertrochanteric					1		1 }		3	0.5
Fatigue fracture				1		2	4		7	1.2
Dislocation fem. diaphysis	1			1						
Knee stiffness						1				
Retained swab	1									
Nerve damage										
a) Fibular	1			1		2	5		9 }	2.0
b) Lat. fem. cutan.						2	1		3 }	
c) Obturator neuritis						1			1	

Table 23. Arthrodesis type and time off work

Arthrodesis type	Time off work (months)														
	1	2	3	4	5	6	7	8	9	10	11	12	up to 18	up to 24	over 24
Freshening					2	15	3	3		7	1				1
Type I				12	13	32	25	24	7	12	1	15	7	3	5
Type II			3	2	3	5	2					1	1	2	1
Type III		4	8	6	20	24	10	8	2	6	6	3	3	7	
Type IV	7	21	39	51	29	48	13	15	8	4	2	12	4		2
Atypical						1	3				1				

Table 24. Association of disability with bone union and PA following HA

Degree of disability	United HA (496)	Pseudarthrotic HA (84)
0–25%	55=11.9%	18=21.4%
25–50%	282=56.8%	2=2.4%
50–75%	99=19.9%	14=16.6%
75–100%	60=12.1%	50=59.5%

accident insurance, life insurance) and sickness funds or on our own assessments at follow-up. Comparison of disability before and after HA cannot be expressed in figures. However, the average reduction in disability thanks to HA amounts to approximately 30%. The correlation between marked disability and radiologically or clinically confirmed PA (Table 24) is particularly noticeable. Disability of 50%–75% occurs in just 20% of cases in which perfect HA union has occurred and disability of 75%–100% in 12% of our cases. In 90% of these cases, however, both hips were affected and the severe degree of disability could not be attributed to the HA alone.

3.3.3 Independence of Patients with Hip Arthrodeses

Answers to our questionnaire and to questions posed at the follow-up examinations also revealed a considerable difference between the patients with united HA and those with PA (Table 25).

Approximately half our patients claimed to be at least partially dependent on others, particularly in pulling on socks and stockings and putting on shoes. In almost all cases they were aided by another member of the family. Persons living on their own had usually made themselves independent using aids which, in some cases, they had constructed themselves. However, in more than 60% of the cases, putting on and tying of shoes on the affected side had already been impossible before the operation.

3.4 Effect of the Arthrodesis on the Contralateral Hip

Detrimental long-term effects following HA have been mentioned by several authors (Conforty; Demigneux et al.; Merle d'Aubigné Fürmaier; Hackenbroch; Hirsch; Hördegen et al.; Maquet; Seewald; Schoenler and others).

Following HA, pelvic tilt occurs on walking. This results in hyperextension of the normal hip. In addition, the weight-bearing phase on the contralateral side during walking is prolonged. This increase in load on the nonarthrodesed side would theoretically affect the joint adversely. For this reason, we followed up our patients who had bilateral arthrosis of the hip 1–10 years following arthrodesis. To our surprise, significant clinical or subjective worsening had occurred in only five cases and in a further five cases subjective improvement was reported with no changes in the radiological appearances of the hips (Table 7). Clearly in many other cases, long-term subjective and objective worsening of the hip arthrosis was observed. However, we have not evaluated these cases since we know from experience that significant worsening over the years may be expected following conservative treatment

Table 25. Association of patients' independence with bone union and PA following HA

	United HA (496)	Pseudarthrotic HA (84)
Unable to dress self	71=14.4%	43=51.2%
Unable to put on shoes	181=36.5%	72=85.7%
Difficulty with sitting	172=34.7%	69=82.1%
Dependent on third party	218=43.9%	68=80.9%

a b c d

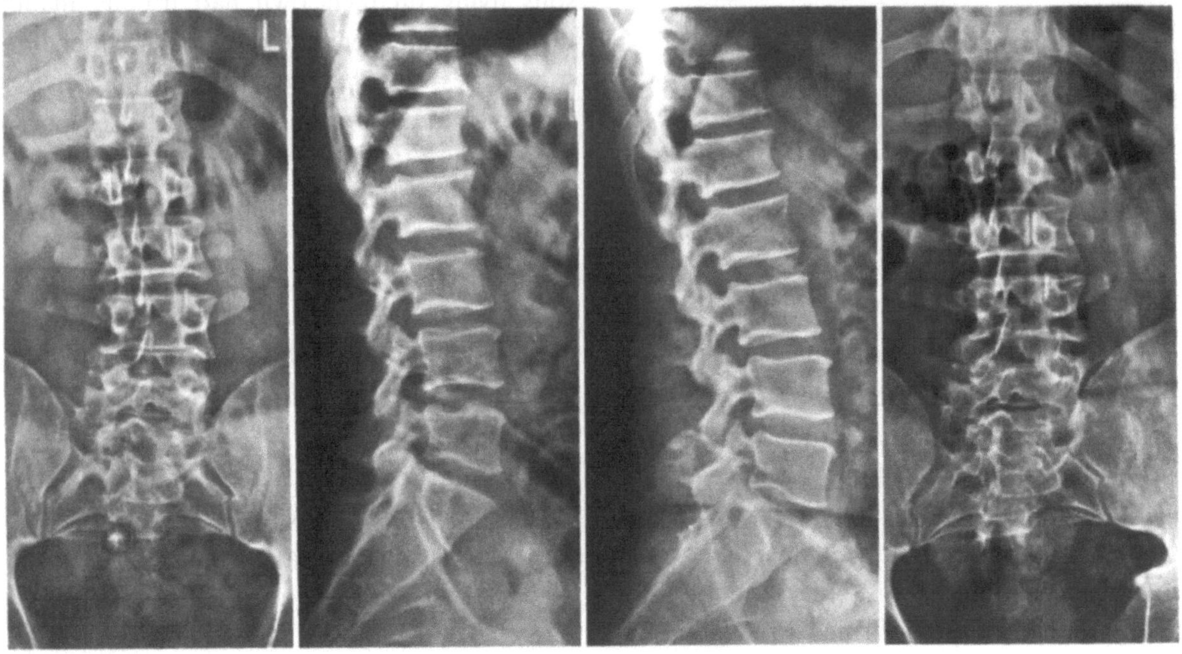

Figs. 115 and 116. *Comparison of LS radiographs taken before and 4 – 6 years after HA*

Fig. 115. F. W., ♂, aged 36 years, No. 135798.
a and b) Prior to HA. Slight torsional scoliosis.
c and d) Four years later. Radiographic appearance unchanged

or operations which preserve joint motion (IO or TP). We believe that HA does not bring about clinically or radiologically noticeable damage in an intact contralateral hip joint. It should be remembered, however, that our series only extends over 10 years but experience has also shown that patients whose hips were arthrodesed 20 or 30 years ago (particularly following trauma) suffer no particular changes in the opposite hip.

3.5 Hip Arthrodesis and Back Complaints

Every normal joint is subjected to body weight and functions on the side as a kind of damper. Arthrodesis of a joint causes transfer of load to the proximally adjacent joint. Thus, HA results at first in increased stress on the SIJ, the lumbosacral joints and, finally, on the lower LS. Theoretically one might expect progressive damage to the LS.

HA frequently causes lumbar pain as a result of the increased load on the LS. This usually regresses, however, after a period of adaptation of 6 – 12 months. In certain cases the pain remains. Here it is necessary to distinguish between complaints which were present *before* arthrodesis and those which arose *after* the operation (Table 26).

Back complaints which were present preoperatively remain unchanged following arthrodesis in 41.8% of cases. They are significantly worsened in 8.8% and significantly improved in 49.4%.

Table 26. Arthrodesis and back complaints

Prior to arthrodesis operation	
Back complaints present	172 = 29%
Following arthrodesis operation	
Occurrence of back complaints	34 = 8.2%
Back complaints unchanged	72 = 41.8%
Back complaints worsened	15 = 8.8%
Improvement in or disappearance of back complaints	85 = 49.4%

Lumbar pain occurred for the first time immediately following the operation or later in 34 patients (8.2%).

Thus, contrary to widespread impression, the operation is seldom solely responsible for the occurrence of spinal complaints.

Radiological investigation of the lumbar vertebral column at an average of 4–5 years following HA showed no significant changes when compared to the preoperative film (Figs. 115, 116).

Unfortunately, back complaints are frequently assumed to be a result of the HA and are treated symptomatically without careful examination by the doctor. Thus in one of our patients, compression of the fourth lumbar root by a vertebral process with an extremely severe medial bulge was diagnosed (Fig. 117). On widening of the foramen and excision of the large chunks of bone which were compressing the root of L4, the patient's symptoms were completely abolished.

3.6 Subjective Results

The answers to the questionnaires sent to our patients and the results of our follow-up examinations have confirmed our clinical impressions. Patients frequently assume at first that the operation will be disabling but the final result shows 90% of them to be completely satisfied. Clearly, active participation and adaptability on the part of the patient is required in order to overcome the difficulties associated with sitting, climbing stairs, automobile driving, bicycle riding, putting on shoes and socks unaided from behind and sexual intercourse. We consider careful preoperative information of the patient and regular postoperative follow-up by the patient's family doctor to be particularly important. More than two-thirds of our patients were able to continue their former job at the same or an improved level of performance. This clearly speaks for HA since, as WITT said, "It is not the range of motion measured on the doctor's couch which is decisive but the effect of the operation on daily life."

In the majority of cases where subjective complaints cause the patient to be dissatisfied with the arthrodesis, the doctor is usually dissatisfied with the poor clinical or radiological result. Of patients with fully united arthrodeses, 89.1% were satisfied with the result and 19% with PA or fibrous ankylosis were satisfied (Table 27). In only one case with

Table 27. Subjective results

Arthrodesis united	Patient satisfied	441 = 89.1%
	Patient more or less satisfied	34 = 6.7%
	Patient dissatisfied	21 = 4.2%
Arthrodesis not united (pseudarthrosis, fibrous ankylosis)	Patient satisfied	16 = 19.0%
	Patient more or less satisfied	10 – 11.9%
	Patient dissatisfied	58 = 69.1%

Table 28. Correlation between subjective results and clinical findings

	Arthrodesis united		Loosening, absence of radiological union		Total	
	Cases	%	Cases	%	Cases	%
Standing on arthrodesed leg impossible	1	0.17	70	12.06	71	12.24
Pain on arthrodesed side	10	1.72	69	11.89	79	13.62

a b c

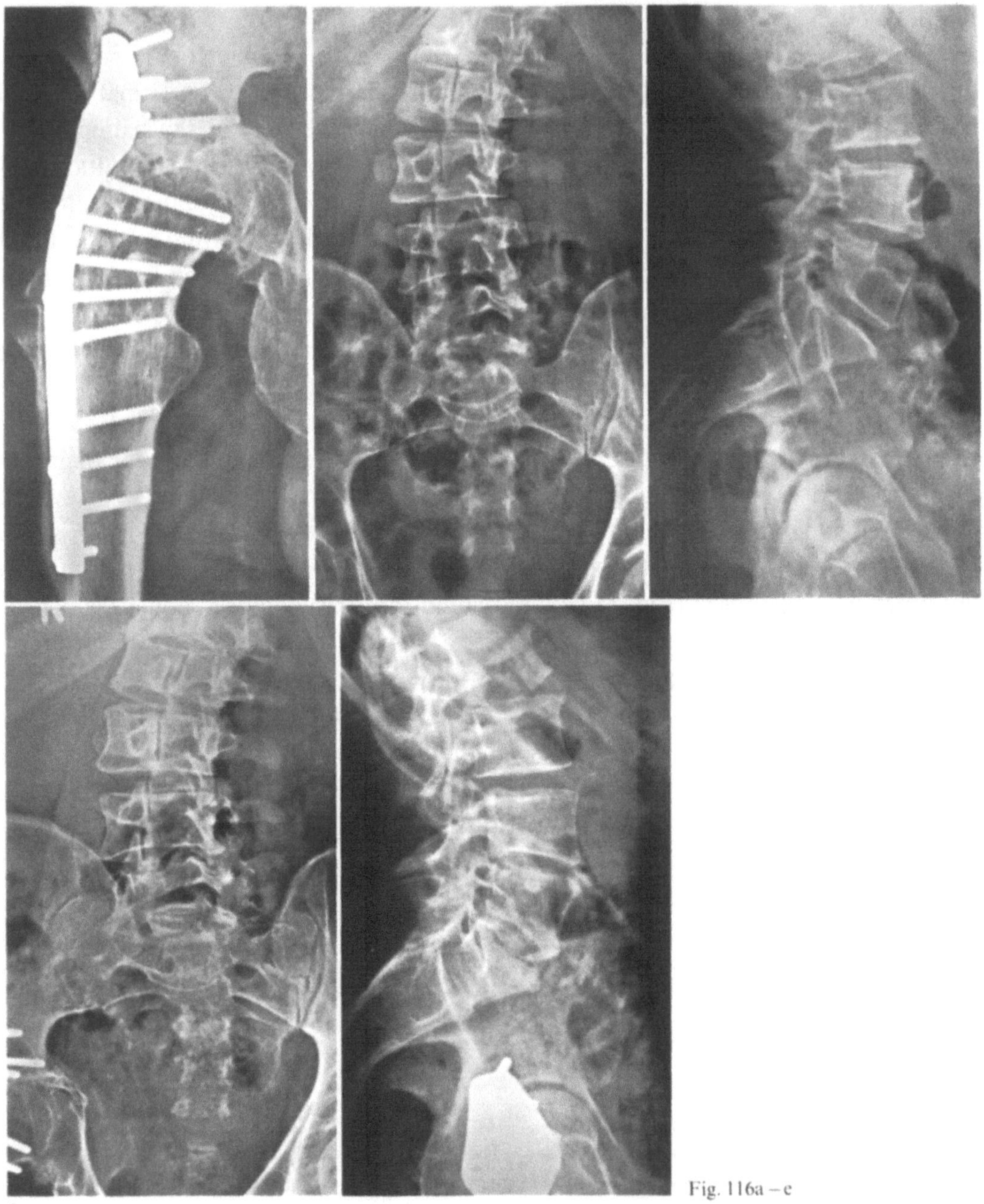

d e

Fig. 116a – e

rigid arthrodesis was the patient unable to stand on one leg. Pain on the arthrodesed side was mentioned in 10 cases (1.7%). Of the 84 patients with PA, 70 (83%) were unable to stand on the arthrodesed side and standing on that side caused pain in 69 (Table 28).

Gait following arthrodesis (Table 29): Of 492 patients with fully united HA, 19 walk with two canes (nine of them because of problems in the opposite hip) and 94 walk with one stick (again, 40 of these on account of disease in the opposite nonarthrodesed hip). Of the 88 patients with PA or fibrous ankylosis following HA, 69 required two canes and 19 only one cane.

We have personally examined more than 300 patients of the total series of 583. We paid particular attention to the 34 persons who were

f g h

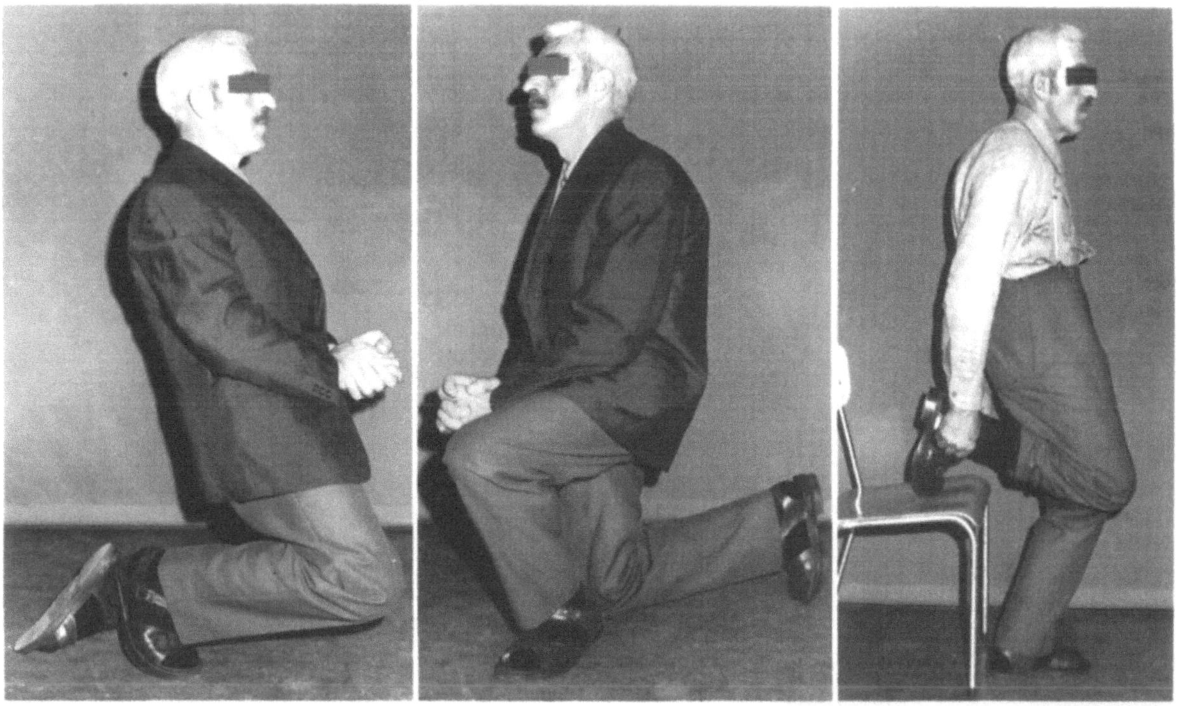

i

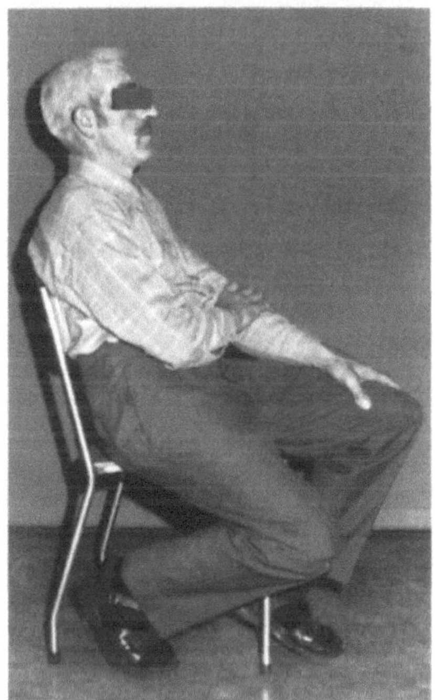

Fig. 116. A. A., ♂, aged 44 years, No. 108310.

a) Five years after cobra-head plate arthrodesis.

b and c) Marked scoliosis and spondyloarthrotic changes prior to HA.

d and e) Five years later. No worsening detectable. No subjective problems.

f–i) The same patient can kneel and put on his shoes without difficulty and sits very well

Table 29. Gait following arthrodesis operation

	United; unilateral disease	United; bilateral disease	Union radiologically absent	PA	Total	%
2 canes	10	9	6	63	88	15.17
1 cane	54	40	7	12	113	19.48
No cane	–	–	–	–	379	65.34
Total	64	49	13	75	580	100.00

Table 30. Patients who were dissatisfied or more or less satisfied with their arthrodesis

Reason	More or less satisfied (34)	Dissatisfied (21)
Pain in:		
Arthrodesed hip	1	2
Back	2	1
Knee	1	2
Knee+back	1	–
Difficulty with:		
Sitting	5	2
Sitting+pain in arthrodesed hip	1	1
Sitting+pain in back	–	1
Sitting+lat. peroneal nerve paresis	–	1
Climbing stairs	1	–
Sexual intercourse	1	–
Sexual intercourse+sitting	–	1
Automobile driving	1	1
Complaints and difficulty with walking because of leg shortening	–	1
Complaints and difficulty with walking because of deformity	1	1
No cogent reason	19	7

only more or less satisfied with the arthrodesis and to the 21 persons who were dissatisfied. In 26 of these patients, no cogent reason could be found or objectively established: frequently the patients wanted their full range of hip motion back, having heard or read a lot about "the new modern prosthetic hip joint." One patient gave his obesity, which he ascribed to the HA, as his reason for dissatisfaction. Another was unhappy because the HA rendered him *capable* of working! The reasons given by the other patients were always credible even if they were not always clinically or radiologically objectifiable (Table 30).

Fig. 117. *Incorrect interpretation of back complaints.* M. J., ♂, aged 52 years, No. 68489.

a and b) Prior to HA.

c and d) Four and a half years later. Osteochondrosis and arthrosis. The complaints were treated symptomatically over a period of 2 years, having been ascribed to the HA.

e and f) Lumbar myelogram. The marked filling defect at the level of L4–L5 is caused by bony compression of the root of L4 by severe medial projection of a vertebral process. Operation resulted in total cessation of complaints

a b c

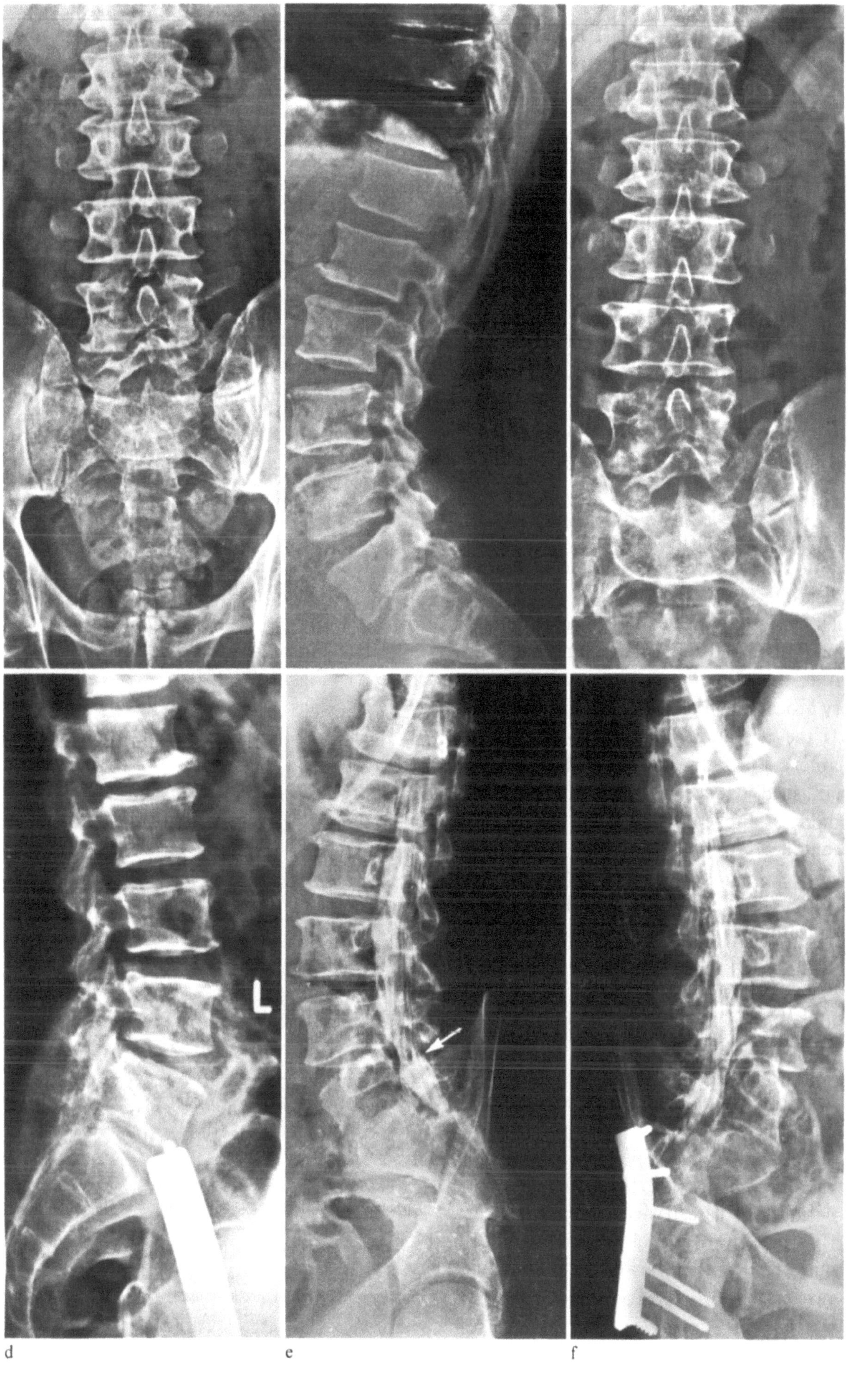

d e f

II. Classification of the Hip Arthrodeses by Indication

1 Hip Arthrodeses for Arthrosis of the Hip and Rheumatoid Arthritis

1.1 Arthrosis of the Hip

1.1.1 Introduction

In our series, the arthroses of the hip and rheumatoid arthritis were by far the commonest indications (391 cases, 67%).

Doctor and patient usually decide on HA if conservative and surgical measures had failed. HA is therefore the one remaining satisfactory procedure in patients with hip arthrosis.

If the operation is indicated (see relevant chapter), the following rules which we have established on the basis of our experience should be applied in choosing the operative technique:

- Type I HA is no longer performed nowadays (frequency of PA, prolonged hospitalisation, early mobilisation impossible because of cast fixation).
- Type II HA with compression-plate fixation and IO is carried out for correction of stiff ankylotic deformity of hip as well as in cases in which leg length is to be increased by upright positioning of the proximal femoral component.
- Type III HA with double-plate fixation offers rigidity comparable to that obtained with the cobra-head plate. It is exceptionally indicated if correct fitting of a cobra-head plate is difficult or impossible for technical anatomical reasons.
- Type IV HA using the cobra-head plate is to be preferred whenever possible (short hospital stay, early mobilisation, lowest frequency of PA).

1.1.2 Case Material

In the following illustrations our HA operations performed between 1961 and 1971 are reviewed.

Type I: Figs. 118 – 123
Type II: Figs. 124 – 128
Type III: Figs. 129 – 131
Type IV: Figs. 132 – 139

Fig. 119. *Type I HA without PO in a case of arthrosis of the hip secondary to subluxation.* C. H., ♀, aged 63 years, No. 71433.

a) Before operation.

b) Two days after operation. During freshening of the joint surfaces and curettage of the cysts in the acetabular roof disintegration of the medial pelvic wall around the acetabulum occurred and resulted in central dislocation of the head.

c) Result $3^1/_2$ years following operation. Perfect healing. Agile gait. Patient works full time as housewife

a b c

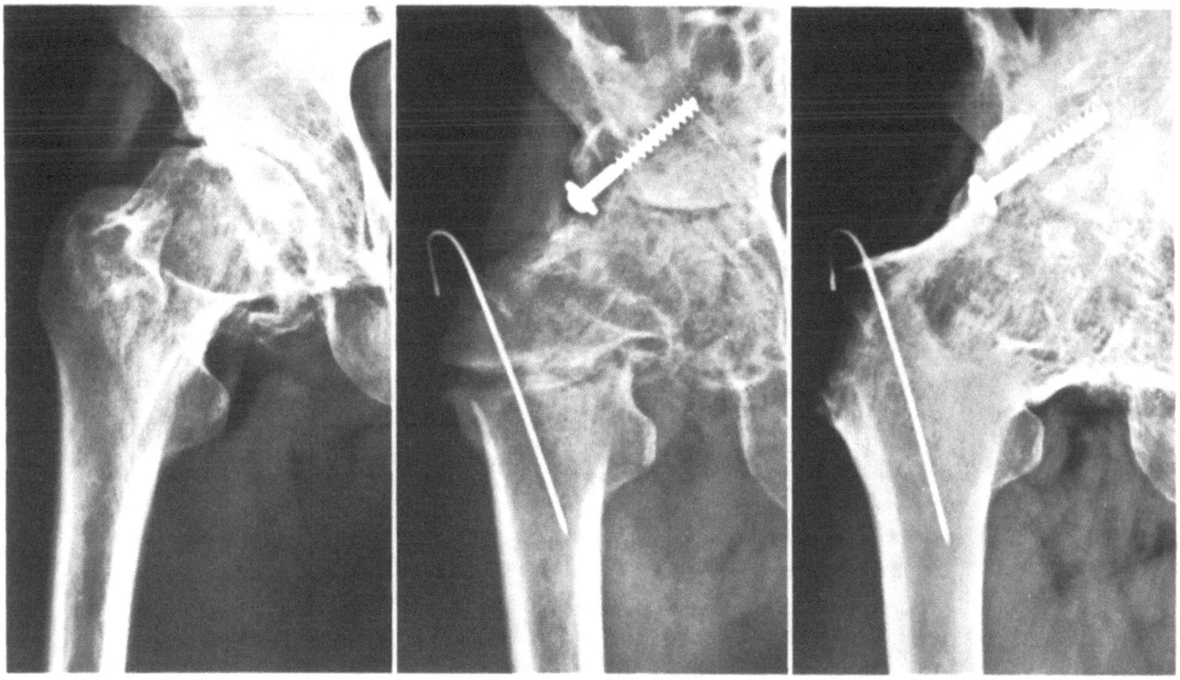

Fig. 118. *Type I HA in a case of severe arthrosis of the hip.* H. H., ♂, aged 37 years, No. 81 720.

a) Eight months prior to operation.

b) Three months postoperative following removal of cast.

Because of the tendency to tilting at the osteotomy a K-wire was driven into the femoral diaphysis from the proximal end.

c) Six and a half years after HA. Perfect healing with correct leg position. Patient well and working full time as a draughtsman

a b c

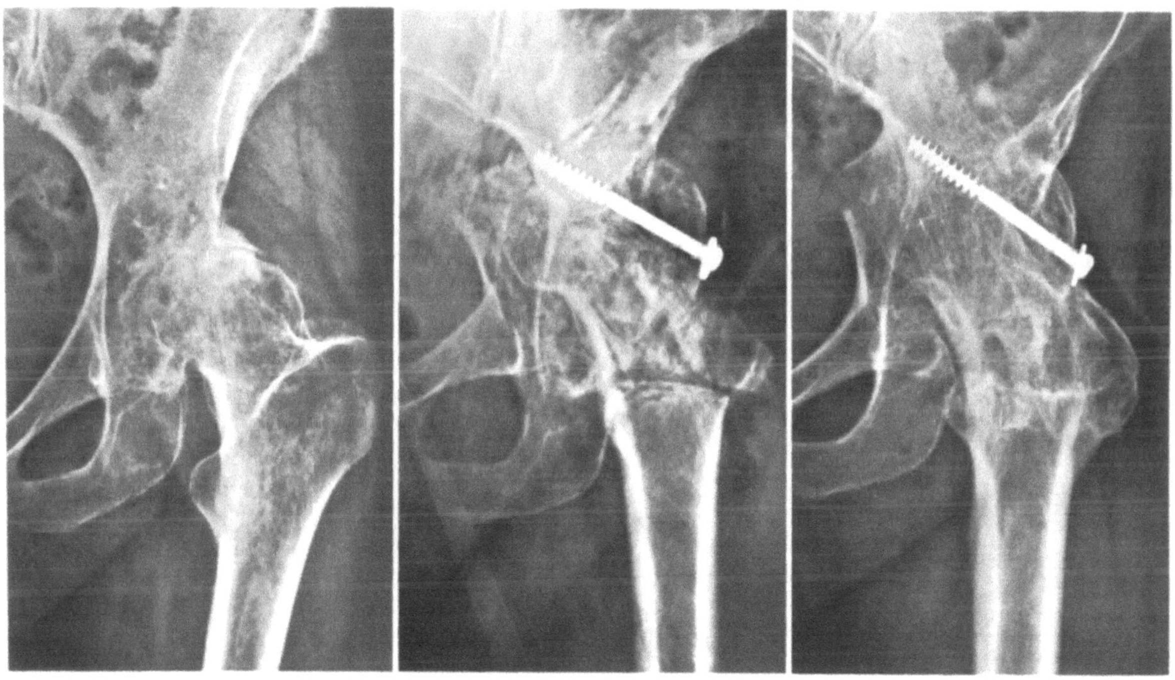

a b c

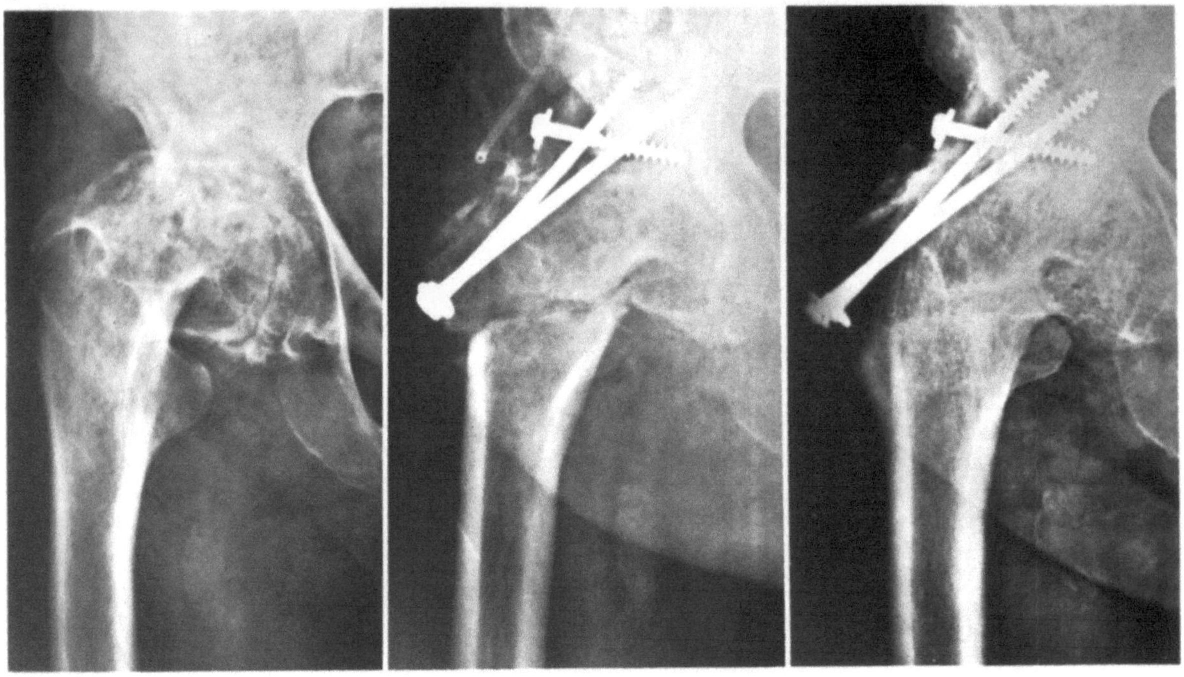

Fig. 120. *Type I HA without PO*. B. W., ♂, male, aged 61 years, No. 71452.

a) Before operation. Partial ankylosis with external rotation deformity.

b) The proximal femur is fixed to the pelvis with two cancellous screws and the greater trochanter is screwed to the pelvis as an iliofemoral graft.

c) Twenty months following HA. Excellent subjective and objective result. Works full time as a storeman

a b c

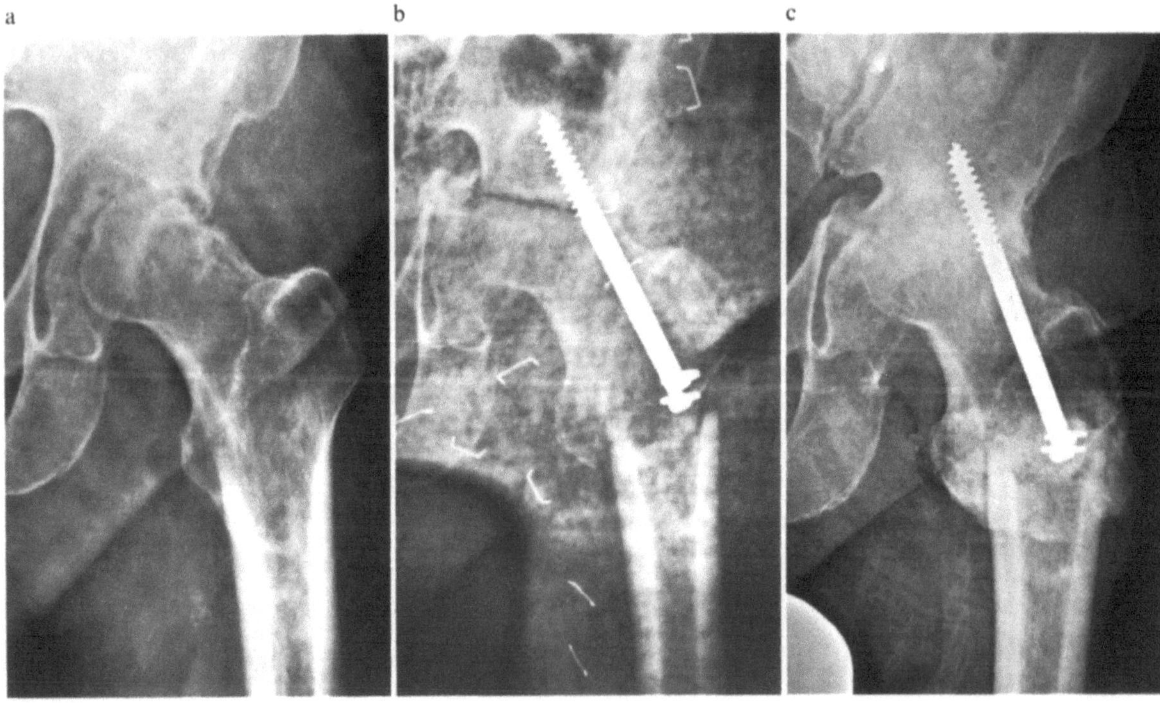

a b c

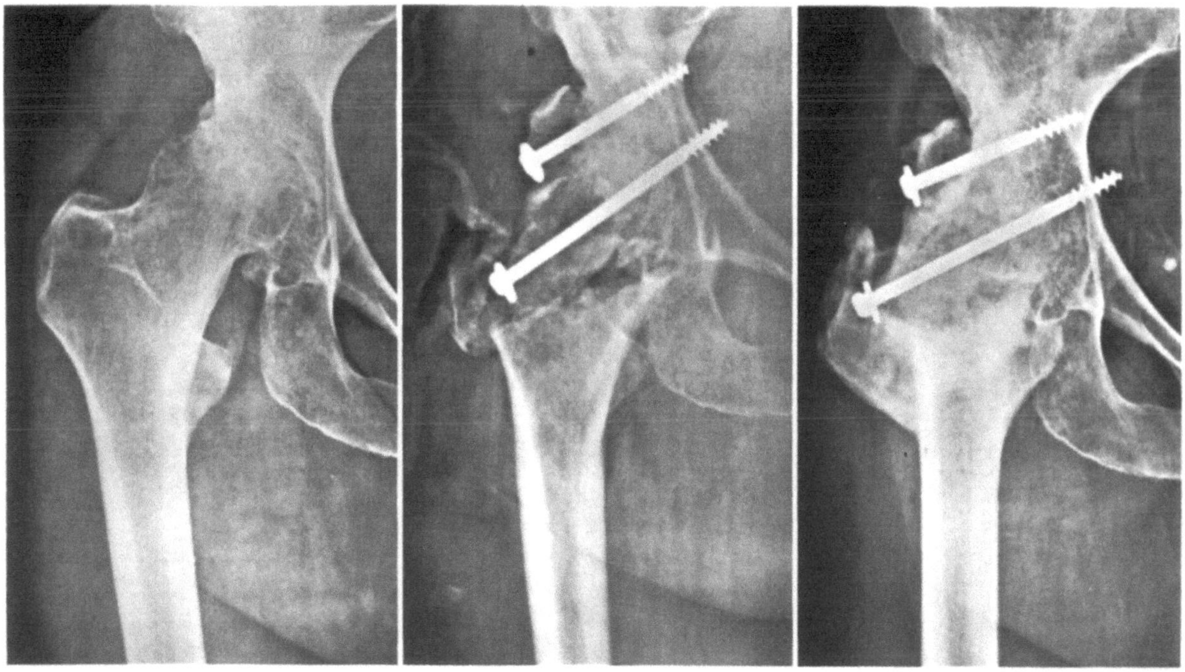

Fig. 122. *Type I HA without PO in a case of severe hip arthrosis.* P. J., ♀, aged 50 years, No. 70953.

a) Almost total painful ankylosis of the hip joint 1 year prior to operation.

b) HA with a very high IO (danger of necrosis due to damage to blood vessels during the operation).

c) Result 1 year later. HA united. Limp due to shortening (functional leg shortening 3 cm). Patient complaint-free

Fig. 121. *Type I HA with PO in a case of hip arthrosis secondary to hip sepsis.* W. K., ♂, aged 44 years, No. 108592.

a) Before operation. Almost total destruction of the hip joint. Flexion/extension 60 – 30 – 0°; all other movement prevented by pain.

b) HA by fixation of the proximal femoral component to the pelvis with two cortex lag screws and subtrochanteric osteotomy.

c) HA clinically and radiologically united. Walks without pain. Works in his hotel with 25% disability

a b c

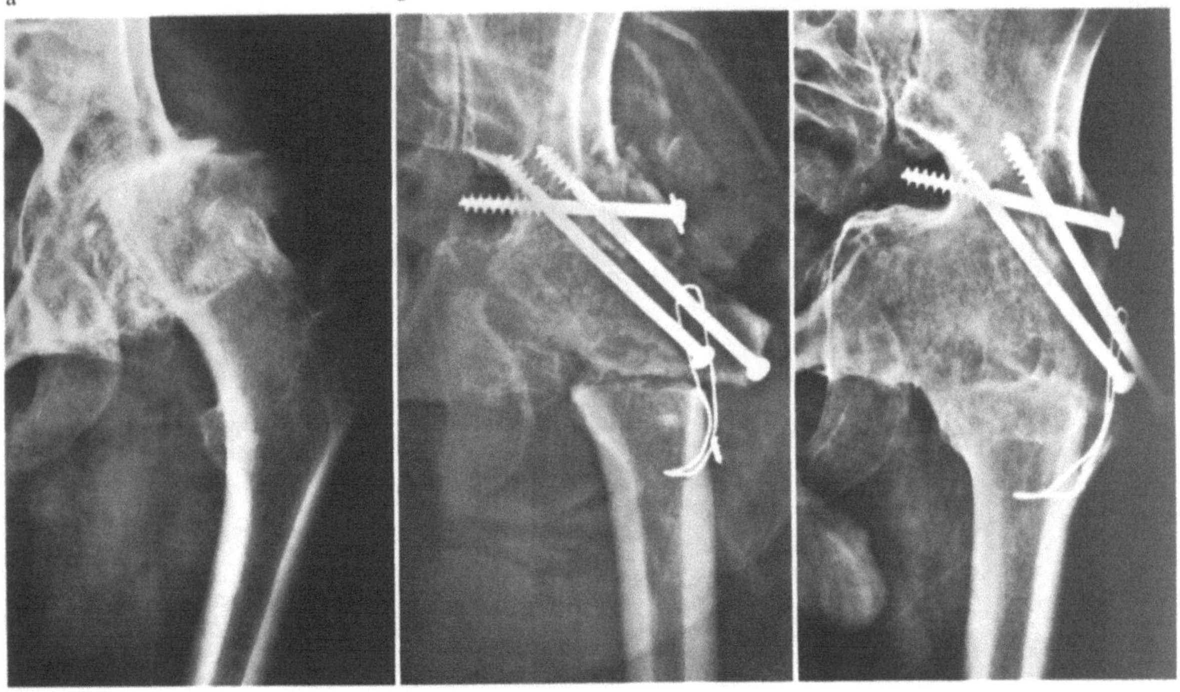

Fig. 123. *Type I HA with PO in a case of secondary arthrosis of the hip with ankylosis (following fracture-dislocation of the hip joint).* Z. E., ♂, aged 49 years, No. 72270.

a) Severe arthrosis of the hip 28 years after fracture-dislocation of the hip joint. Subluxation of the hip.

b) Good contact surfaces as a result of large medial displacement following PO. The IO is secured by a tension-band wire loop.

c) Four years following operation. Good subjective and objective result, no complaints. Works as labourer with no disability

a b c

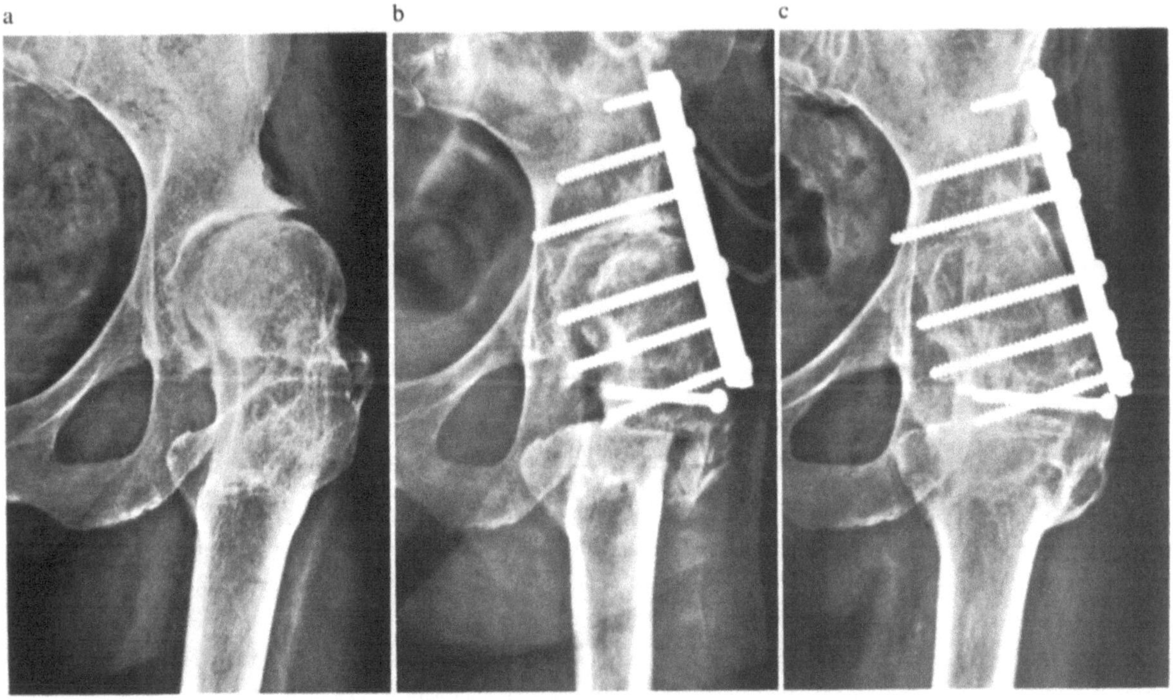

a b c

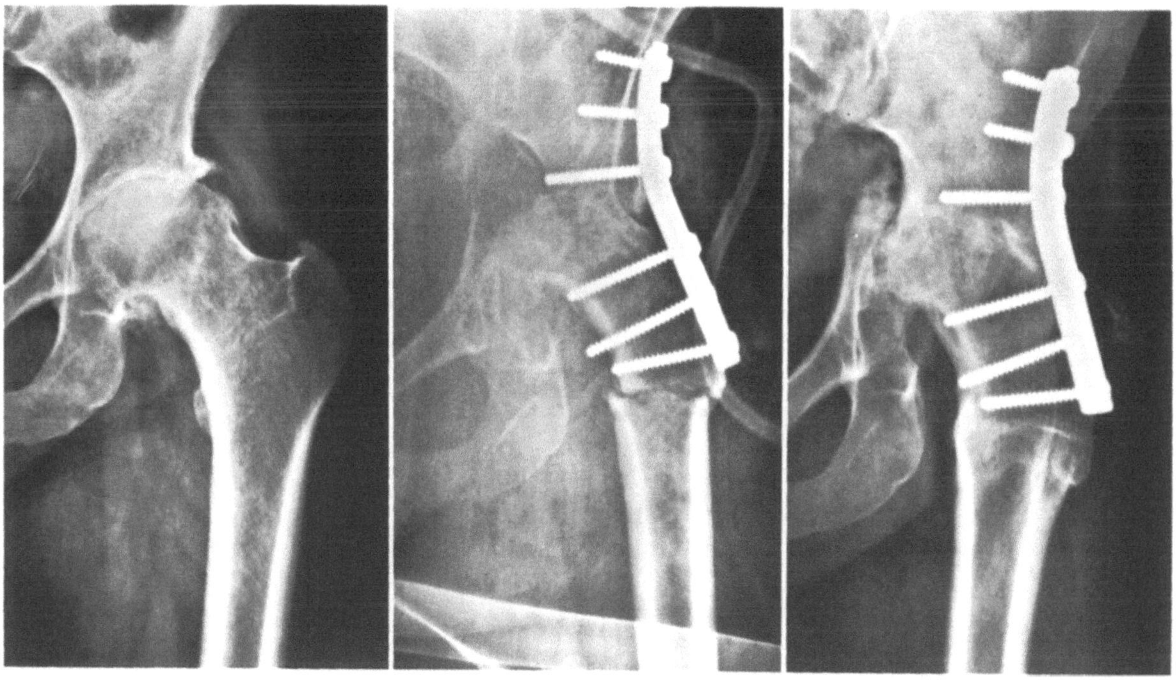

Fig. 125. *Type II HA with pelvic osteotomy*. S. G., ♀, aged 50 years, No. 95050.

a) Before operation.

b) HA with 6-hole plate following PO with moderate displacement. Transverse osteotomy underneath the plate.

c) Four years after operation. HA united. Hip limp on the left side with 2 cm functional leg shortening. Works full time as housewife

Fig. 124. *Type II HA in a case of ankylosing arthrosis of the hip*. S. H., ♀, aged 65 years, No. 73690.

a) Three years following subtrochanteric osteotomy with adductorotomy, excision of cysts and cancellous bone plasty. Severe complaints.

b) HA with 6-hole plate. A graft taken from the greater trochanter was fixed over the IO with a screw.

c) Result 5 years after operation. HA united with 15° adduction deformity and functional leg shortening of 2 cm

a b c

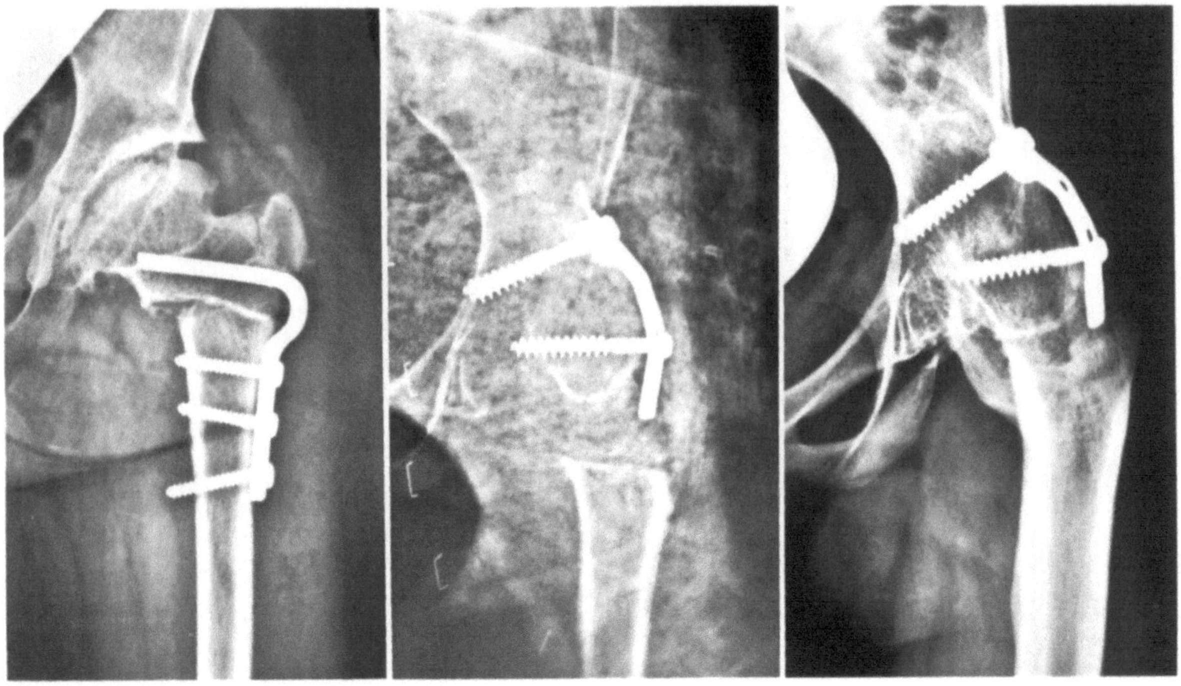

Fig. 126. *Type II HA with PO in a case of hip arthrosis.* L. L., ♂, aged 55 years, No. 99885.

a) Left hip fixed in 45° external rotation and neutral abduction/adduction position.

b) HA with 6-hole plate following PO with small medial displacement and IO.

c) Eighteen months later. HA and IO united. Patient complaint-free. Works as farmer with 50% disability

a b c

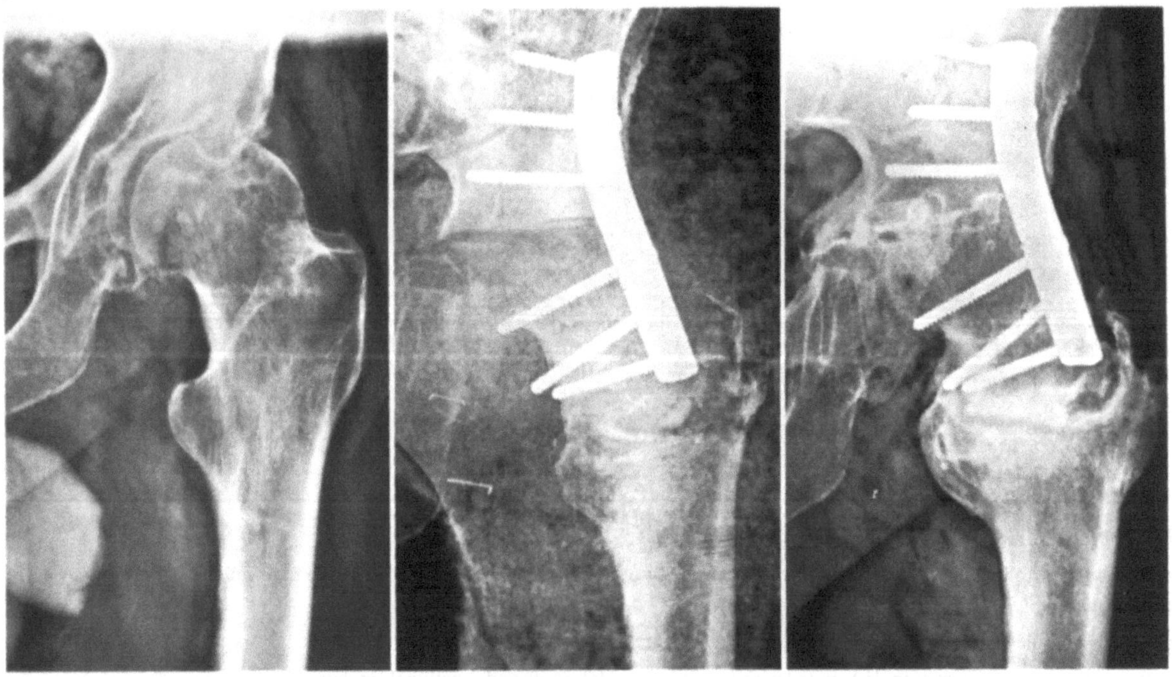

a b c

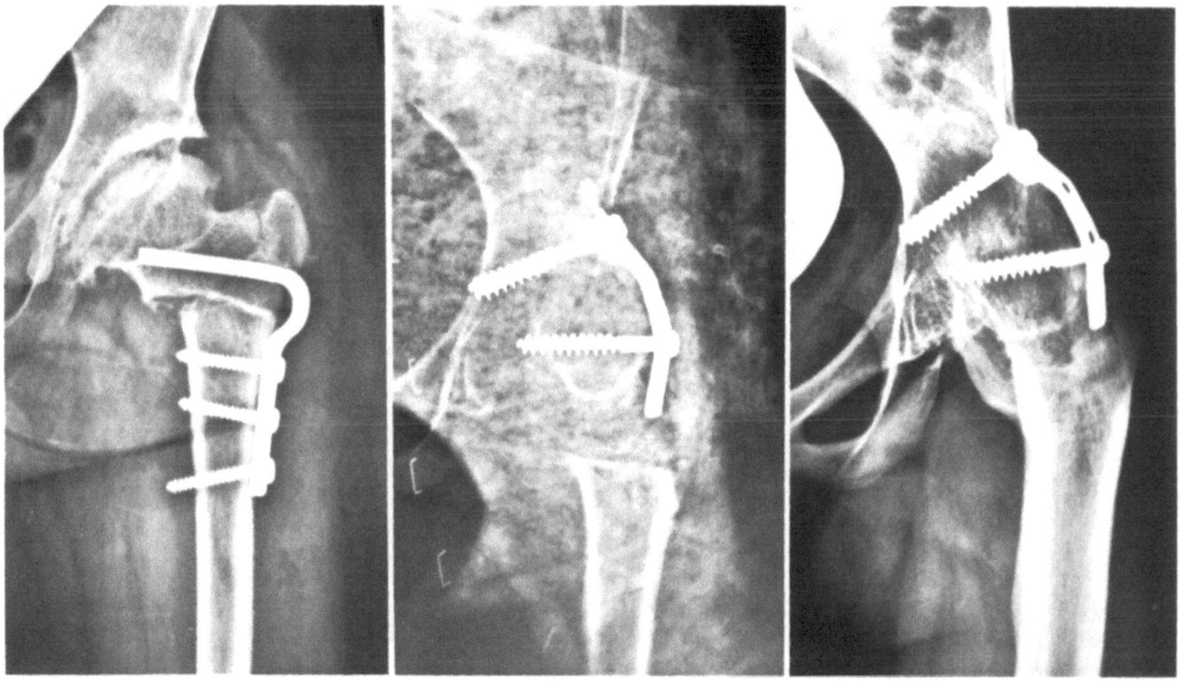

Fig. 128. *Type II HA for suspected infection secondary to IO in an old CDH.* S. Y., ♀, aged 13 years, No. 90325.

a) Six weeks after osteotomy. Suspected postoperative infection. Severe limitation of hip joint movement.

b) HA using a shoulder plate which was bent to shape.

c) Two years later. HA united in ideal position following osteotomy 1 year previously to correct 12° adduction deformity and 4.5 cm functional leg shortening. Patient complaint-free

Fig. 127. *Type II HA in a case of hip arthrosis secondary to congenital subluxation.* B. H., ♀, aged 56 years, No. 97891.

a) Subluxation of the hip which is fixed in 70° external rotation. (Radiograph: protrusion of the lesser trochanter.)

b) Type II HA. Cobra-head plate arthrodesis was technically impossible because of the short femoral neck, the marked anteversion of the head and the external rotation deformity.

c) Thirteen months following HA. Bone union complete with 8° abduction deformity. Patient complaint-free. Walks with a cane to reduce load on the left hip (arthrosis secondary to high dislocation on the left side)

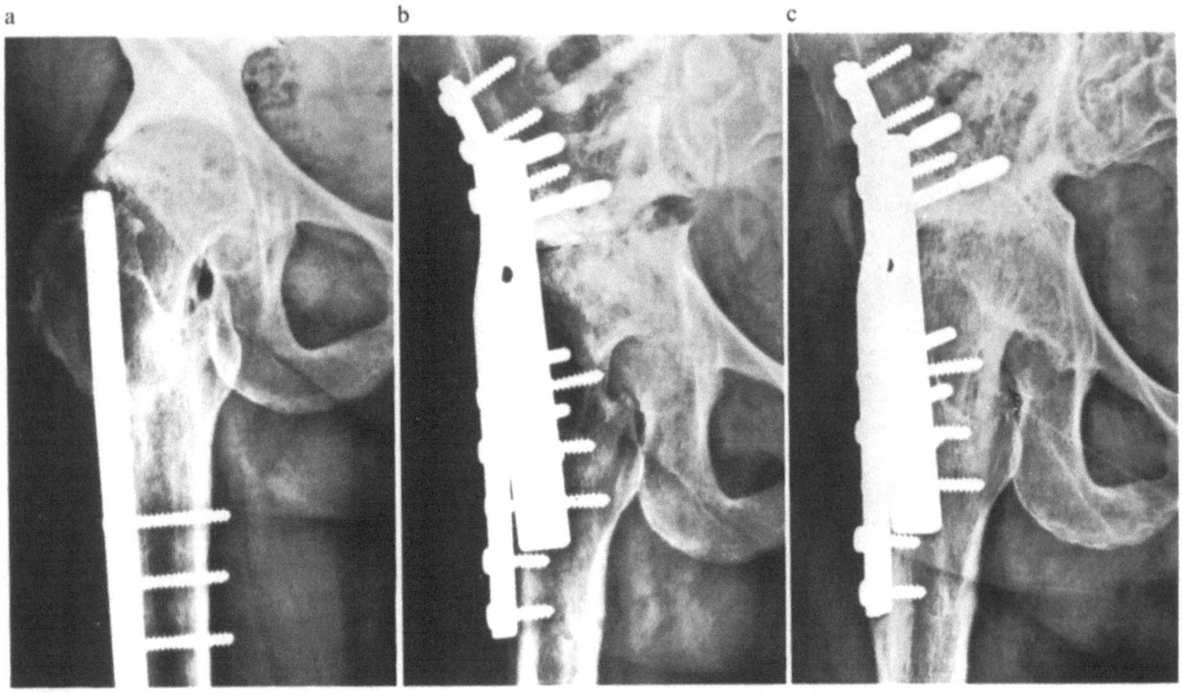

Fig. 129. *Type III HA with PO following IO in a case of hip arthrosis*. S. E., ♀, aged 61 years, No. 64493.

a) Two years following IO. Extensive ankylosis with flexion and external rotation deformity.

b) Double plate arthrodesis following PO osteotomy and moderate medial displacement.

c) Two years following operation. Right hip fixed in ideal position. Patient complaint-free and working full time as housewife

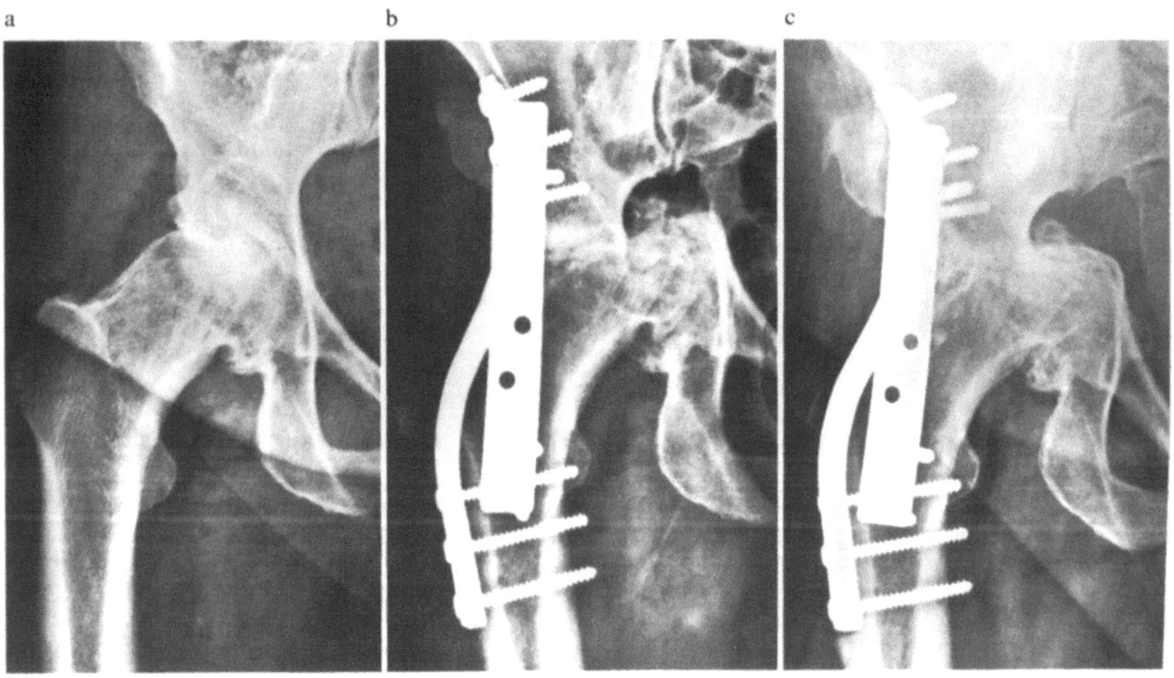

Fig. 130. *Type III HA with PO in a case of hip arthrosis*. E. E., ♀, aged 49 years, No. 83134.

a) Before operation.

b) Double plate arthrodesis with extreme medial displacement following PO.

c) Two years after HA. Free painless gait without cane. Works full time as housewife

a b c

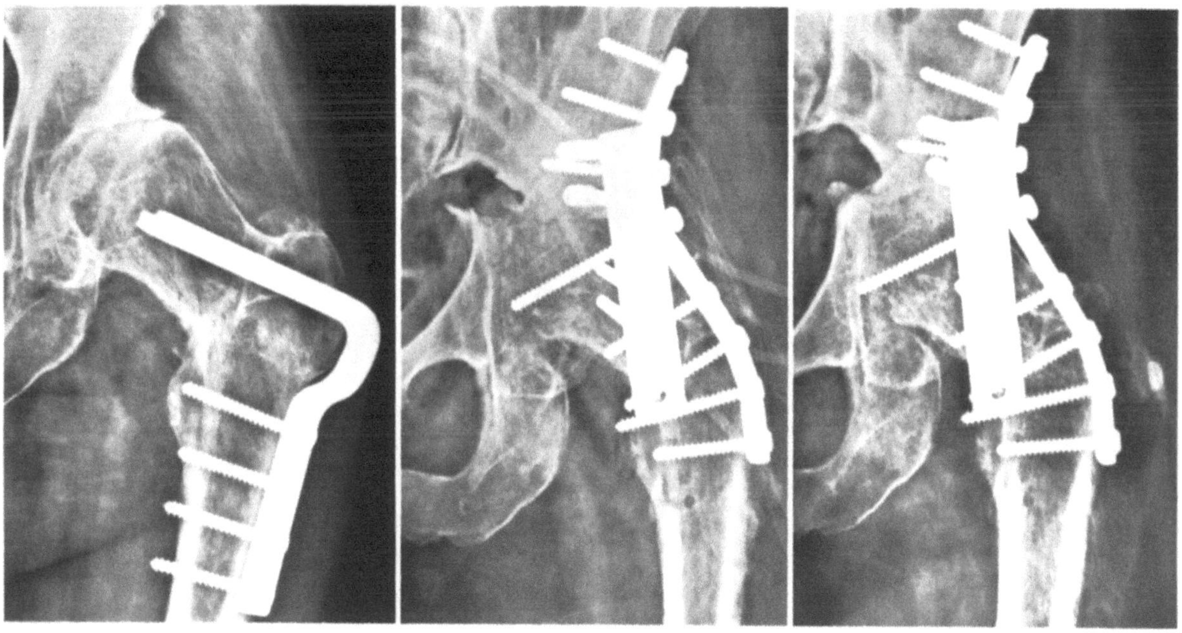

Fig. 131. *Type III HA with PO in a case of hip arthrosis (valgus subluxation of the hip)*. T. M., ♀, aged 50 years, No. 77450.

a) Fifteen months following varus IO. Completely united with 20° adduction deformity.

b) Double plate arthrodesis with PO and moderate medial displacement.

c) Four months following operation the HA is united in ideal position. Painless gait without cane. Patient has recovered her independence around the house

a b c

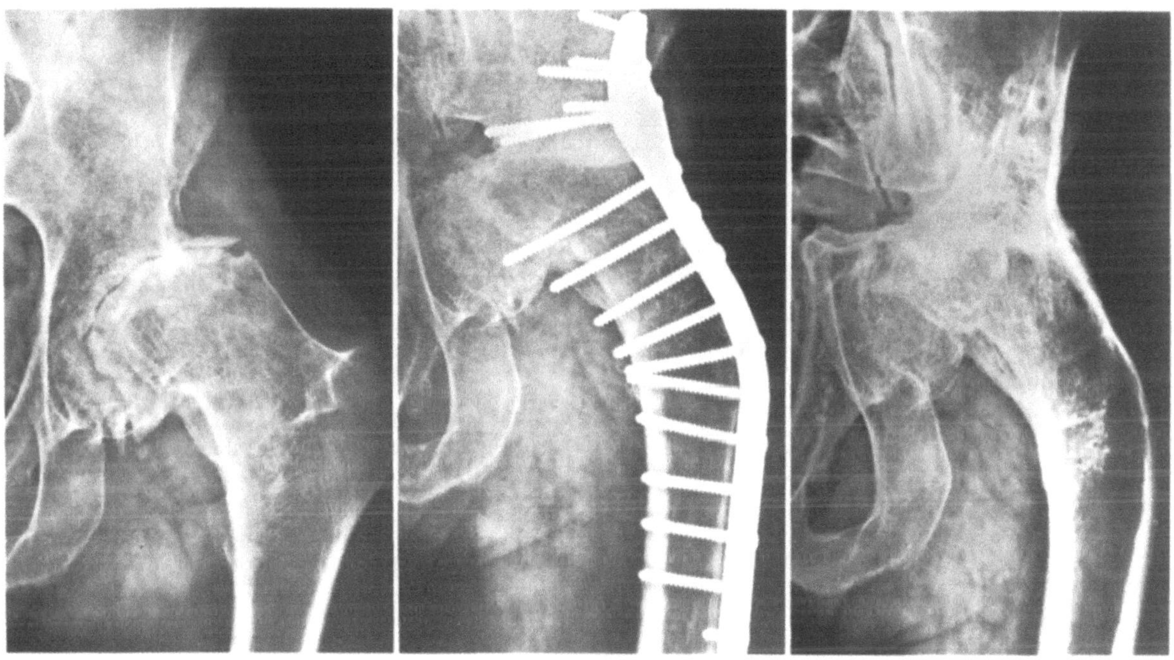

Fig. 132. *Type IV HA with PO in a case of hip arthrosis*. W. H., ♂, aged 62 years, No. 113835.

a) Severe arthrotic hip changes. Hip fixed in full extension, 25° abduction, 15° external rotation.

b) Four months after operation. HA united in good position. Patient has returned to his work as an engineer; no disability.

c) Two years following implant removal (requested by the patient). Incipient column formation

a b c

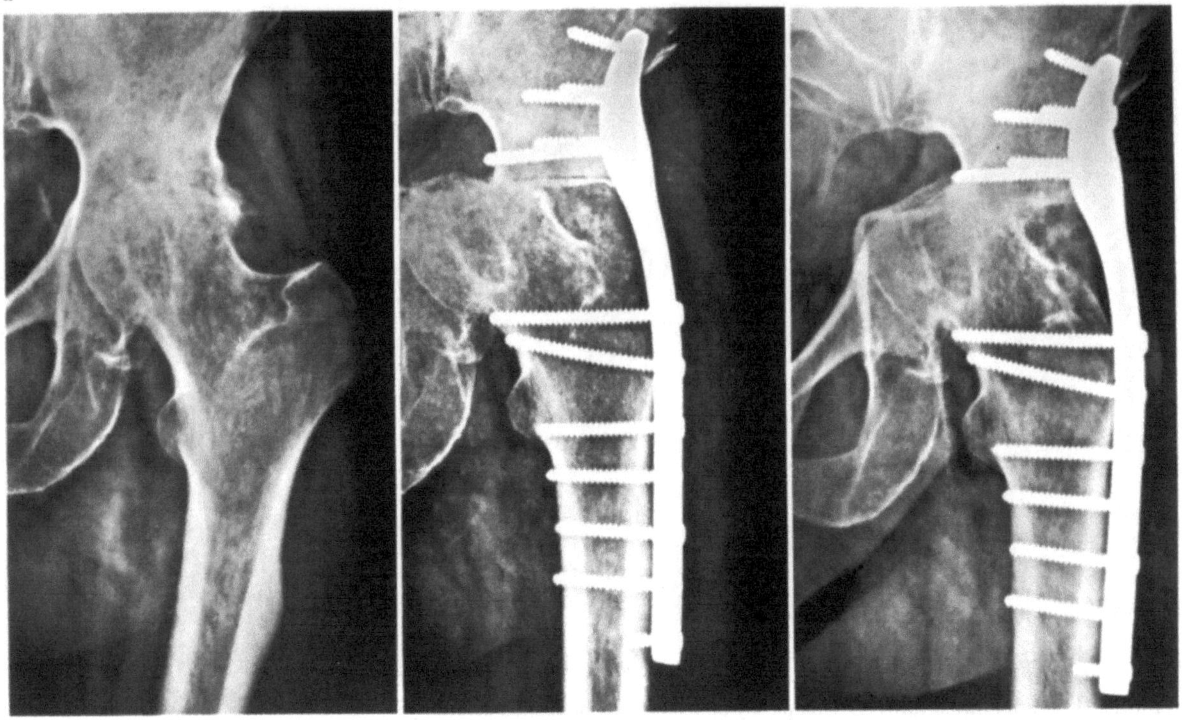

Fig. 133. *Type IV HA with pelvic osteotomy in a case of severe arthrosis of the hip*. H. K., ♀, aged 55 years, No. 149980.

a) Very painful and almost totally stiff hip (flexion/extension 30 – 10 – 0°).

b) Cobra-head plate arthrodesis with PO and very large degree of medial displacement.

c) Four months after operation. HA in ideal position. Patient is complaint-free and works full time as housewife without residual disability

a b c

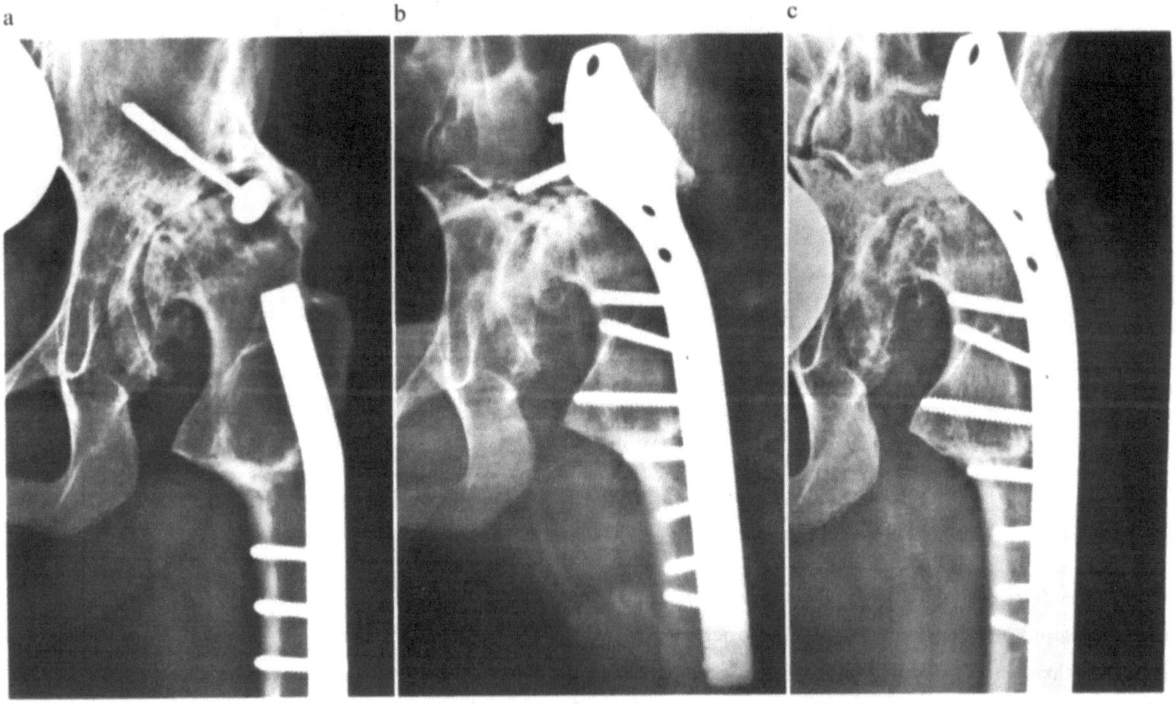

d e f g

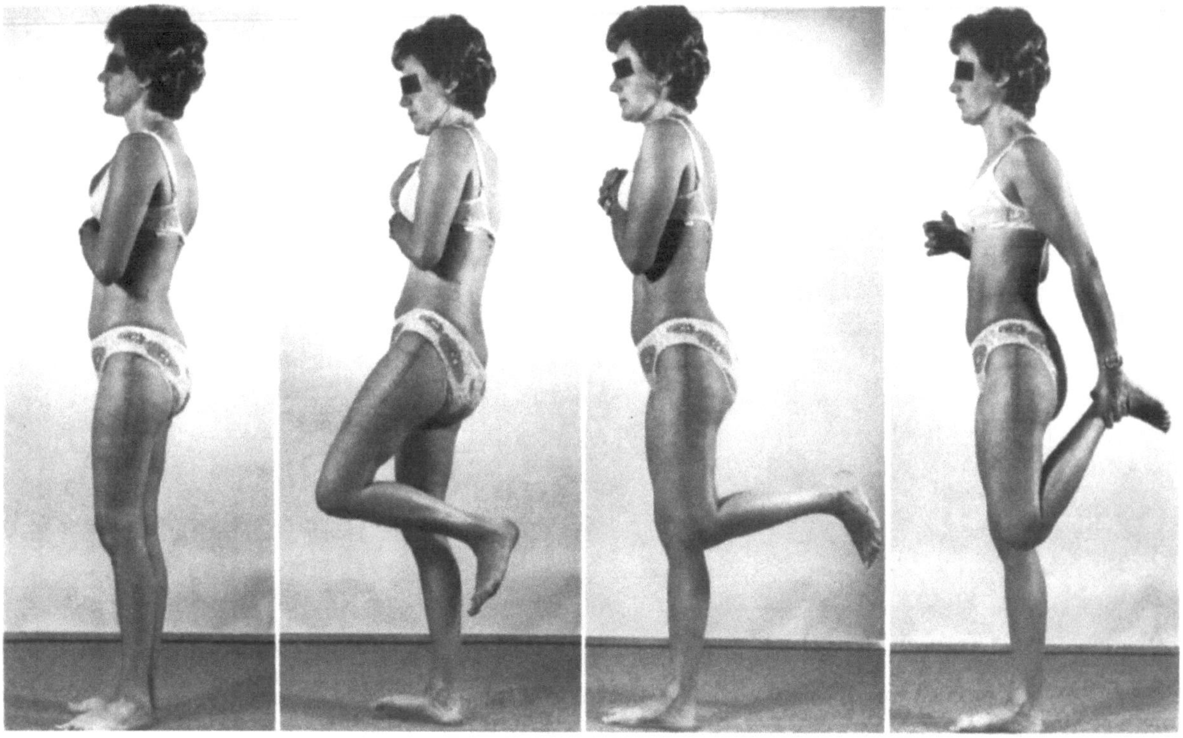

h

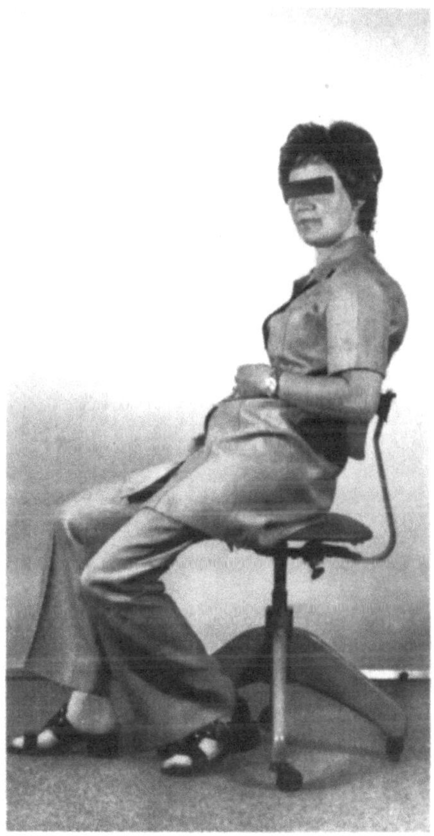

Fig. 134. *Type IV HA in a case of hip arthrosis secondary to CDH.* D. A., ♀, aged 35 years, No. 154934.

a) Following valgus IO and acetabular roof plasty. Severe complaints; hip hardly capable of bearing weight.

b) Immediately following Type IV HA with PO and moderate medial displacement. The most proximal screw was removed as the pelvis afforded it insufficient hold. Postoperative cast for 10 weeks.

c) Following removal of the hip spica. Position of the arthrodesis clinically and radiologically ideal.

d – g) Radiographs taken at time of cast removal.

d) Standing on both legs.

e) Reduced lordosis on "flexion" of the hip.

f and g) Good range of knee movement (no problems with putting on shoes).

h) Comfortable sitting possible

a b c

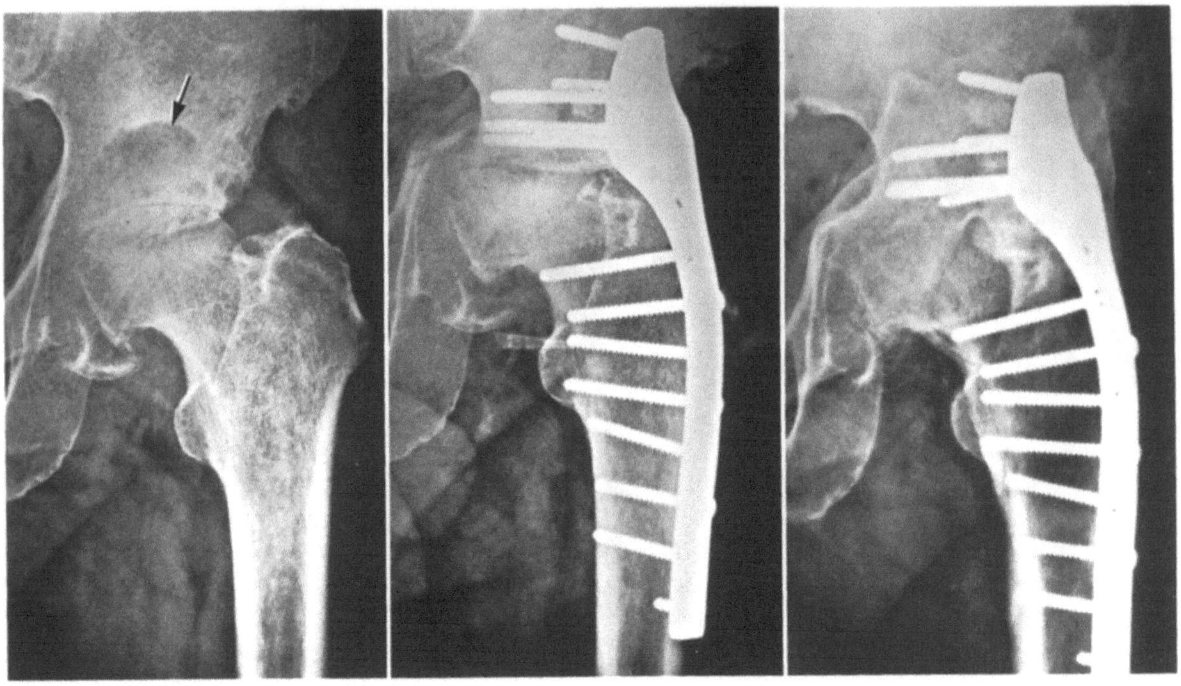

Fig. 135. *Type IV HA with PO in a case of hip arthrosis*. M. G., ♂, aged 62 years, No. 107200.

a) Flattening of the head, severe narrowing of the joint space, large cyst in the acetabular roof.

b) Cobra-head plate arthrodesis. The large cyst in the acetabular roof has been filled with cancellous bone taken from the inner surface of the ala iliaca.

c) Follow-up $4^1/_2$ years after the operation. Ideal union. Patient working full time as buyer

a b c

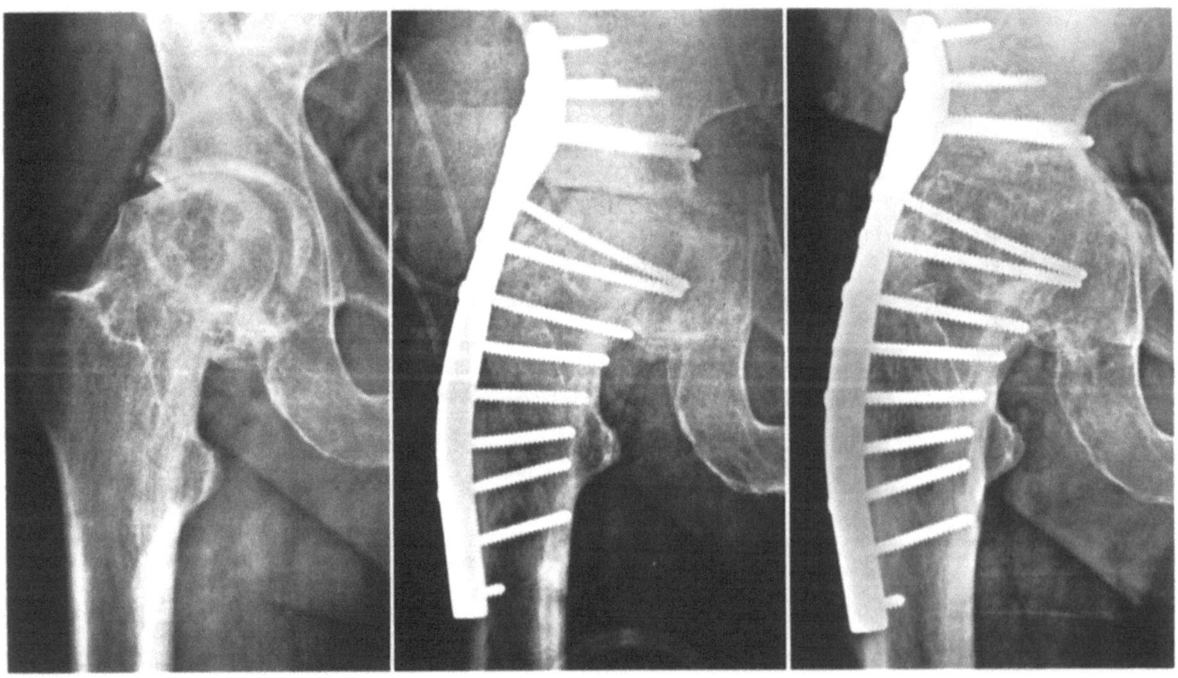

a b c

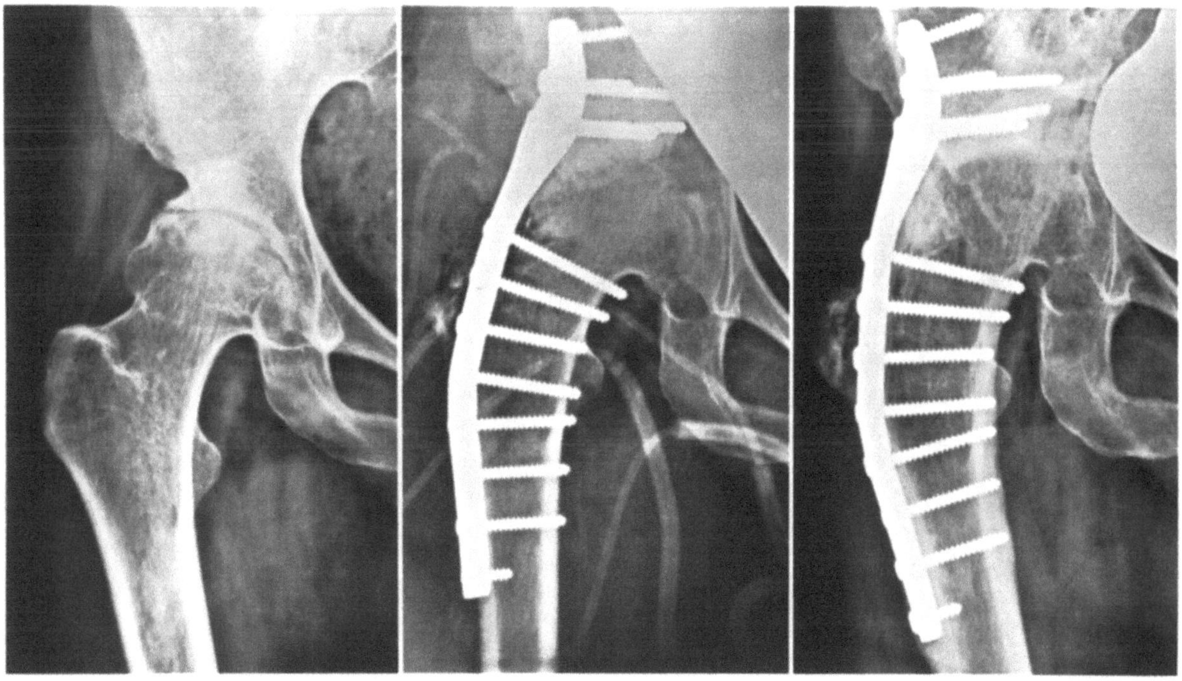

Fig. 137. *Type IV HA with PO in a case of secondary hip arthrosis.* S. R., ♀, aged 36 years, No. 81621.

a) Severe secondary arthrosis of the hip with ankylosis (bilateral hip infection when aged 12 years; pus was aspirated from left side).

b) Cobra-head plate arthrodesis following PO with moderate medial displacement.

c) Four and a half years following HA. Hip arthrodesed with 12° adduction deformity. With 2.5 cm leg shortening. Excellent subjective result. Complaint-free and working full time as housewife

Fig. 136. *Type IV HA with PO in a case of hip arthrosis.* S. W., ♂, aged 42 years, No. 115426.

a) Before operation.

b) Cobra-head plate arthrodesis with PO and moderate medial displacement.

c) Four years after HA. Hip united in ideal position. Change of job (from foundryman to office worker) because of painful arthrosis on the left side. No disability

a b c

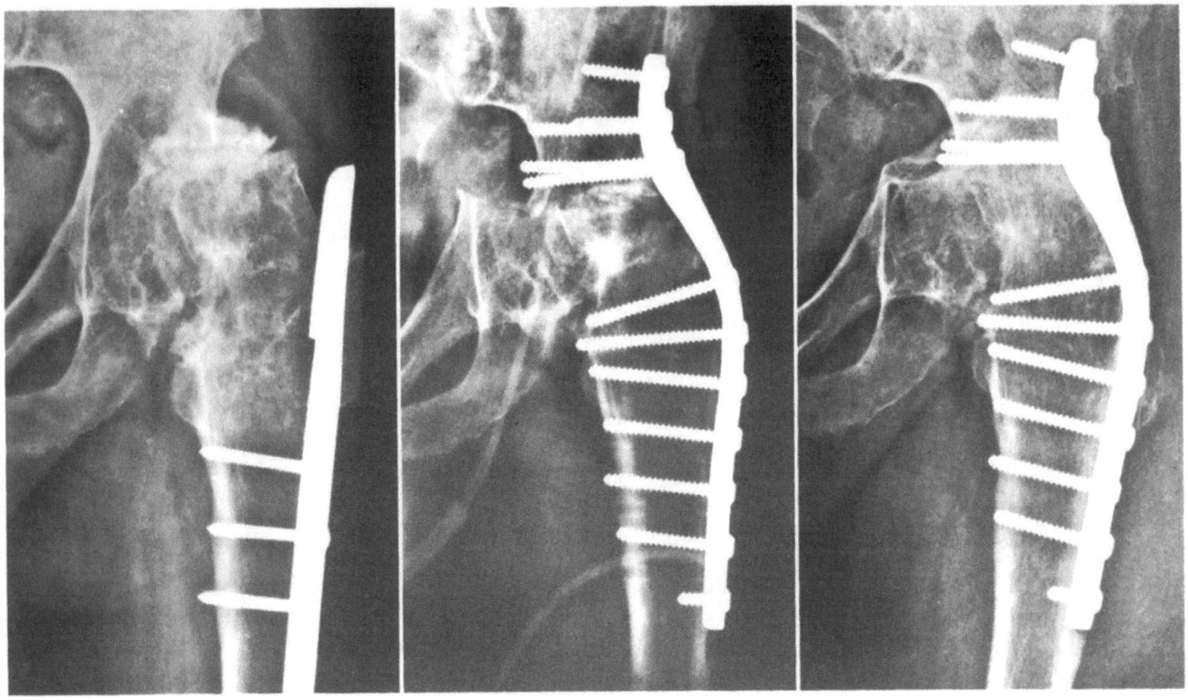

Fig. 138. *Type IV HA with PO in a case of hip arthrosis.* K. H., ♀, aged 68 years, No. 133498.

a) Eleven years following IO. Very severe hip arthrosis with subluxation of the femoral head.

b) Cobra-head plate arthrodesis with PO and large medial displacement.

c) One year after HA. Hip united in ideal position. Symptom free with cane-free and almost limp-free gait. Works full time as housewife

a b c

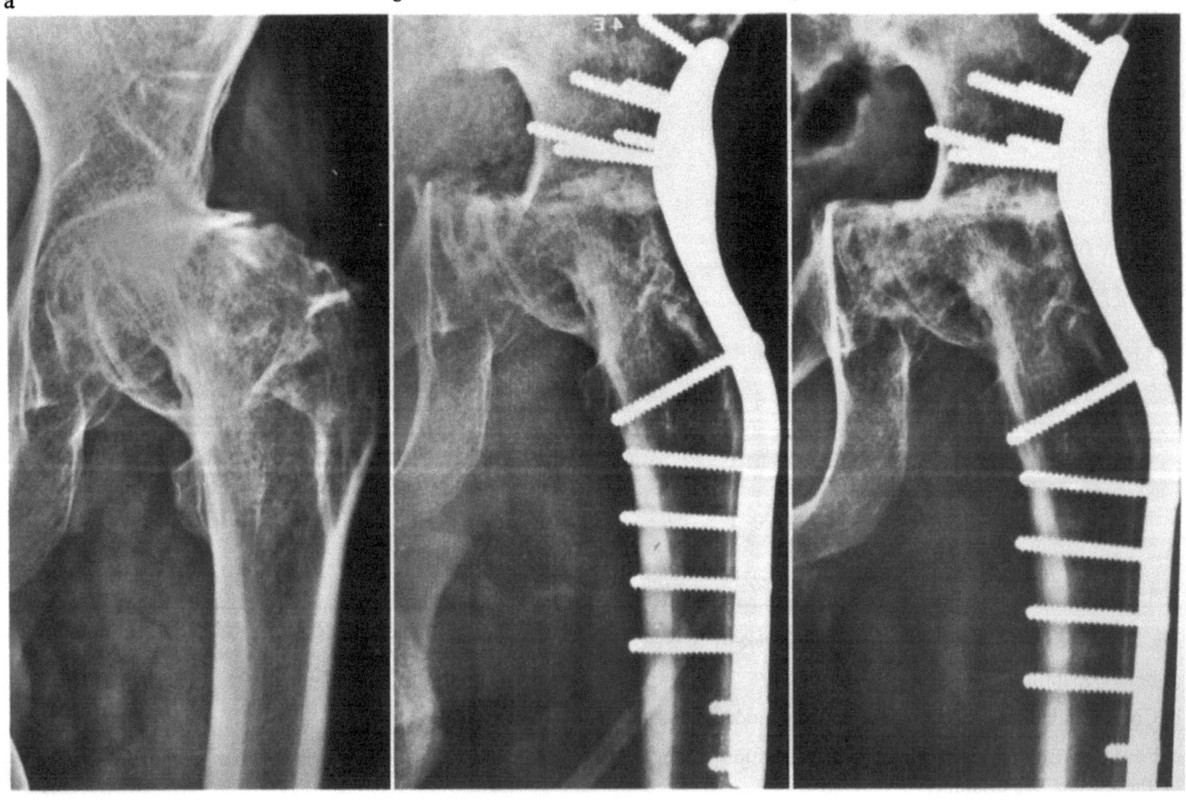

1.2 Rheumatoid Arthritis

1.2.1 Introduction

Involvement of the hip joint in rheumatoid arthritis is relatively rare (only 10% of cases according to VAINIO and PULKKI).

Monoarthritic rheumatoid arthritis may be incorrectly diagnosed as primary arthrosis of the hip unless a careful history is taken and backed up by the relevant laboratory tests. This error is sure to have occurred in our series during classification of the hip arthroses. Since it is frequently impossible to obtain the relevant data retrospectively from the case history or radiographs, we have combined the cases of rheumatoid arthritis and primary arthrosis of the hip for statistical purposes.

Radiographically rheumatoid arthritis of the hip is accompanied by more pronounced osteoporosis than arthrosis but, conversely, the former shows little or no osteophytic reaction. Also one frequently sees the tendency to central dislocation described by GSCHWEND, which should be regarded as preliminary to central dislocation. Narrowing of the joint space particularly occurs centrally.

Severe destruction of the hip joint is being observed with increasing frequency and is associated with long term corticosteroid therapy (EDSTRÖM). The spectrum of changes ranges from central dislocation to subluxation.

The indication for HA in the treatment of rheumatoid arthritis may still be justified alongside the other procedures such as early synovectomy, IO, release of the hip adductors, hip flexors and hip abductors (the Voss operation), resection of the proximal femur (Girdlestone) with or without subtrochanteric osteotomy (MILCH-BATCHELOR), and TP. Total prosthesis is the procedure of choice for advanced rheumatoid destruction of the hip joint since it brings about both abolition of pain and restoration of joint function. It is undoubtedly to be preferred to all other operative procedures in older patients or in younger patients with bilateral destruction of the hip joint or involvement of the knee joints.

For the latter reasons, HA is indicated with decreasing frequency in the rheumatoid hip. It may still be indicated in young patients with severe monoarticular arthritis of the hip. The chief advantages of HA lie in the freedom from pain, the complete rigidity and the capacity for weight bearing. Furthermore, canes may be dispensed with after approximately 8 weeks which is particularly important if there is simultaneous involvement of the joints of the upper extremities.

At this point, a condition should be mentioned which did not occur in our series, namely that described by GSCHWEND as "adult van Neck disease." This little-known complication of HA consists of fatigue fracture at the junction of the ischial and pubic bones in the region of the obliterated ischiopubic synchondrosis. It is probably brought about by abnormal loading of the bones anterior to the obturator foramen with concomitant osteoporosis resulting from long-term administration of corticosteroids.

In cases of rheumatoid arthritis we primarily perform cobra-head plate arthrodesis with or without PO in order to allow early mobilisation of the patient. The prerequisites are: disease confined to one hip; slowly evolving disease; an intact knee joint on the side which is to be arthrodesed.

1.2.2 Case Material

(Figs. 140 – 144).

←

Fig. 139. *Type IV HA with PO in a case of hip arthrosis secondary to slipped epiphysis.* B. C., ♂, aged 42 years, No. 159646.

a) Before operation.

b) Immediately following cobra-head plate arthrodesis. PO with particularly large degree of medial displacement.

c) Three months later. HA clinically and radiologically united. Patient has returned to full-time work as an executive

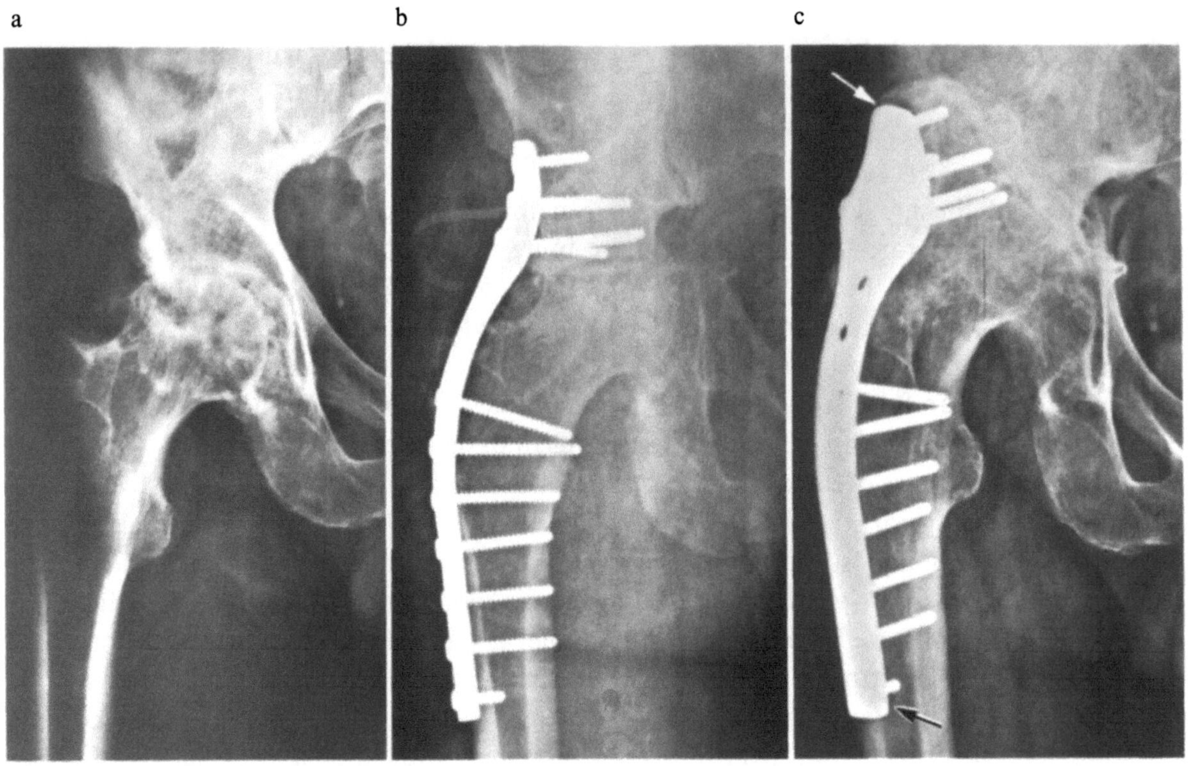

Fig. 140. *Type IV HA in a case of rheumatoid arthritis*. N. A., ♂, aged 56 years, No. 114556.

a) Severe destruction of the hip joint with severe reduction in range of motion (flexion/extension 70 – 30 – 0°).

b) Cobra-head plate arthrodesis with PO and moderate degree of medial displacement.

c) Four and a half years following HA. HA united with 13° adduction deformity. With 4 cm functional leg shortening (2.5 cm shoe correction). Patient works full time as a warehouse worker and is very satisfied with the result. Note the small area of translucency around the head of the cobra-head plate and at the end of the proximal screw. This is a sign of implant loosening which explains the clinically and radiologically observed increase in adduction

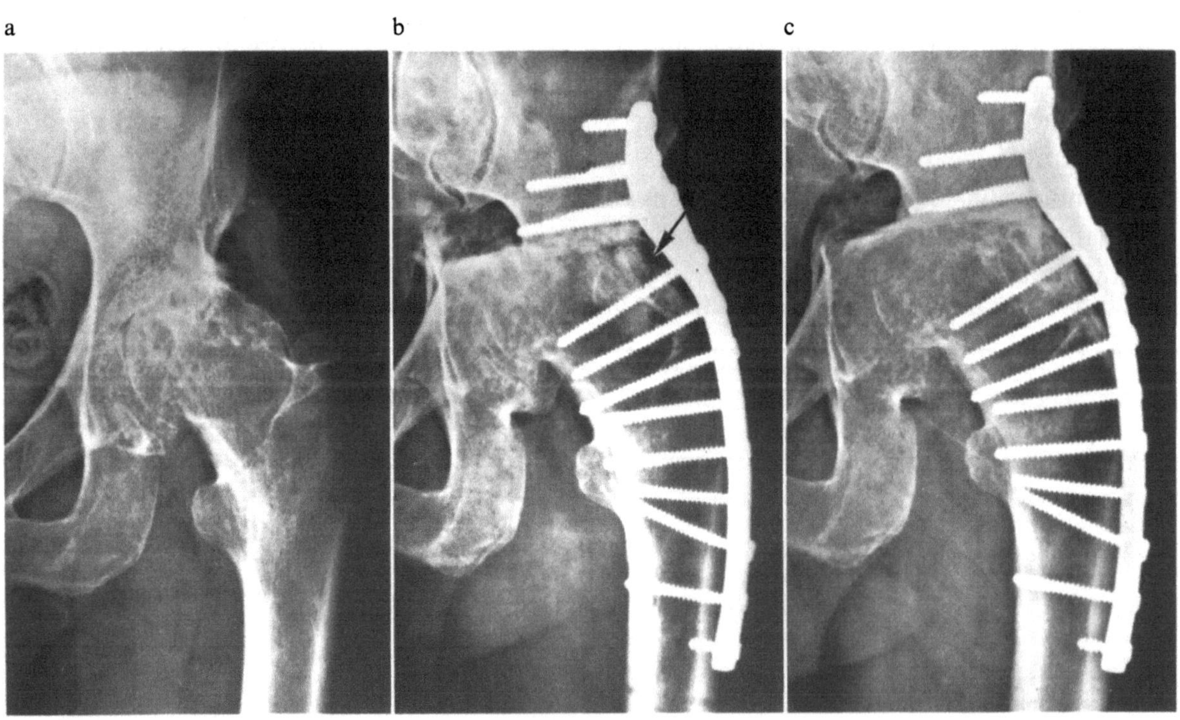

a b c

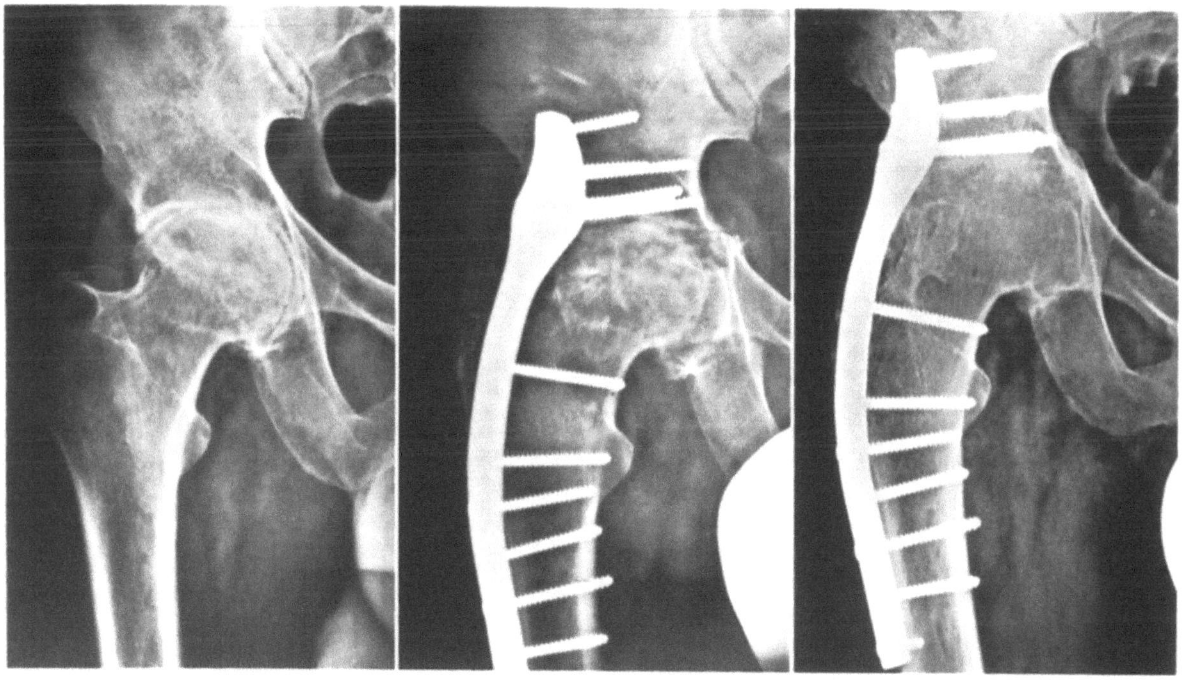

Fig. 142. *Type IV HA with PO in a case of arthrosis of the hip secondary to rheumatoid arthritis.* B. R., ♂, aged 31 years, No. 111670.

a) Arthrosis of the hip with narrowing of the joint space particularly in the centre.

b) Cobra head plate arthrodesis with PO and minimal degree of medial displacement.

c) Eleven months following HA. Hip united in ideal position with 1.5 cm functional leg shortening. Patient complaint-free; works full time as agent

←

Fig. 141. *Type IV HA in a case of rheumatoid arthritis.* L. F., ♂, aged 56 years, No. 119126.

a) Severe arthrotic changes. Joint space obliterated in the weight-bearing area with casts in the femoral head and loss of head sphericity. Small osteophyte in the lateral acetabulum.

b) Cobra-head plate arthrodesis with PO and large degree of medial displacement. The greater trochanter was clamped between the femoral neck and the plate (see arrow).

c) Result 22 months following HA. Left hip arthrodesed in good position with 1.5 cm functional leg shortening. Ideal subjective result. Patient works full time as woodworker

a b c

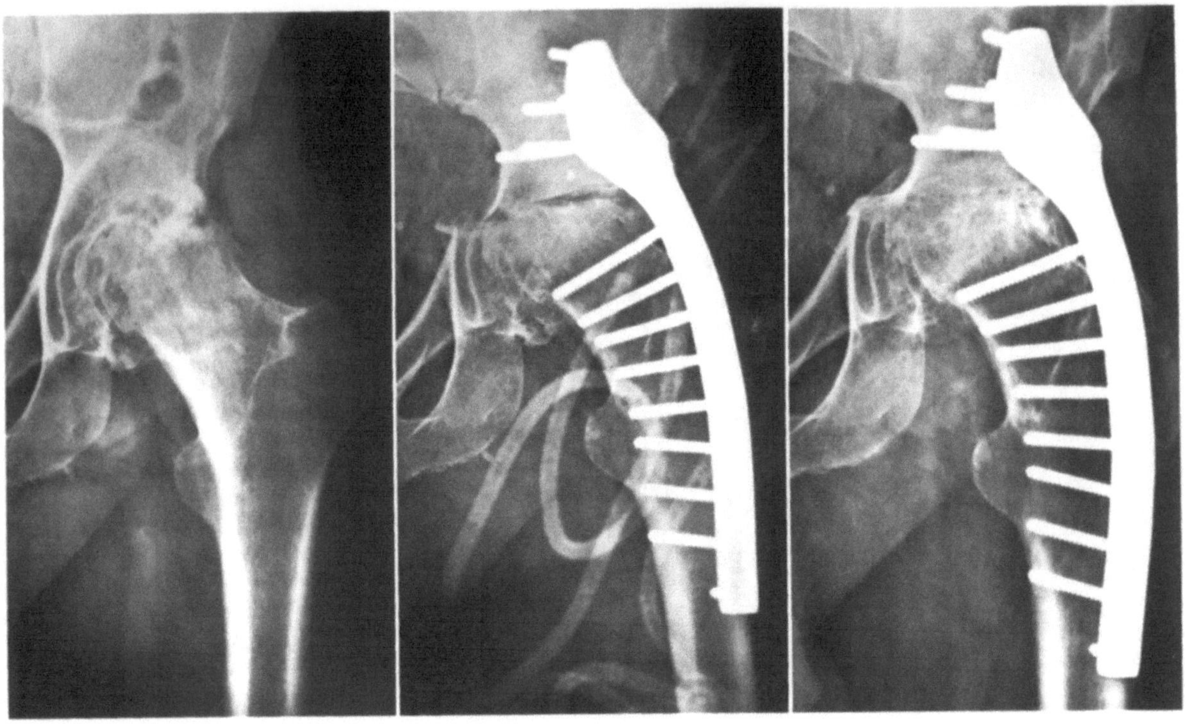

Fig. 143. *Type IV HA in a case of hip arthrosis with rheumatoid arthritis*. P. A., ♂, aged 53 years, No. 118980.

a) Severe destruction of the hip joint with large cysts in the femoral head and acetabular roof.

b) Cobra-head plate arthrodesis with PO and small degree of medial displacement.

c) Two years after HA. Bone union with somewhat increased external rotation (35°). Patient has returned to full-time work as a fisheries overseer

a b c

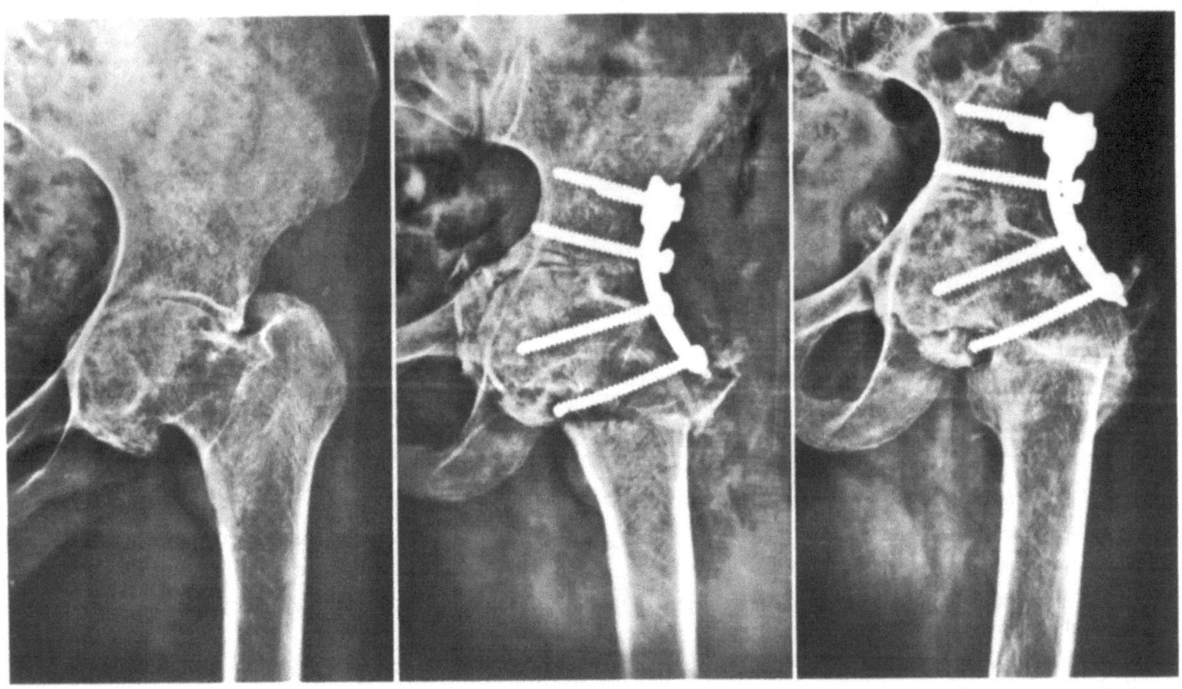

2 Hip Arthrodeses in Cases of Hip Dysplasia

2.1 Introduction

We have performed 81 HA operations in cases of hip dysplasia (19.9%). Only cases of high congenital dislocation of the hip and varus hip are discussed since these present particular problems for arthrodesis.

2.2 Hip Arthrodeses for High Congenital Dislocation of the Hip

HA may be indicated in cases of unilateral dislocation of the hip if:

a) The increase in leg length produced by HA results in a significant equalisation of leg length.
b) Arthrotic changes in the secondary joint are present.

2.2.1 Increasing Leg Length by Hip Arthrodesis

The joint surface of the dislocated hip is resected and the head is reduced into the original deepened acetabulum. Ten to fourteen days preoperative traction and subcutaneous tenotomy of the shortened adductor muscles simplify reduction. Following the latter, the femoral head is kept in place with a buttress plate.

Apart from increased hip stability the leg may be lengthened by 3 – 5 cm using this technique (Figs. 145, 146).

2.2.2 Hip Arthrodesis for Arthrosis of the Secondary Acetabulum

These arthroses always cause pain. The aim of the operation is not lengthening of the extremity but rather the creation of a painless hip which is capable of weight bearing. Arthrodesis is carried out at the level of the secondary joint. PO is always carried out. If technically possible, the HA is stabilised with a cobra-head plate (Fig. 147).

As regards the operative technique, we differentiate between cases in which angulation osteotomy has been performed and high dislocation with formation of a new joint.

a) Hip Arthrodesis Following Angulation Osteotomy

In cases where there is severe angulation following osteotomy of the proximal femur, thus making corrective osteotomy necessary, a short plate is used (Figs. 148, 149).

b) Hip Arthrodesis in the Presence of High Dislocation with Formation of a New Joint

In these cases, PO at the level of the new joint is technically no longer possible. In one such case we have resected the femoral head, performed PO at the original level of the acetabulum roof, wedged the proximal femur under the osteotomy and completed the operation with a subtrochanteric osteotomy. Internal fixation was rejected in favour of cast fixation because of extensive osteoporosis (Fig. 150).

Fig. 144. *Type II HA without PO in a case of hip arthrosis with rheumatoid arthritis and coxa vara.* F. M., ♀, aged 56 years, No. 92308.

a) Marked protrusio.

b) HA with small shoulder plate which has been bent to shape. Exceptionally, the use of the compression instrument was unnecessary as the femoral head was particularly well wedged into place.

c) Result 3 months following operation. Bone union. Patient complaint-free and working full time as housewife

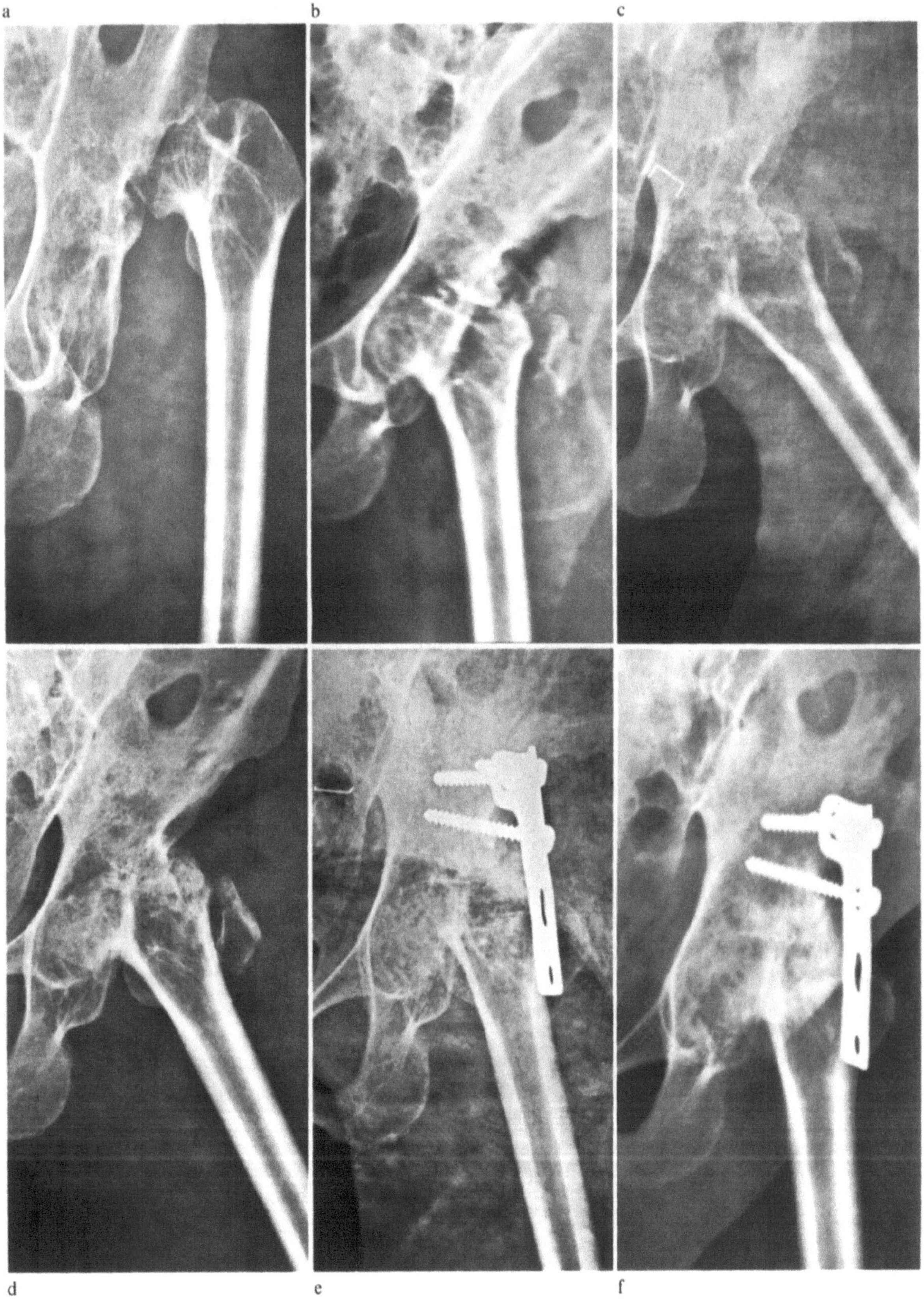
a
b
c
d
e
f

a b c

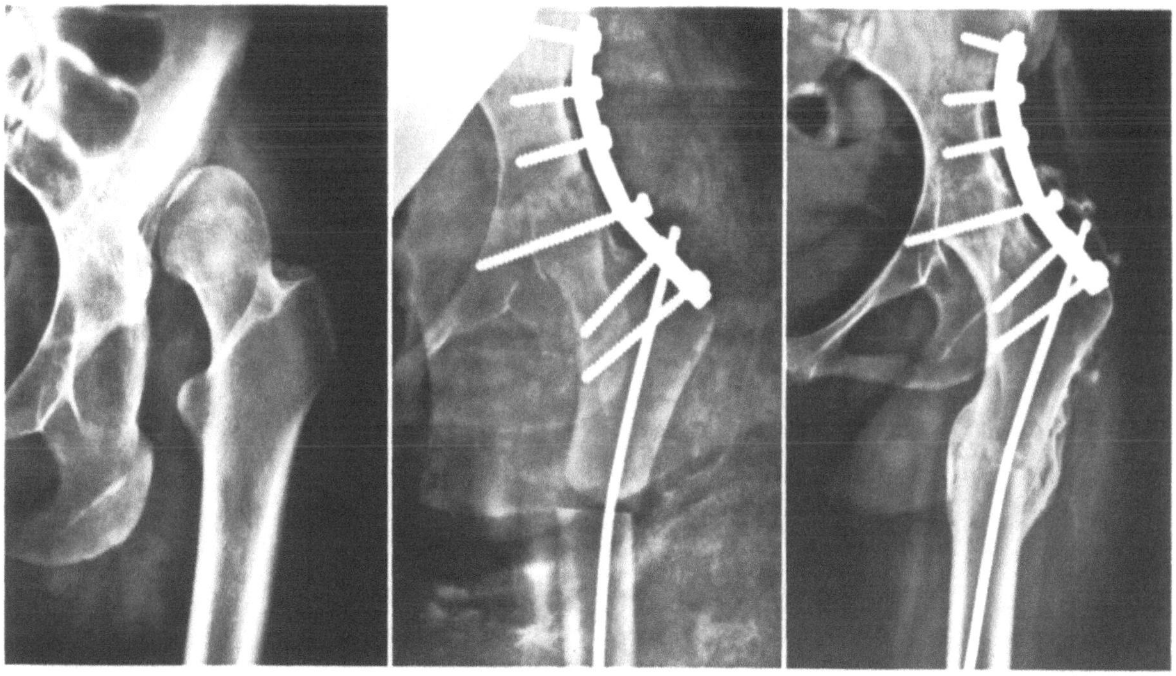

Fig. 146. *Type II HA in a case of late CDH with dysplastic femoral head.* S. D., ♀, aged 27 years, No. 150399.

a) High dysplastic femoral head. With 4 cm leg shortening.

b) Eleven days following HA. Leg in cast. An Oberholzer nail was used to stabilise the subtrochanteric osteotomy.

c) Four months later. HA and subtrochanteric osteotomy united with 1.5 cm leg shortening

Fig. 145. *Atypical HA in an old case of high dislocation on the left side.* S. N., ♀, aged 36 years, No. 97468.

a) High dislocation of a severely deformed femoral head. With 6.5 cm of shortening.

b) First stage of HA. Bringing the head into the true acetabulum.

c) Hip spica in abduction and slight internal rotation.

d) Five and a half weeks later. The HA is already clinically and radiologically united.

e) Second stage. The abduction is corrected by a femoral osteotomy 1 cm below the arthrodesis. A shoulder plate is used which has a pure buttress function and is therefore only fixed to the pelvis.

f) Five months following second stage. Perfect healing. Only 3 cm leg shortening remains (corrected with orthopaedic shoe)

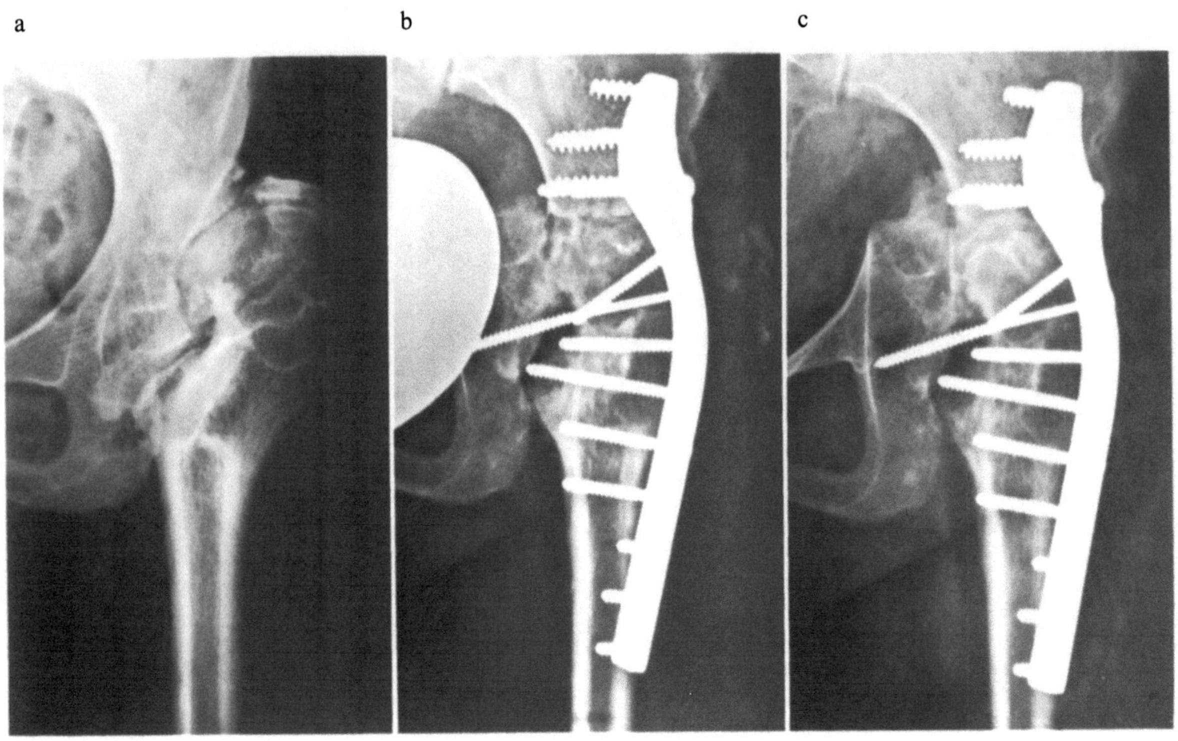

Fig. 147. *Type IV HA in a case of late CDH.* U. N., ♀, aged 50 years, No. 139701.

a) Sixteen years following Schanz osteotomy. Arthrosis in the secondary acetabulum.

b) Six weeks following Type IV HA with PO and large medial displacement.

c) Eight months later. HA united in good position. With 3 cm leg shortening (corrected with orthopaedic shoe)

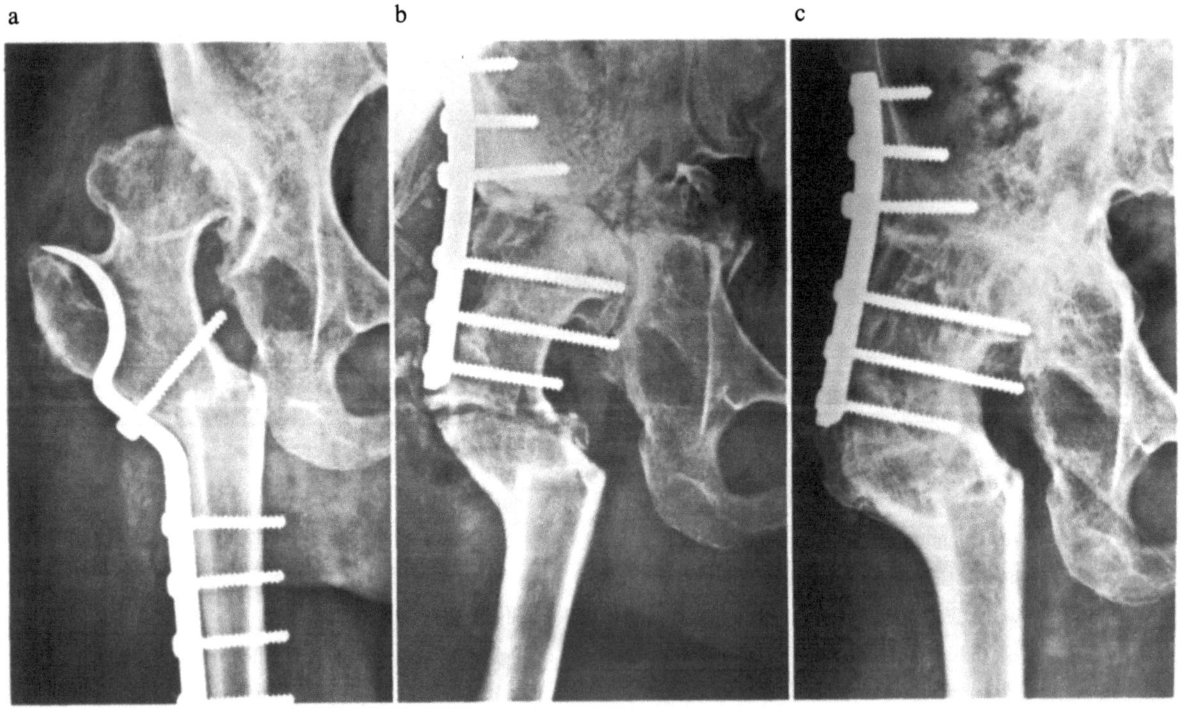

a b c

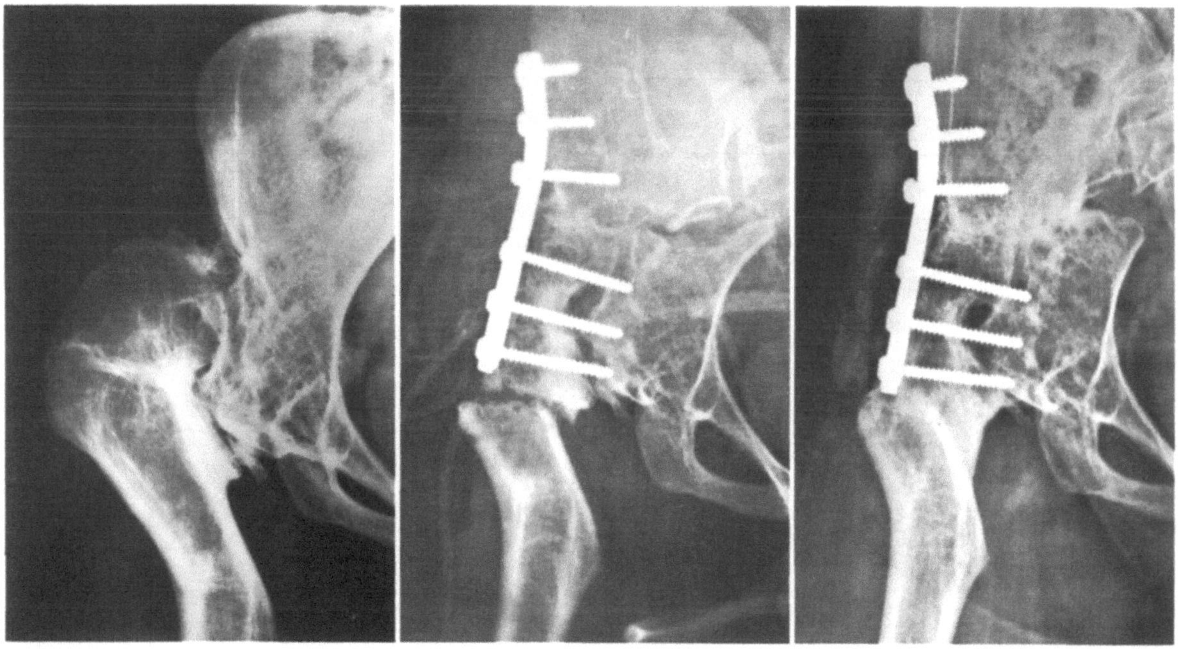

Fig. 149. *Type II HA following angulation osteotomy*. D. F., ♀, aged 42 years, No. 47972.

a) Following Schanz osteotomy for CDH.

b) Type II HA with PO and large medial displacement. Osteotomy has been performed 1 cm distal to the plate to correct the marked angulation of the proximal femur.

c) Two years later. HA and osteotomy united. Trouble-free gait without cane. With 2 cm residual leg shortening; 1 year previously a 7 cm difference in leg length had been corrected by a shortening IO (5 cm)

Fig. 148. *Type II HA following angulation osteotomy in a case of late CDH*. D. M., ♀, aged 58 years, No. 64463.

a) One year following Schanz osteotomy.

b) Type I HA with PO.

c) Seven years later. Trouble-free gait without pain. With 4 cm leg shortening corrected by raising heel. HA united in ideal position.

a b c

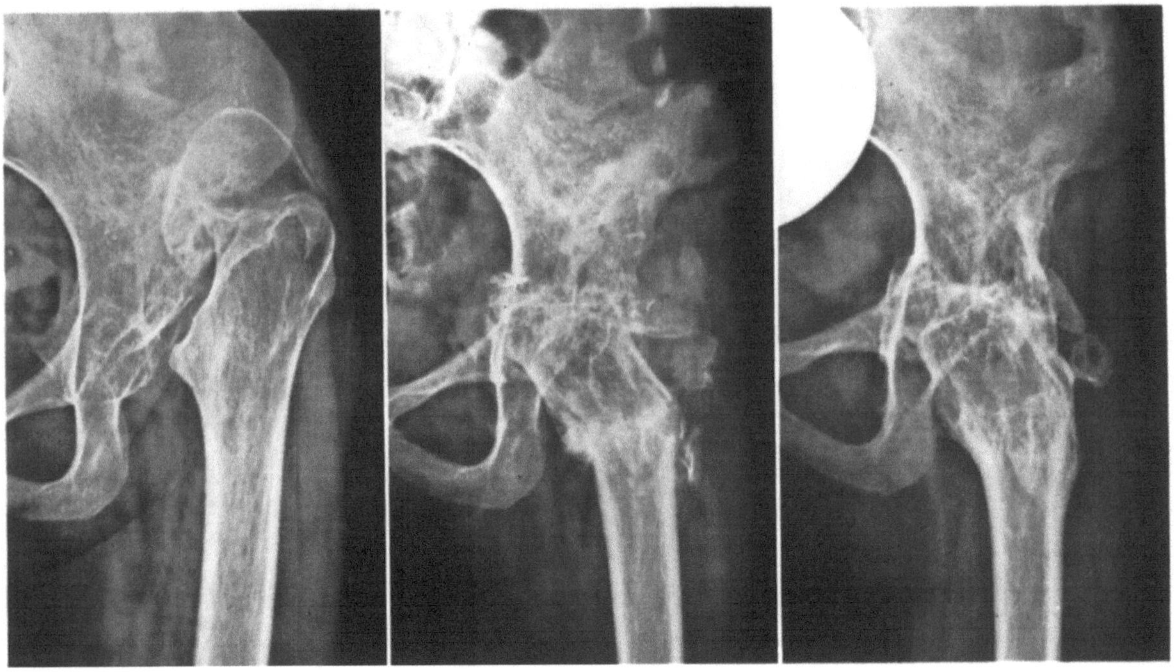

Fig. 150. *HA in a case with high secondary acetabulum.* H. H., ♀, aged 34 years, No. 85741.

a) CDH with hip arthrosis. With 5 cm leg shortening.

b) Eleven weeks following HA. The femoral head has been returned to the true acetabulum. Then HA with leg in 130° abduction. Six weeks later adjustment of leg position by IO. HA and IO union almost complete.

c) Twenty months following HA. Complete union with 7° abduction. With 1 cm leg shortening. Trouble-free gait without cane

a b c

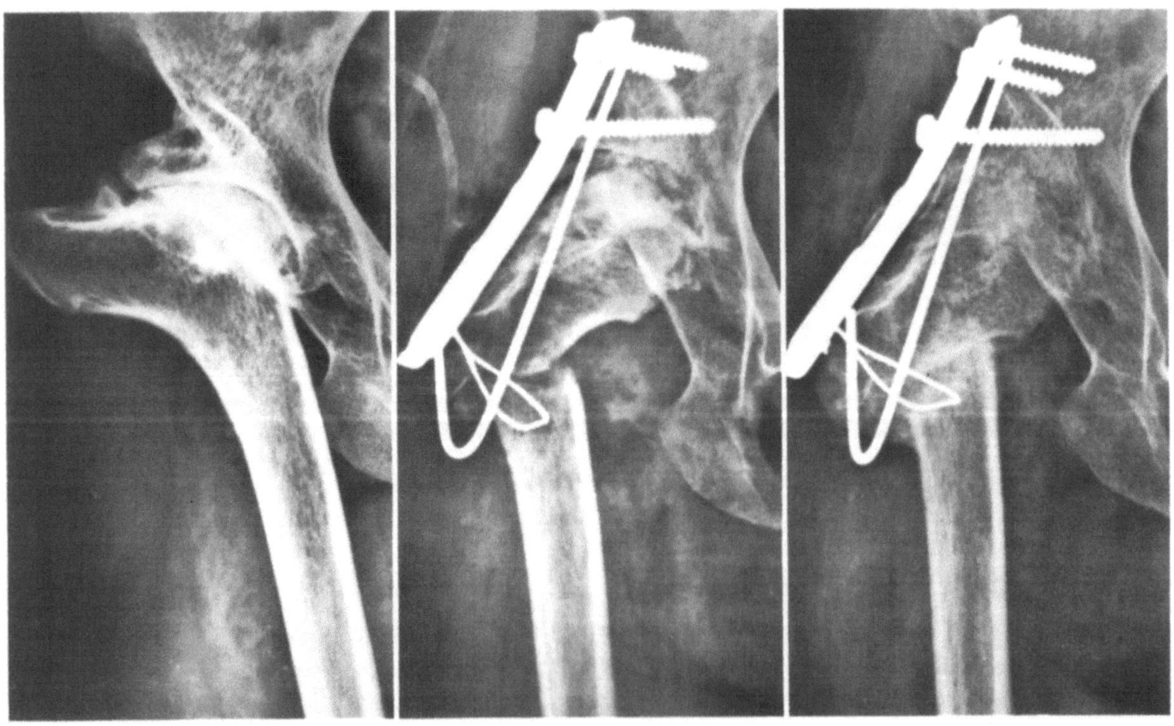

2.3 Hip Arthrodeses for Varus Hip

In varus hip the high trochanter has to be osteotomised.

This is followed by the usual arthrodesis with a cobra-head plate or with a short plate and additional IO (Figs. 151 – 153).

3 Hip Arthrodesis for Posttraumatic Hip Disease

3.1 Introduction

The majority of HA operations in this group are performed for femoral neck fracture. Partial or total necrosis of the head of the femur following nailing of a femoral neck fracture occurs in 35% – 40% of cases (SCHÖRNER 37%, BÖHLER 34%).

Acetabular fractures and hip dislocations are, however, becoming more frequent as a result of high-energy highway accidents (Table 31).

Table 31. Post-traumatic cases

Femoral neck fracture (and necrosis of the femoral head)	38
Pelvic and acetabular fracture	28
Dislocation of the hip	7
Total	73 (12.5%)

Nowadays, the majority of the fracture dislocations of the pelvis are operated on. Perfect reduction is an essential prerequisite to good function. Often, during the operation the femoral head is found to be more extensively damaged than had been expected from the radiograph. Operative reconstruction is usually difficult since the high-speed fractures are frequently impacted or multifragmented. Although in such cases the functional results are not always satisfactory the situation is improved for a subsequent HA.

Fig. 151. *Type II HA in a case of varus hip*. K. G., ♀, aged 39 years, No. 104203.

a) Before operation.

b) At operation. Type II HA. Buttress plate and K-wire fixation of the proximal femoral component which has been brought into a vertical position, thus increasing leg length.

c) Five months later. HA and subtrochanteric osteotomies united

3.2 Subsequent to Fractures of the Femoral Head

Only in a few cases where a small distal head fragment has broken off can a partial necrosis of the head be prevented by internal fixation. If the fragment is in the weight-bearing area, the prognosis is hopeless.

If such a situation occurs in a young patient, early HA is indicated. The technique described on p. 75 is recommended in order to bring about valgus correction of the proximal femur (Figs. 154, 155).

3.3 Posttraumatic Necrosis of the Femoral Head

This does not only occur following fracture of the femoral neck but also subsequent to dislocation of the hip or pelvic fracture with impaction of the femoral head (frequently without a radiologically visible lesion). The frequency of NHF following union of an undislocated femoral neck fracture lies between 10% – 20% in the majority of statistics and over 30% in dislocated fractures (BÖHLER 34%, BOYD 33%, CLAFFEY 19%, CLEVELAND 17%, FIELDING 43%, FLATMARK 44%, MERLE D'AUBIGNÉ 50%, MITTAG 25%, RUSSE 35%, SALEM 20%, SCHÖRNER 37%). Dislocation of the hip is accompanied by tearing of the capsular vessels and of the vessels in the round ligament and this leads to ischemic necrosis. The femoral neck fractures cause necrosis by interruption of the

a b c

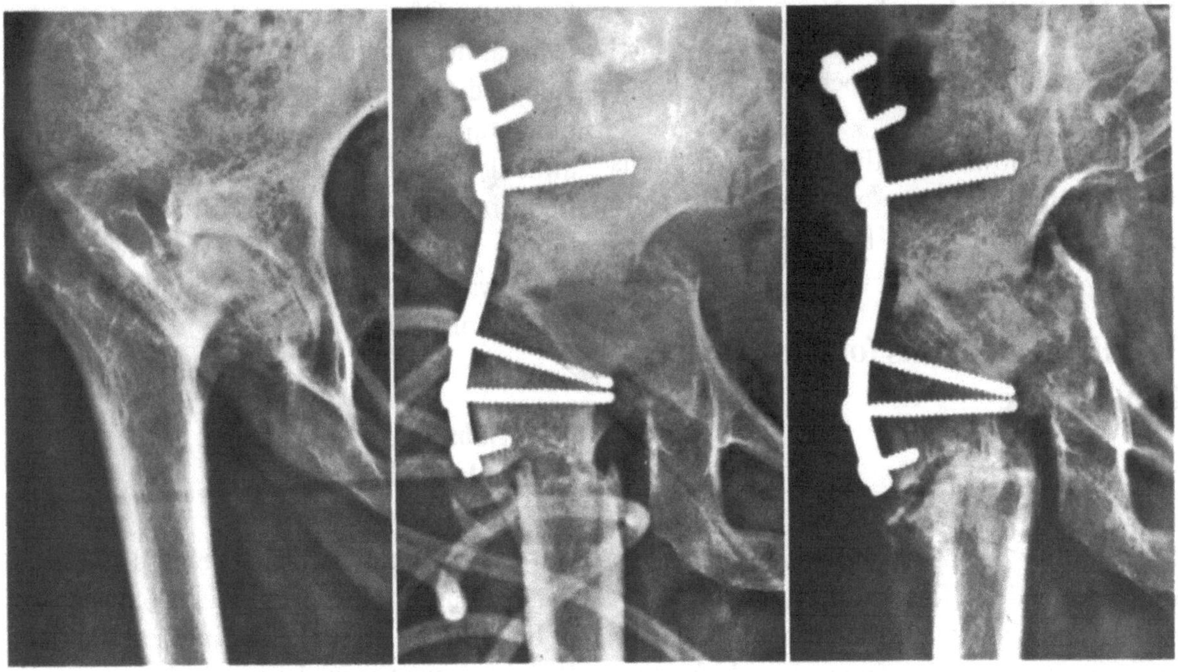

Fig. 152. *Type II HA in a case of varus hip*. P. R., ♀, aged 47 years, No. 106809.

a) Varus hip with secondary arthrosis (accident at age 7 months with injury to right hip) with 5 cm leg shortening.

b) Increase in leg length by sliding the transected trochanter laterally under the proximal pelvic component. Type II HA.

c) Three months later following cast removal. HA and osteotomy largely united. HA clinically united in good position. Only 1 cm leg shortening remains

a b c

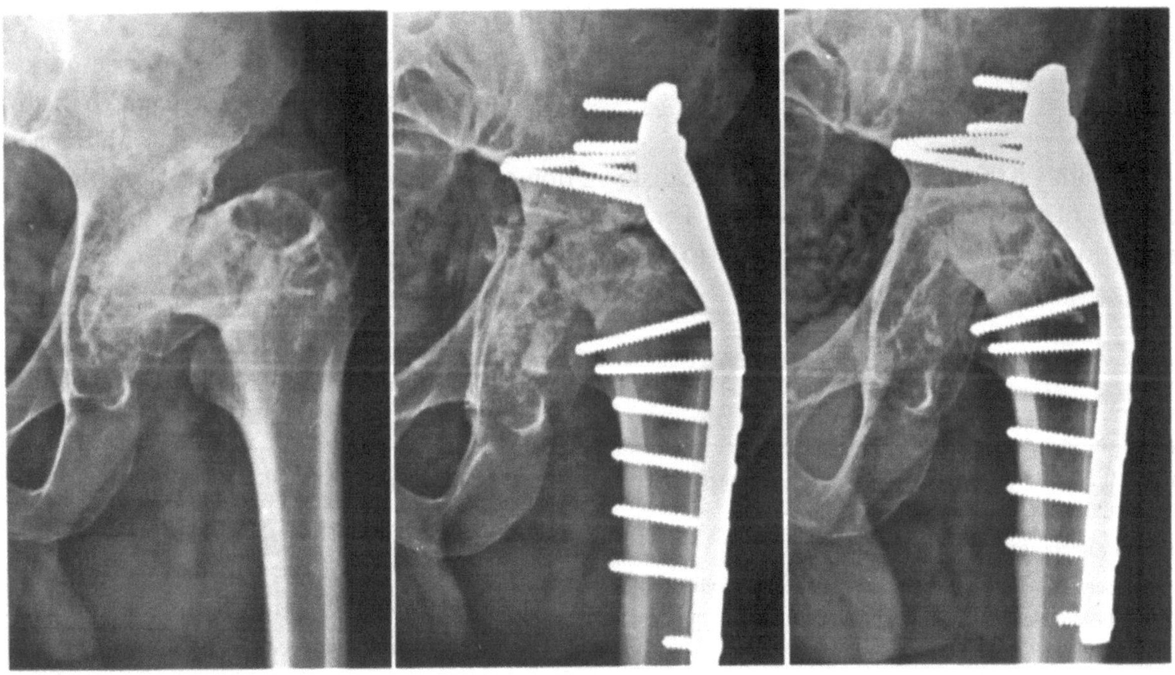

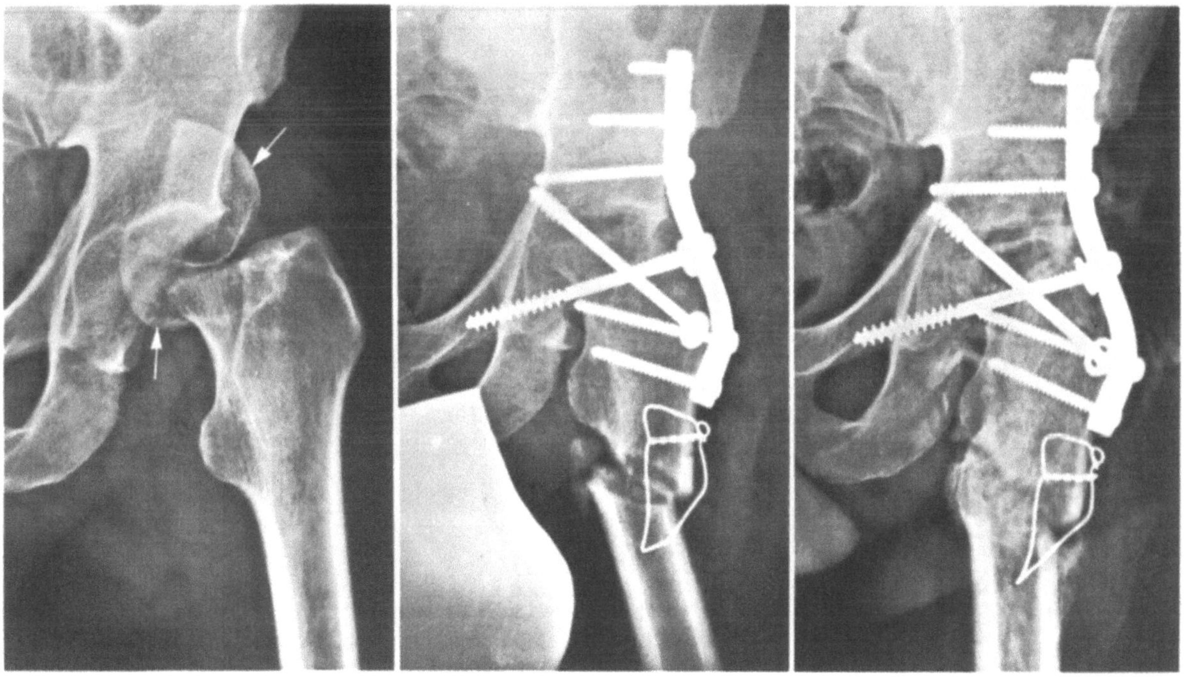

Fig. 154. *Primary arthrodesis of the hip following dislocation with fracture of the femoral head in two fragments*. Z. H., ♂, aged 41 years, No. 151 715.

a) Four days following accident. The two fragments which have broken off the femoral head are clearly visible

b) One month following primary HA. The abduction deformity was corrected by applying a new hip spica.

c) Four months after operation. The HA and the subtrochanteric osteotomy are uniting. Patient still requires crutches; 50% weight bearing with no subjective problems

Fig. 153. *Type IV HA in a case of advanced arthrosis of the hip secondary to Perthes disease*. R. J., ♂, aged 52 years, No. 145 725.

a) Severe hip arthrosis secondary to Perthes disease with 2 cm leg shortening.

b) Fourteen days following cobra-head plate arthrodesis with PO and small medial displacement of the distal pelvic component.

c) Twenty months after HA. Full bone union with leg in ideal position with 1 cm leg shortening. No complaints. Patient works full time as farmer

a c d

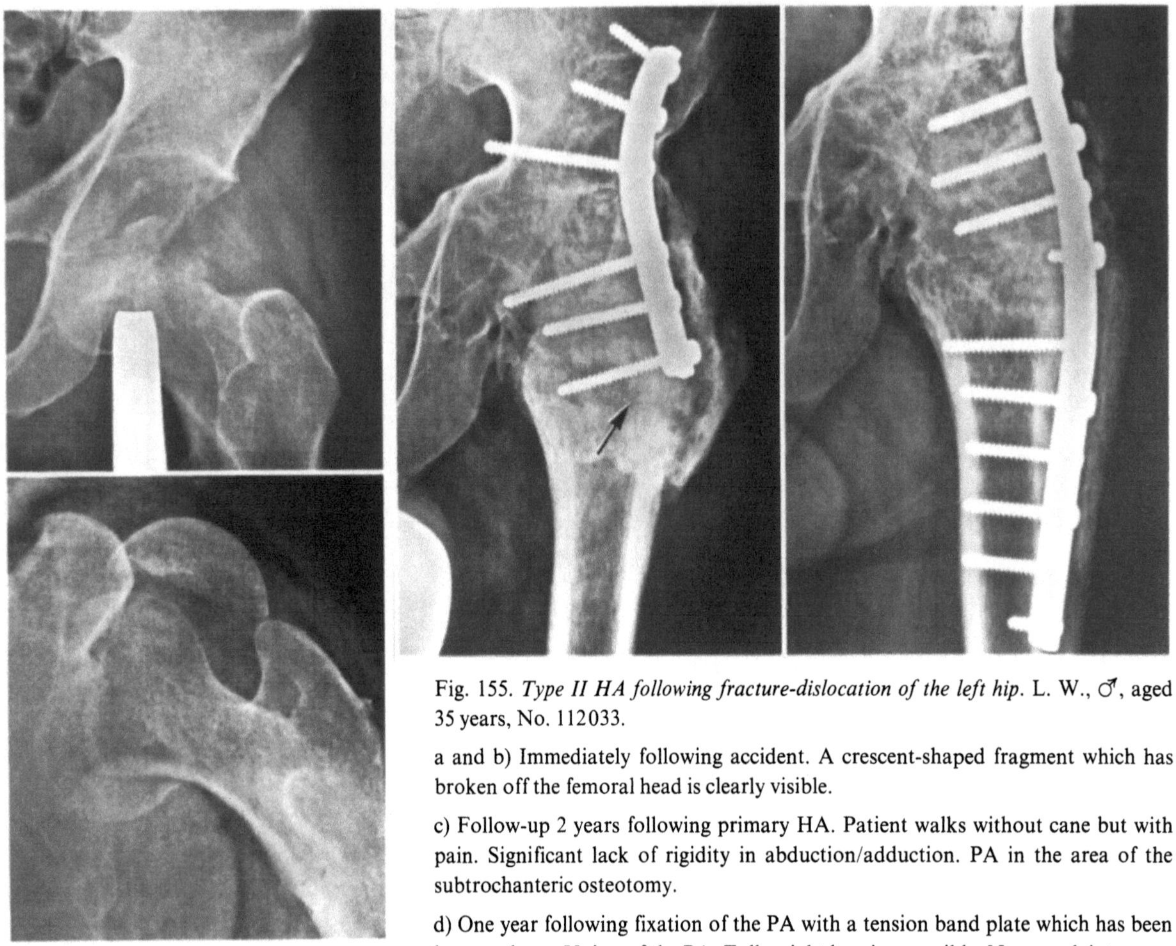

b

Fig. 155. *Type II HA following fracture-dislocation of the left hip.* L. W., ♂, aged 35 years, No. 112033.

a and b) Immediately following accident. A crescent-shaped fragment which has broken off the femoral head is clearly visible.

c) Follow-up 2 years following primary HA. Patient walks without cane but with pain. Significant lack of rigidity in abduction/adduction. PA in the area of the subtrochanteric osteotomy.

d) One year following fixation of the PA with a tension band plate which has been bent to shape. Union of the PA. Full weight bearing possible. No complaints

a b c

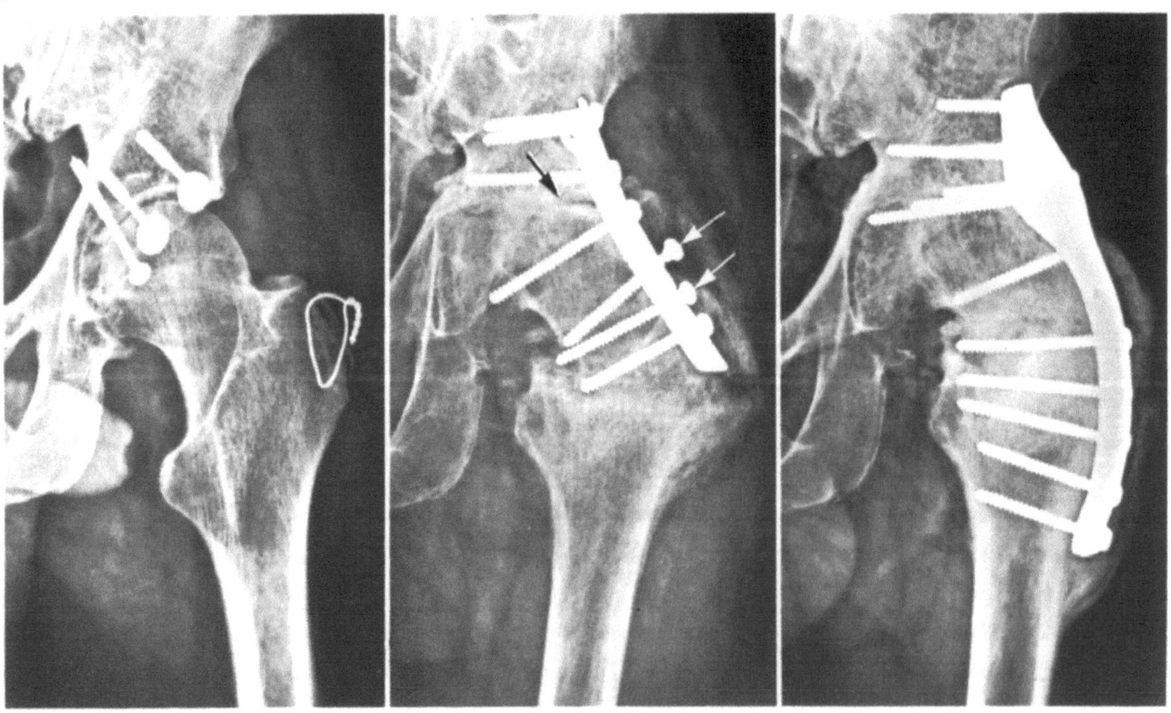

intramedullary blood supply. The frequency of necrosis following traumatic dislocation is directly proportional to the energy of trauma and the time interval between trauma and reduction. According to the nature of the force, the vessels are partially or completely destroyed, thus explaining the localisation of the necroses (necrosis of the lateral part of the weight-bearing area of the head; necrosis of the whole head).

In fracture of the femoral neck, the femoral head is still supplied with blood from the vesels in the ligament of the head and also to a certain extent by the capsular vessels. If the fracture is not impacted and is not reduced, radiologically visible necrosis is usually present at 6 – 8 weeks. By impaction of the fracture and rigid internal fixation, the vessels are given a better chance of growing in from the distal side of the fracture and revitalising the head.

In post-traumatic NHF, HA is indicated in young patients and prosthetic replacement in older patients. It has been stated that union is difficult to bring about in the presence of NHF (PHEMISTER, HOFMEISTER, GILL, NIGST). Our results do not confirm this. Following HA with rigid internal fixation the frequency of PA and fibrous ankylosis was the same in the patients with post-traumatic arthrosis and NHF as in the primary hip arthrosis group.

Fig. 156. *Type II HA in a case of post-traumatic arthrosis of the hip*. R. J., ♂, aged 51 years, No. 80154.

a) Fracture dislocation of the left hip. Reduction and fixation of the acetabular fragments with malleolar screws. Cerclage fixation of the gluteal muscles to the greater trochanter.

b) HA 2 years following internal fixation of the acetabular roof because of painful post-traumatic arthrosis. Nine months following HA there is loosening of the metal, particularly of the distal screws. There is PA of the PO and union of the IO.

c) Result 29 months after rearthrodesis with a cobra-head plate. The PA has united

The case material can be found in the chapter "HA in idiopathic and posttraumatic necrosis of the femoral head."

3.4 Dislocation of the Hip with or without Fracture of the Acetabular Roof

Reduction is urgently required following traumatic dislocation of the hip. If the acetabular margin is broken off it is reduced and fixed with screws at the same time. Head necrosis results, despite adequate treatment, in approximately 20% of cases according to STEWART and MITFORD.

Where dislocation has occurred, stretching of the circumflex vessels may lead to gradual restriction of the blood supply and this is followed by stasis and thrombosis (WEIL). This process may be reversible and this, in turn, may be the reason why NHF occurs more frequently following dislocations which were not immediately reduced. MERLE D'AUBIGNÉ has estimated the frequency of head necrosis as follows:

If a simple dislocation of the hip is reduced within 24 h necrosis does not occur; reduction later than 24 h results in 66% necroses. Reduction within 24 h of a dislocation which is accompanied by fracture of the acetabular roof is associated with a necrosis rate of 30%; the latter rises to 100% if reduction is carried out more than 24 h later. If simple post-traumatic dislocation of the hip results in NHF, the guide lines given for idiopathic NHF (Fig. 156) apply.

If the posterior fracture of the acetabular margin is not treated operatively, instability of the hip results with posterior subluxation. In such cases arthrodesis of the hip is performed at a later date (Figs. 157 – 160).

3.5 Pelvic Fractures with Central Dislocation of the Hip

These complex fractures pass transversely through the acetabulum and pelvis and fre-

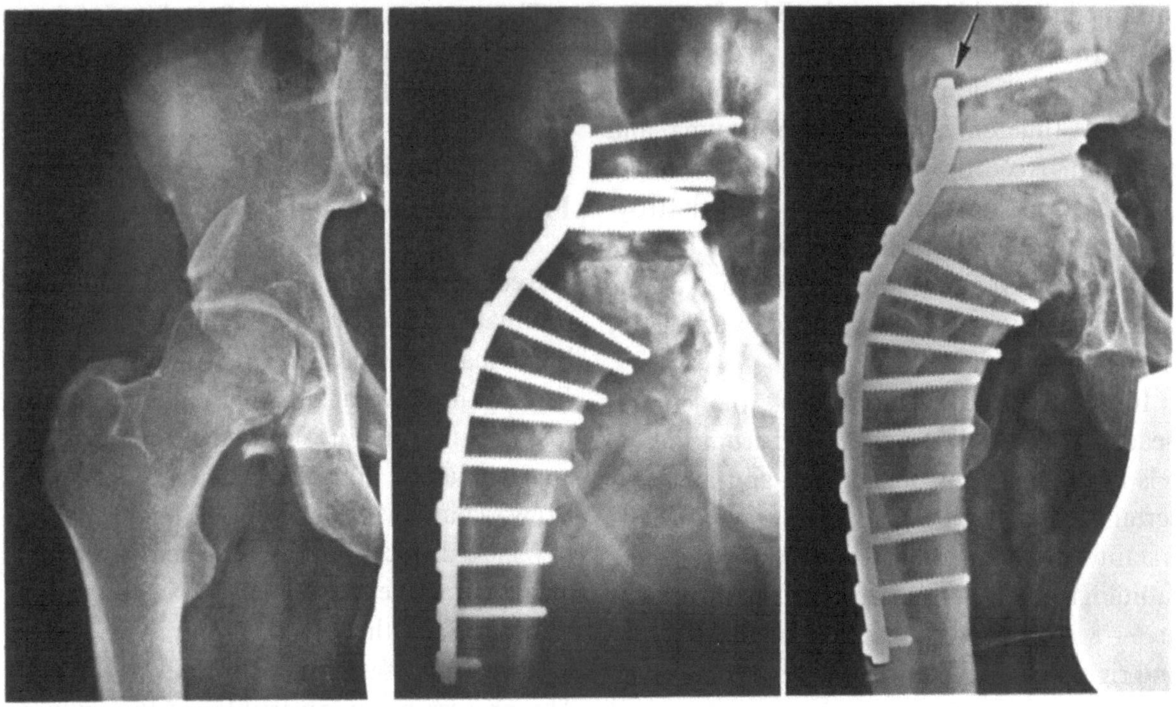

Fig. 157. *Type IV HA in a case of fracture dislocation of the hip.* S. G., ♂, aged 25 years, No. 140625.

a) This posterior fracture of the acetabular roof with dislocation of the impressed head was first diagnosed 1 month after the accident.

b) Cobra-head plate arthrodesis with PO.

c) Eighteen months later. Medial osteotomy gap still visible with union on the lateral side. Small area of radiotranslucency around the head of the plate, probably as a result of loosening of the proximal screw. All other screws tight. HA clinically united in ideal leg position. Patient complaint-free and has returned to full-time work

quently result in post-traumatic NHF as a result of contusion of the femoral head. *Restoration of the original anatomy should always be attempted if possible* since one loses nothing by it. Even if the functional result is bad, the situation has been improved for a subsequent HA.

In our series, the head necrosis referred to had always occurred. Due regard must be paid to the special features of these cases in choosing the HA technique, as is shown in the cases illustrated. Here too, the cobra-head plate offers optimum rigidity.

3.5.1 Case Material

(Figs. 161 – 166)

3.6 Summary

Immediate HA is only seldom indicated in cases of hip trauma (fractures of the femoral head in the weight-bearing area). On the other hand, later HA may be indicated in post-traumatic necrosis of the femoral head or if hip function is poor. Restoration of the original anatomy by immediate internal fixation of comminuted or impacted fractures allows later HA without technical difficulties.

a b

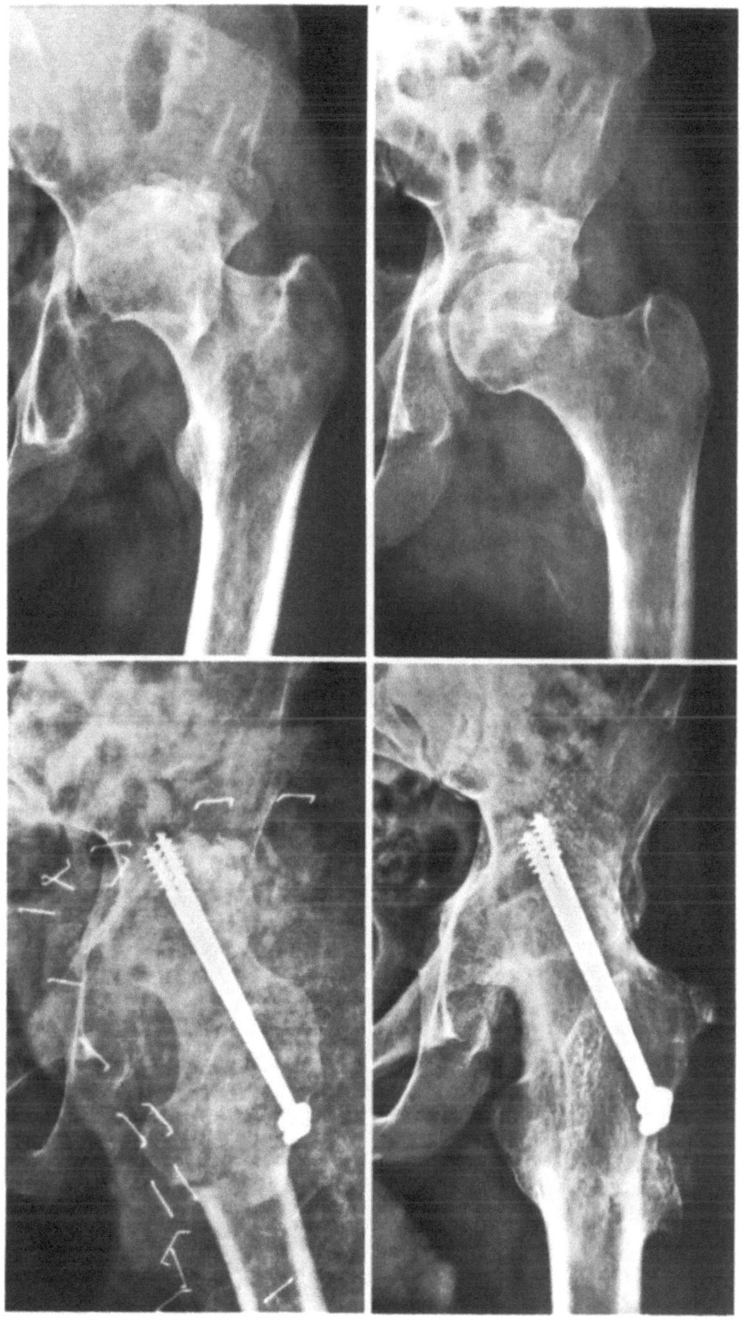

c d

Fig. 158. *Type I HA in a case of post-traumatic arthrosis of the hip*. A. H., ♂, aged 31 years. No. 125141.

a) One year after accident. The fracture dislocation of the hip in this multiple-injured patient was not diagnosed.

b) Ten days before the intended HA 15 kg supracondylar traction was applied with a Steinmann pin in order to facilitate reduction of the head during the operation. The head of the femur now seems to be at the level of the true acetabulum.

c) HA by double axial screw fixation using cancellous bone screws driven in from the direction of the innominate tubercle. The head of the femur was in a secondary acetabulum approximately 6 cm above and behind the true acetabulum. A third of the femoral head was resected. The femoral head was then reduced with marked adduction of the leg. A suitable iliac site for plate fixation could not be found and double-screw fixation was therefore carried out. Subtrochanteric osteotomy to correct the adduction deformity

d) Thirty months following operation. HA united with good leg position. Painless gait

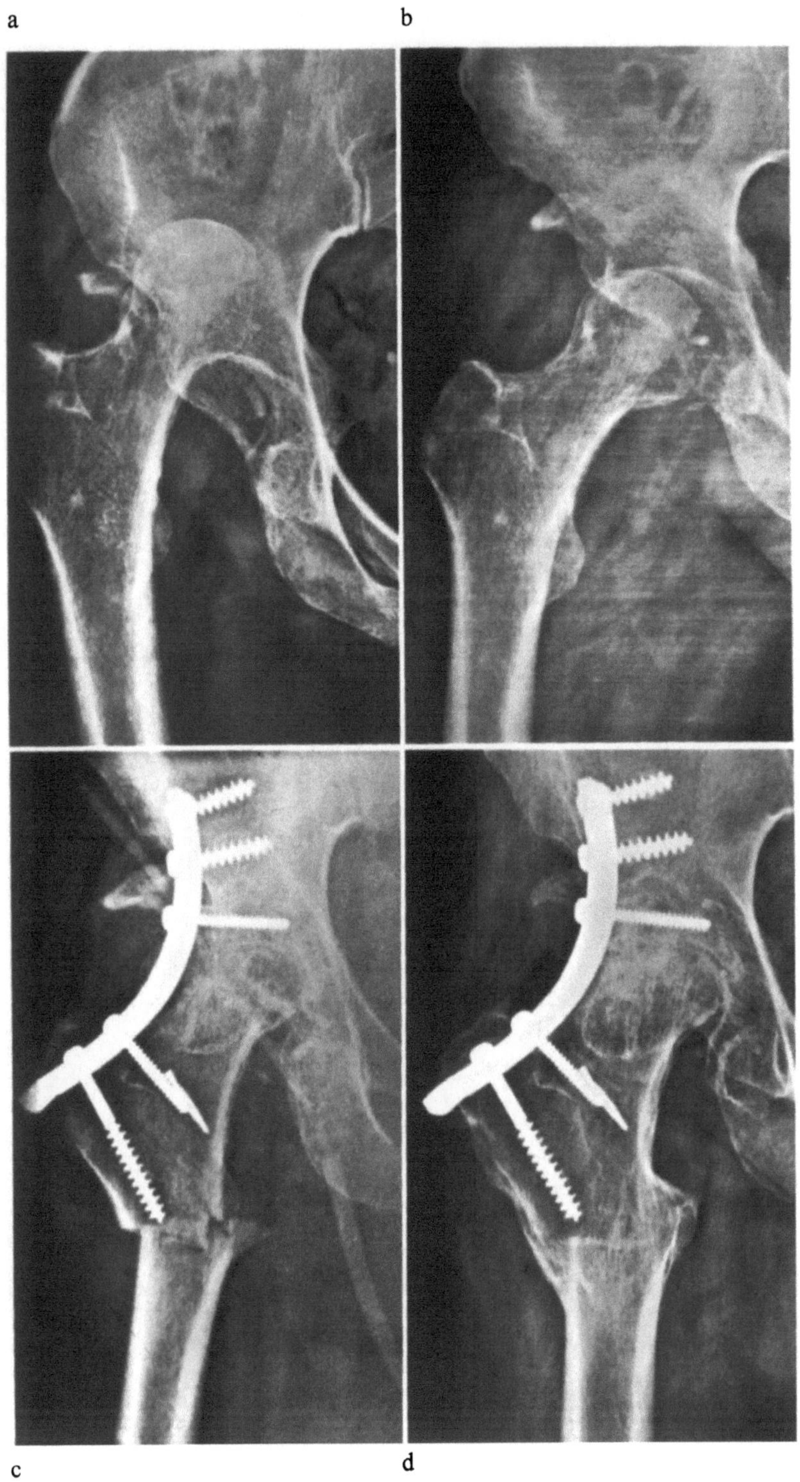

Fig. 159. *Type II HA in a case of post-traumatic arthrosis of the hip*. B. M., ♂, aged 57 years, No. 138634.

a) Old traumatic dislocation of the hip with acetabular fracture (radiological diagnosis 3 months after accident).

b) Fourteen days after 20 kg supracondular traction with Steinmann pin.

c) HA. The femoral head was dislocated dorsally and the acetabulum was completely filled with connective tissue. The head was reduced and fixed in the acetabulum with a Steinmann pin. The plate was then fitted and screwed into place (drill fractured on coming into contact with the Steinmann pin).

d) HA and subtrochanteric osteotomy both united with ideal leg position. Leg shortening 0.5 cm

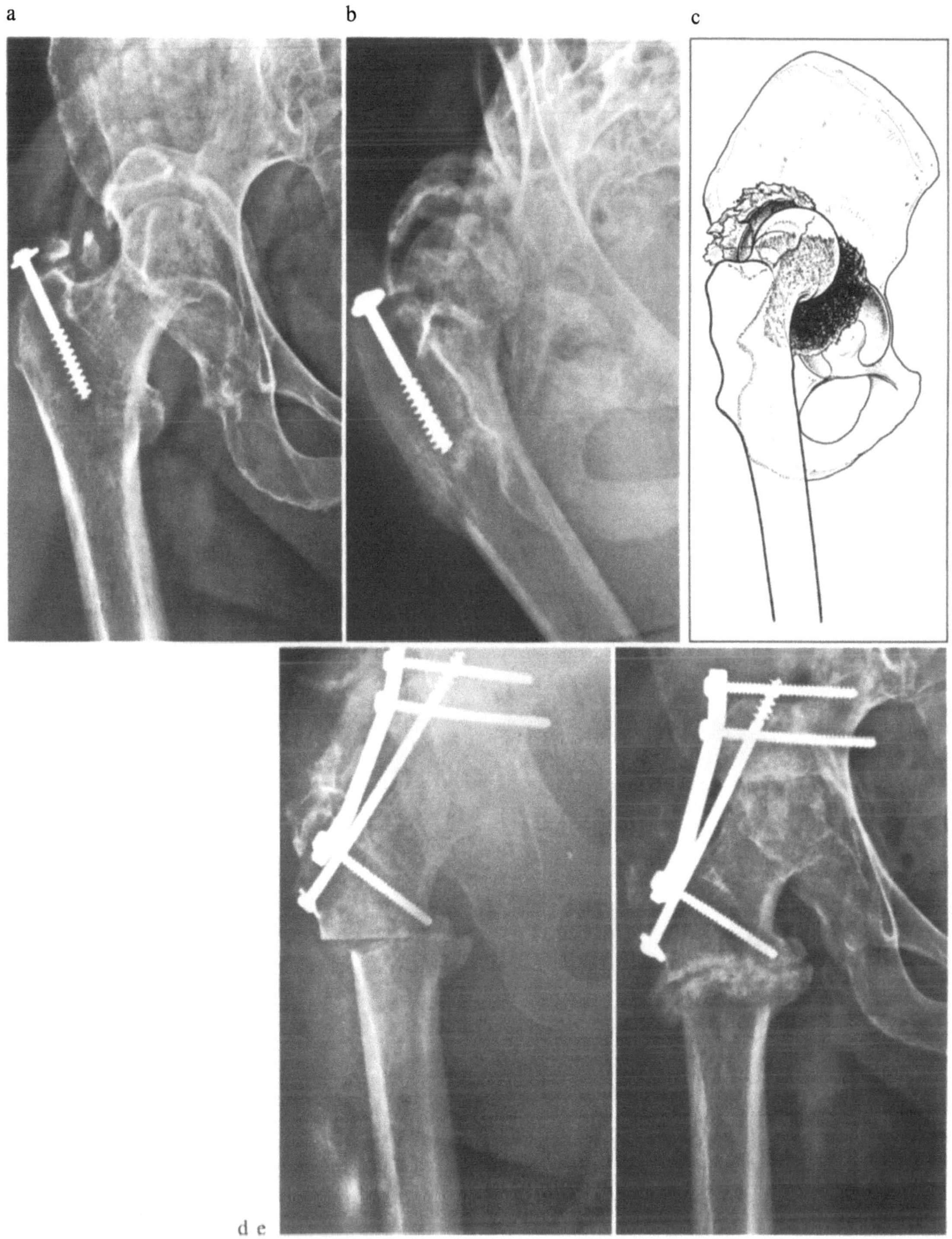

Fig. 160. *Type II HA in a case of post-traumatic arthrosis of the hip.* W. N., ♀, aged 61 years, No. 164556.

a and b) Sixteen months following posterior dislocation of the hip with fracture of the acetabular roof and following fixation of the transected greater trochanter with a cancellous screw in another hospital.

c) Diagram of the anatomy in Figures a) and b). A large fragment has broken off the acetabular roof and was driven upwards and backwards by the dislocated femoral head. Residual dislocation with formation of a secondary acetabulum. The hip remains unstable and incapable of bearing weight.

d) Immediately following arthrodesis of the hip. The femoral head has been fixed to the pelvis with a cancellous compression screw inserted from the direction of the innominate tubercle. The 5-hole plate prevents any tendency to varus; in fact the hip is in valgus. IO to prevent transmission of load to the hip. Eight weeks bed rest followed by painless walking with two canes.

e) Four months following HA. Advanced union of the HA and IO. HA clinically united; full weight bearing possible.

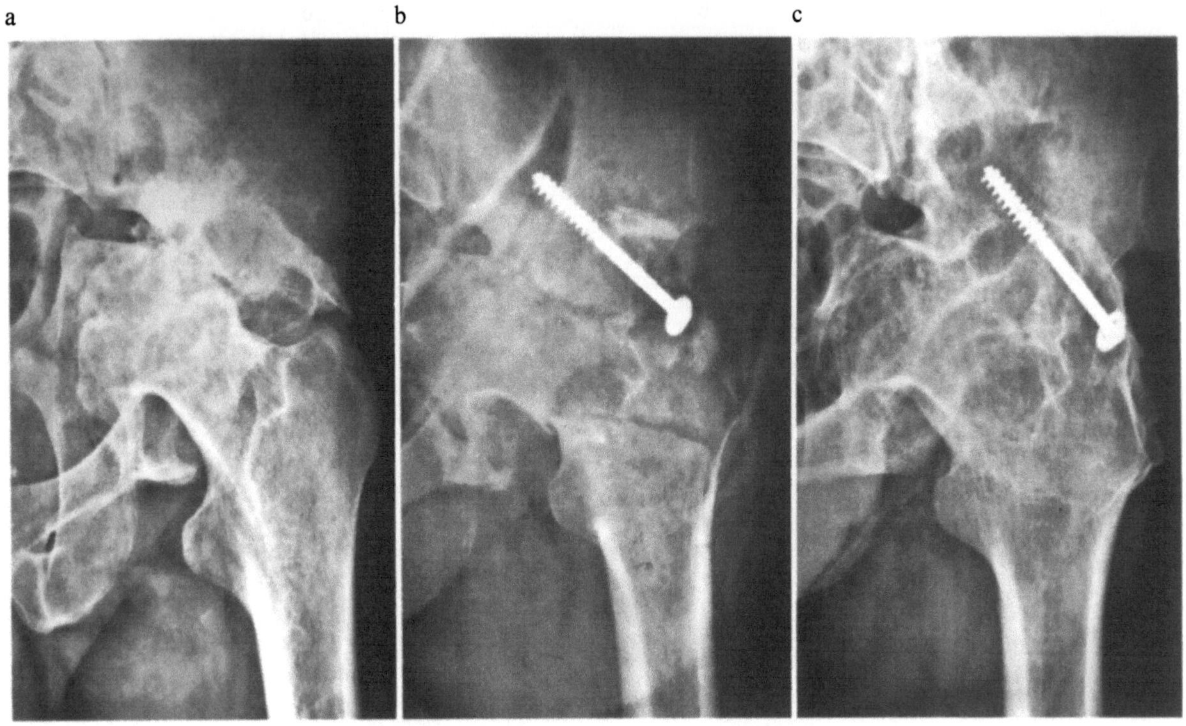

Fig. 161. *Type I HA in an old case of central dislocation of the hip.* J. A., ♂, aged 26 years, No. 84900.

a) Fifteen months after accident. Central dislocation of the femoral head with break-through of the whole ischial bone.

b) Type I HA. Cancellous bone grafts were taken from the iliac crest and inserted between the freshened acetabular roof and the freshened femoral neck.

c) Eighteen months later. HA united with good leg position. Patient has returned to full-time work as miner

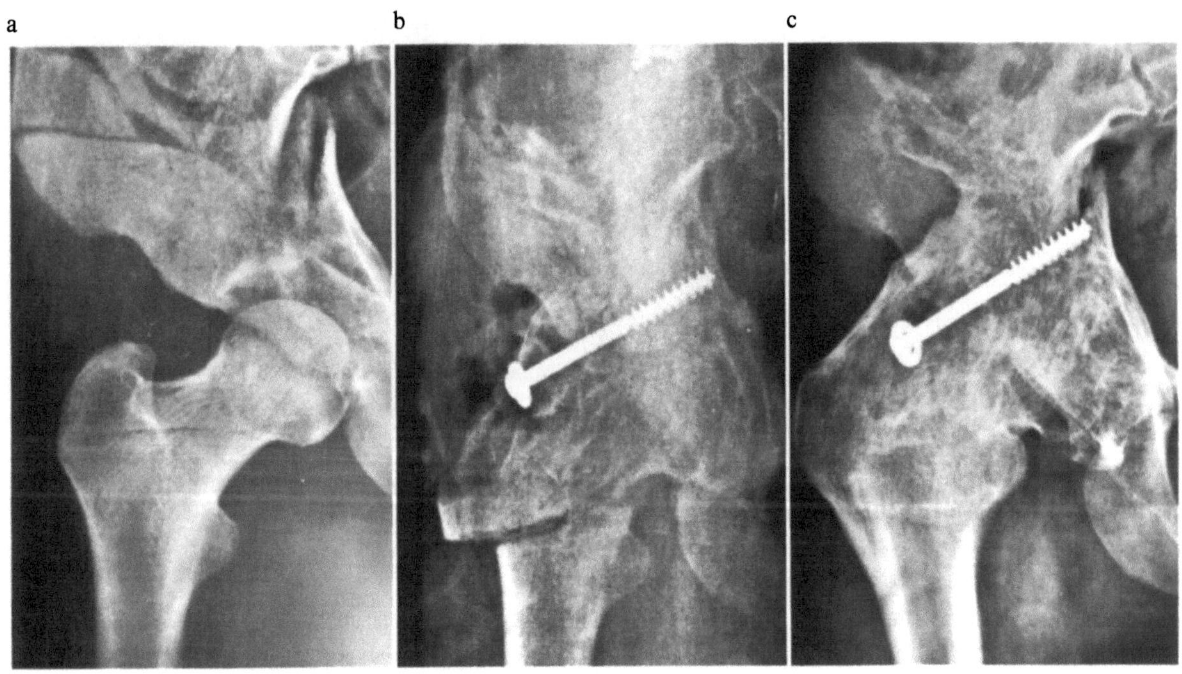

Fig. 162. *Late HA in a case of post-traumatic arthrosis of the hip.* B. A., ♀, aged 30 years, No. 74117.

a) Two weeks after accident. Fractures of the pelvis and acetabulum.

b) HA 1 year after accident.

c) Two years later. HA united with ideal leg position and 3 cm leg shortening. Pain-free gait without cane

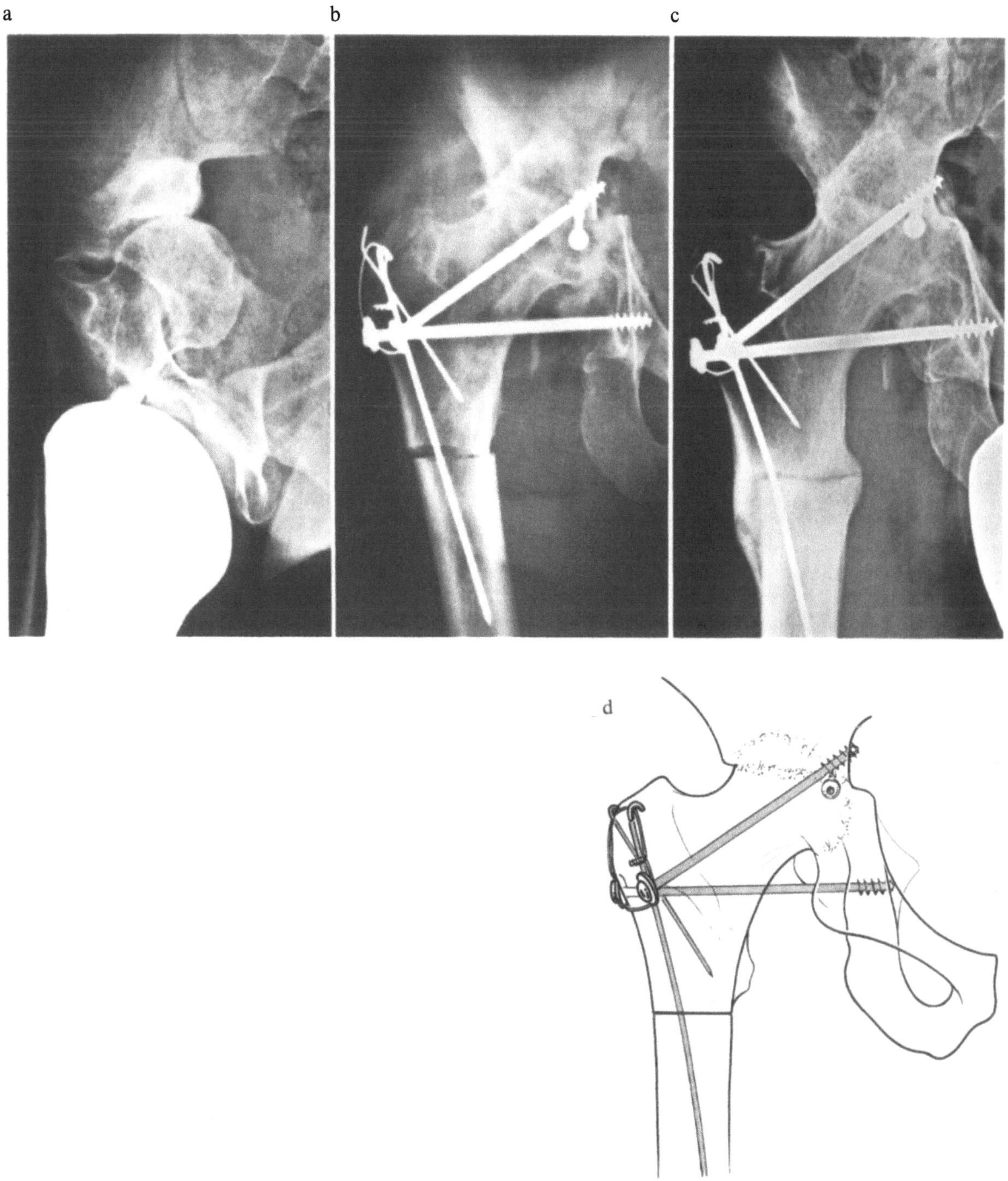

Fig. 163. *HA in a case of posterior hip dislocation with acetabular fracture.* S. W., ♂, aged 24 years, No. 146706.

a) Seven months after accident. Residual posterior dislocation of the hip; the large fragment has broken off the acetabulum. Sciatic nerve pain and partial paresis of the common peroneal branch.

b) HA. Cobra-head plate arthrodesis could not be performed because the posterior superior segment of the acetabulum was missing. Transverse PO. Screw fixation of the acetabular fragment. Fixation of the HA with two cancellous screws. Freeing of the sciatic nerve which was surrounded by connective tissue below the infrapiriform foramen.

c) Four months later. HA united with good leg position and 3 cm leg shortening. Electromyographic evidence of reinnervation of the most proximal lower leg muscles which are supplied by the peroneal nerve.

d) Diagram of the HA. Stabilised by cancellous screws which fix the proximal femoral component to the pelvis. Additional K-wire to prevent displacement at the level of the subtrochanteric osteotomy

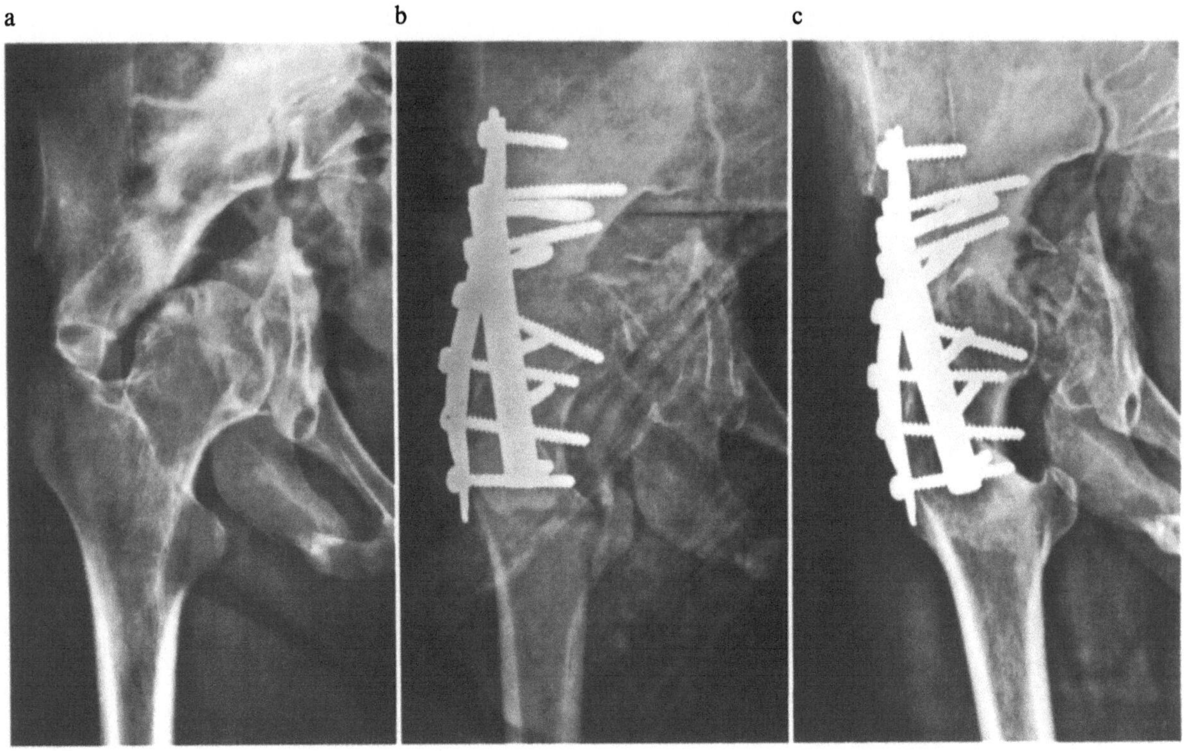

Fig. 164. *Type II HA in an old case of central fracture dislocation of the hip.* L. M., ♀, aged 37 years, No. 93952.

a) Seventeen months after accident.

b) HA with rigid internal fixation following reduction of the femoral head.

c) Nineteen months later. HA united with good leg position and 1.5 cm leg shortening

Fig. 165. *Type IV HA in a case of post-traumatic arthrosis of the hip.* C. G., ♀, aged 29 years, No. 89861.

a) Pelvic fracture with central dislocation of the hip. Open reduction of the fracture followed by 5 weeks traction.

b) Six months later. Very severe pain on weight bearing. Pain elicited on testing function but range of movement almost normal.

c) Eleven months following cup plasty.

d) Cobra-head plate arthrodesis with PO.

e) Fatigue fracture at distal end of plate.

f) Result 5 months following internal fixation with two plates. Fracture healed. HA united with good leg position

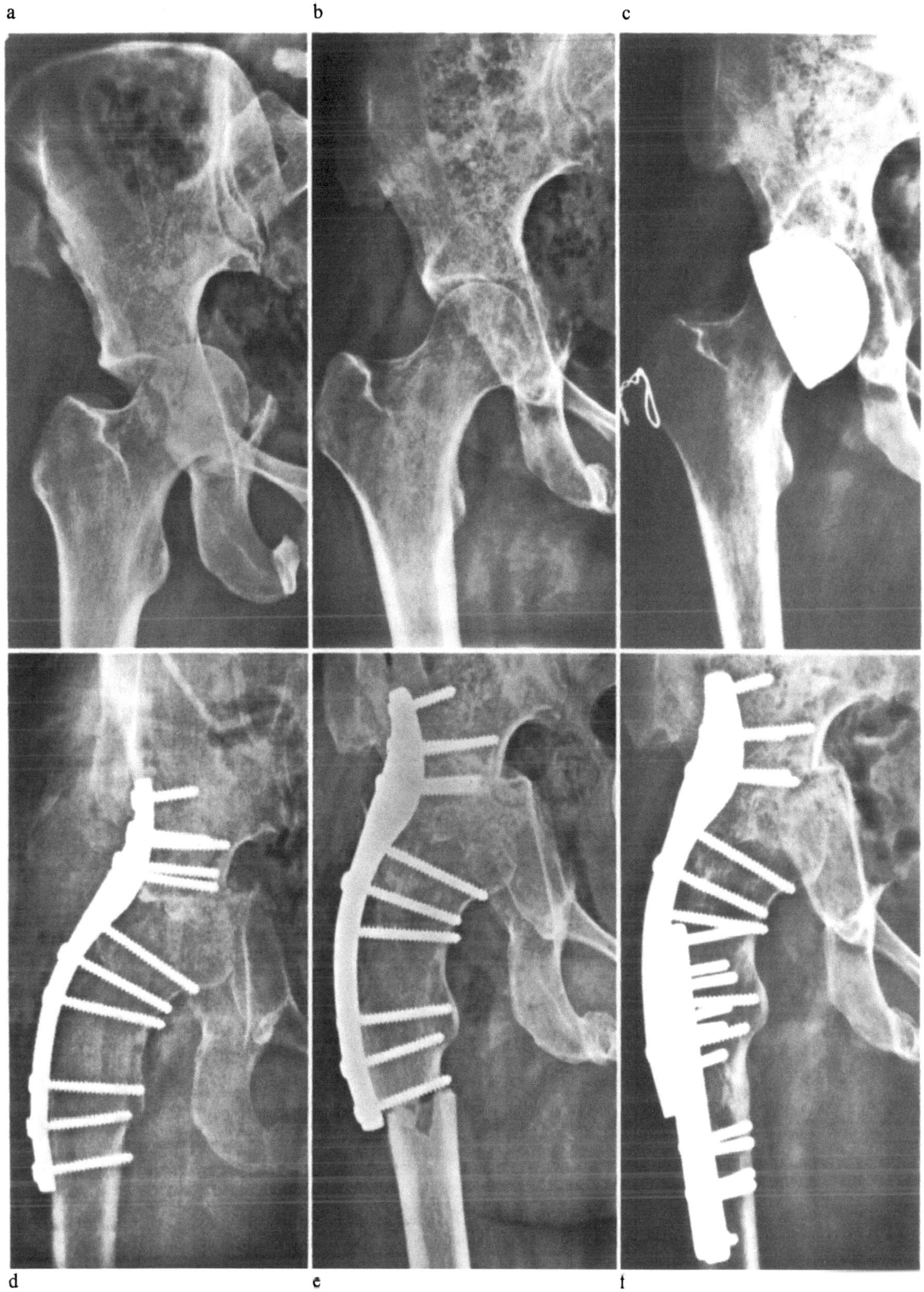

a b

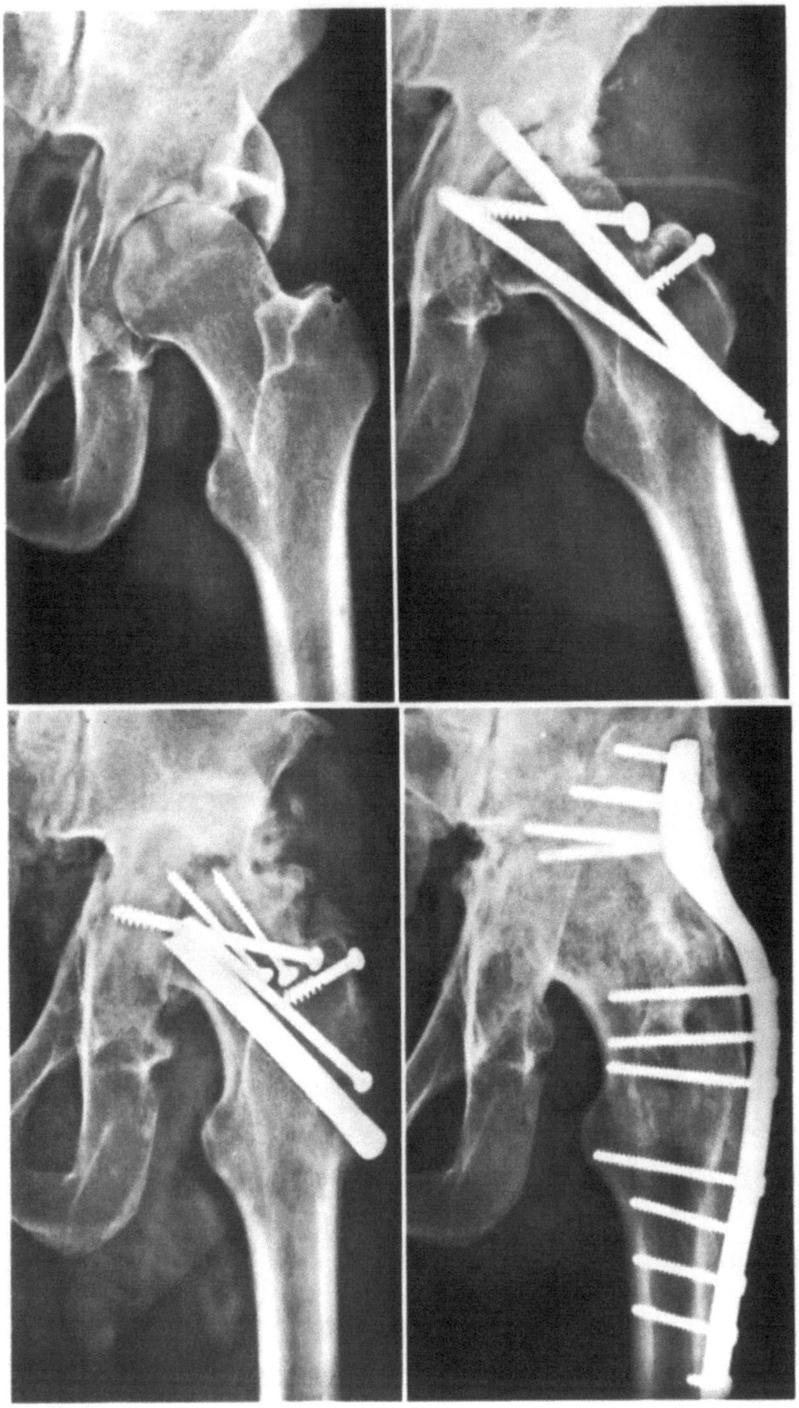

c d

Fig. 166. *Type IV HA following fractures of the acetabulum; arthrodesis had twice been attempted in another hospital.* L. A., ♂, aged 55 years, No. 102056.

a) One month following accident.

b and c) Failed HA performed in another hospital (insufficient rigidity as a result of inadequate technique).

d) Three and a half years following cobra-head plate arthrodesis without PO, the PA and osteotomy are almost united. Full pain-free weight bearing possible with 2.5 cm leg shortening

4 Arthrodesis of Infected Hips

4.1 Introduction

In our series, ten HA (1.7%) were performed for tuberculosis of the hip and 19 HA (3.3%) for nontuberculitic infection. Of the latter, 16 were iatrogenic (Table 32).

The guide lines on page 79 apply to nontuberculitic hip infection, i.e., the acute infection should either be eradicated or rendered quiescent. A quiescent infection allows a HA to be performed with minimal internal fixation. HA is the treatment of choice in Tb of the hip joint which has passed the acute phase.

Table 32. Infected hips

Tuberculous hip infection	10	29
Nontuberculous hip infection	19	
16 cases were iatrogenic, thus:		
Subsequent to intra-articular injections	1	16
Subsequent to orthopedic operations	8	
Subsequent to internal fixation (post-traumatic)	7	

4.2 Tuberculosis of the Hip

4.2.1 General Guide Lines

HA is the treatment of choice in Tb of the hip in young patients as well as in adults for the following reasons:

a) In the tuberculitic hip, the partial ankylosis which results from more or less severe destruction of the joint is usually fibrous rather than bony. A recurrence of the Tb is always possible if increased stressing of this ankylosis occurs.

b) In old cases, the patients frequently complain of continuous pain in the presence of hip joint deformity which results from the almost total destruction of the joint with concomitant reduction in range of movement.

HA may be performed and should be performed when the acute stage is passed, when destruction has ceased and repair has commenced (reduction in osteoporosis, change in blood film and sedimentation rate), and where joint destruction is so extensive that there is no hope of retaining adequate joint function.

In one case we have operated in the acute phase. Radical extirpation of the infected tissue was carried out and followed by compression-plate arthrodesis despite the fistulae. If the tuberculosis is inactive the usual HA with rigid internal fixation is performed.

4.2.2 Case Material

(Figs. 167 – 170)

4.3 Nontuberculitic Infection

4.3.1 Introduction

HA is recommended in adults with nontuberculitic hip infection with destruction (and perhaps subluxation) of the joint.

HA is almost always performed by screw fixation and IO immediately above or at the level of the lesser trochanter. Radical excision of joint cartilage, radical débridement and, if indicated, suction or perfusion drainage are all important here.

4.3.2 Case Material

(Figs. 171 – 175).

a b c

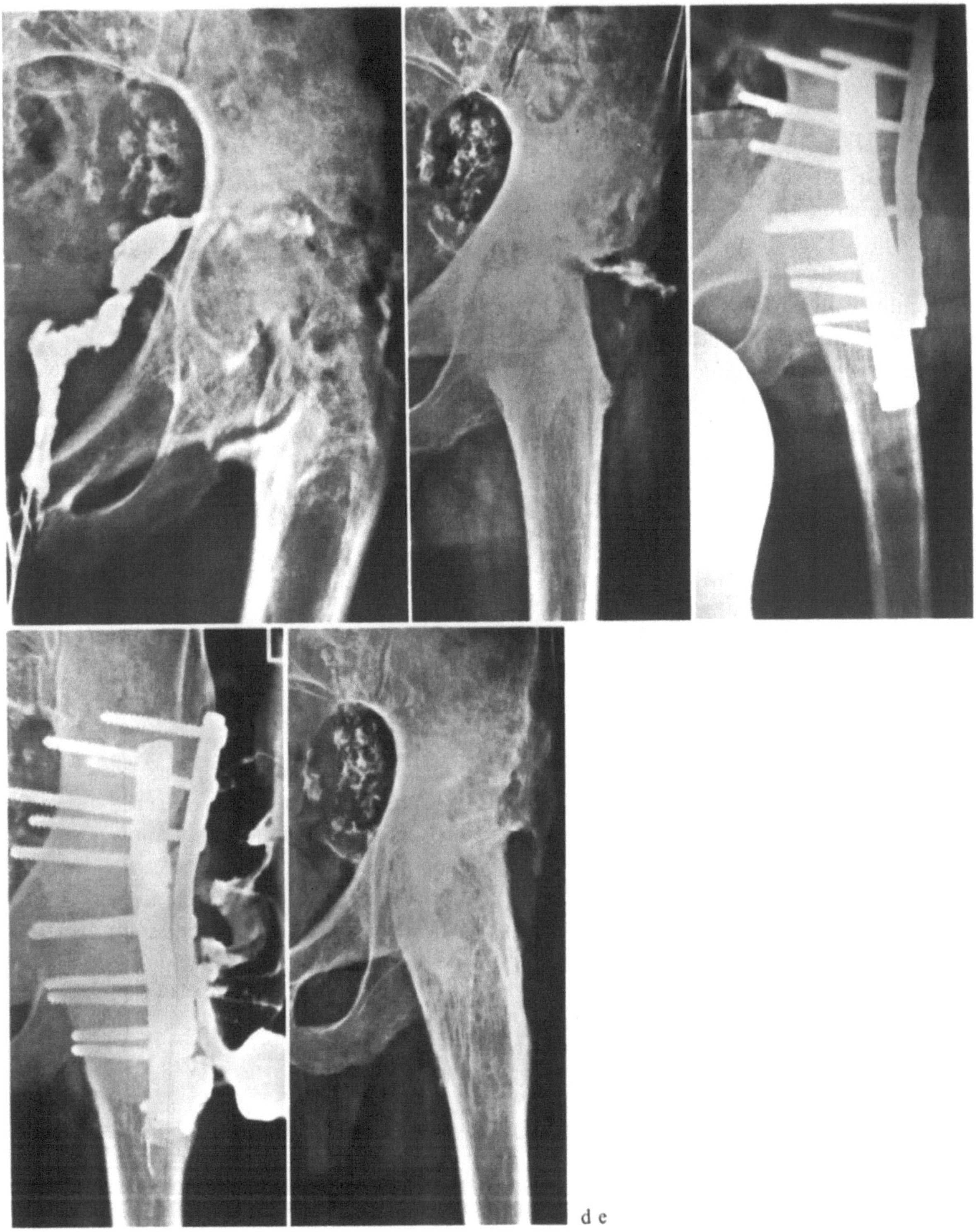

d e

Fig. 167. *Type III HA without PO in an old tuberculous hip.* L. Ch., ♂, aged 43 years, No. 98635.

a) 35-year old tuberculous hip infection with fistulae. This radiograph was taken 5 months after surgical excision of the infected tissue and cancellous bone plasty. Injection of contrast medium shows the fistula running between the greater trochanter and the perianal area (tuberculosis with simultaneous Proteus infection).

b) Infected PA 24 months after attempted HA (freshening arthrodesis).

c) Excision of the fistula and Type III HA without PO

d) Fifteen months later. HA united. Residual fistula down to the metal.

e) Ten months after implant removal and excision of the fistula. HA united with good leg position and 4 cm leg shortening

a b c d

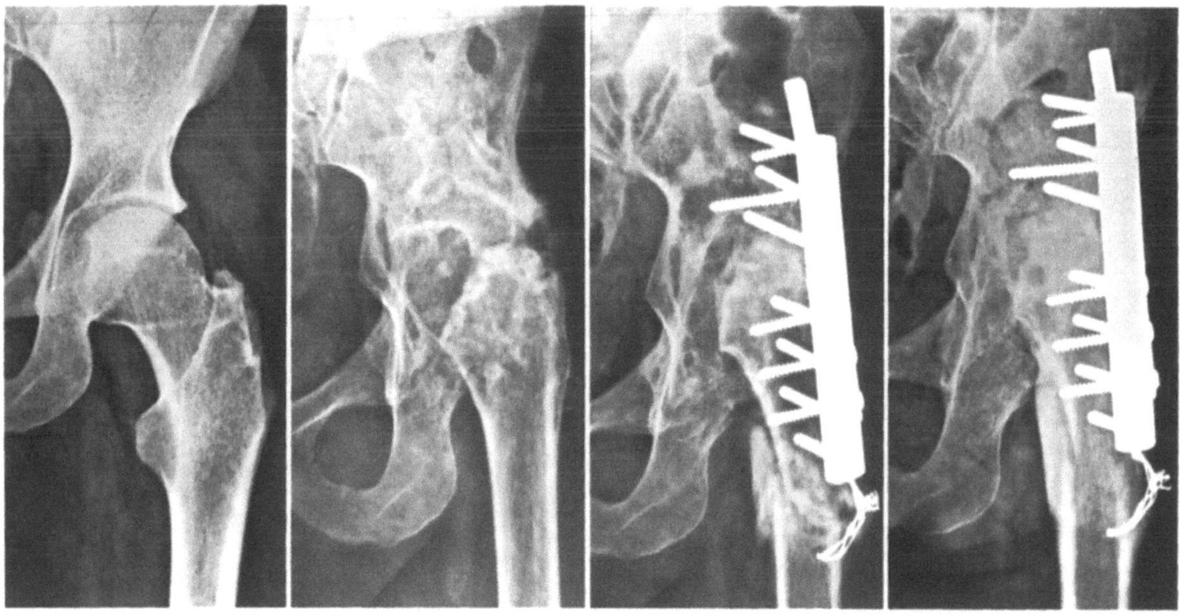

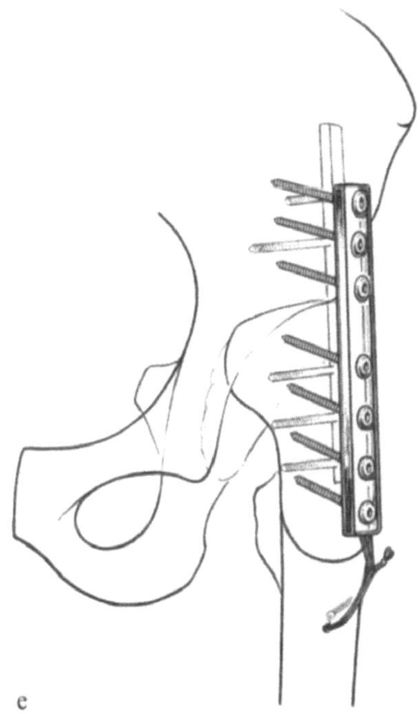

e

Fig. 168. *Type II HA in a case of PA following two arthrodesis attempts in an old tuberculous hip.* R. H., ♂, aged 48 years, No. 400168.

a) Radiograph taken 20 years previously following multiple drainage procedures, curettages and osteotomy of tuberculous bone around the greater trochanter.

b) Radiograph taken 5 and 6 years, respectively following two attempts at arthrodesis in another hospital. Femoral head missing.

c) Four months following Type II HA and following cast removal. Advanced bone union in the HA and the osteotomy.

d) Sixteen months following HA. HA, PA and osteotomy are all healed. No subjective problems. Good gait without pain. Correction of 5 cm leg shortening with orthopaedic shoes.

e) Diagram of the arthrodesis. Perfect rigidity is assured by the two plates which lie vertical to each other. Displacement of the distal femur at the level of the IO is prevented by the wire loop which is secured by the lowest screw

a b c

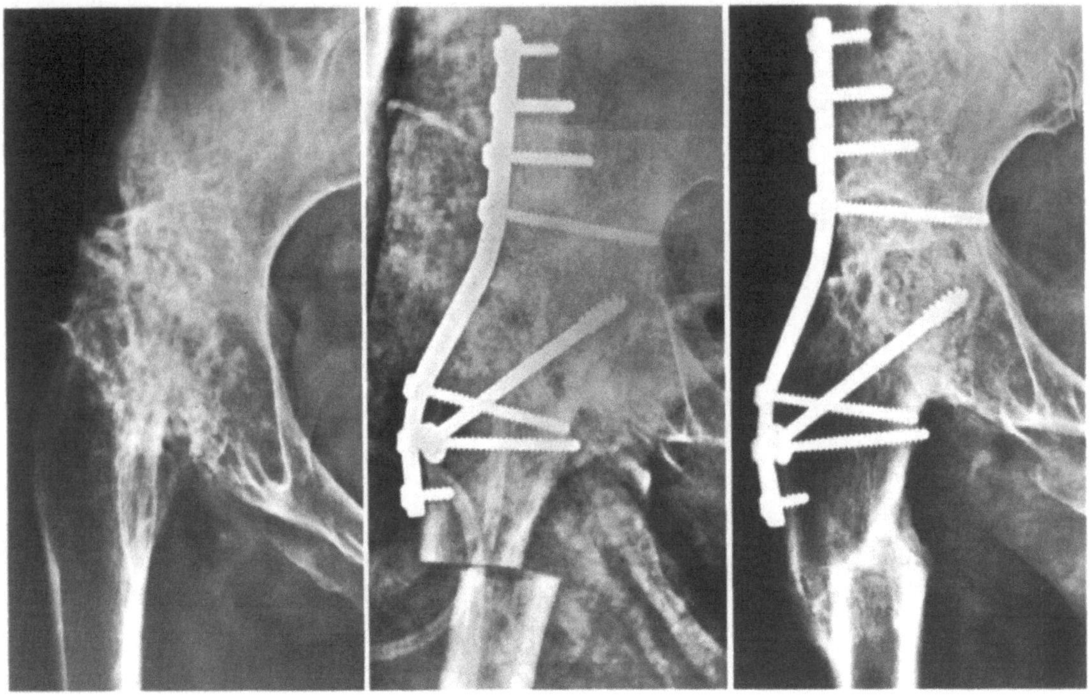

Fig. 169. *Type II HA in a case of fibrous ankylosis secondary to joint infection.* S. S., ♂, aged 48 years, No. 144707.

a) Painful fibrous ankylosis with severe adduction deformity and *10 cm* leg shortening (35 years after tuberculosis of the hip).

b) Type II HA following removal of caseous material from the head and acetabulum. Subtrochanteric osteotomy. Pelvic cast.

c) Follow-up 24 months later. HA and subtrochanteric osteotomy united with ideal leg position. Normal scar. Patient complaint-free and working full time in a factory. Only 4 cm residual leg shortening (corrected with orthopaedic shoe)

a b c d

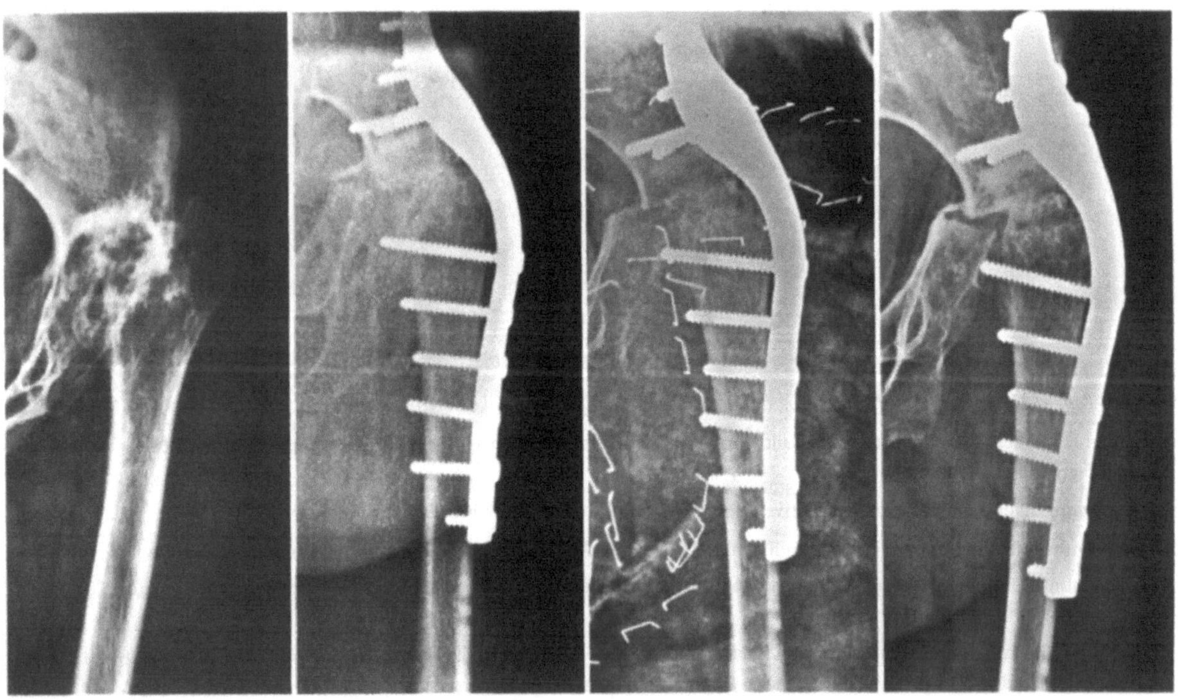

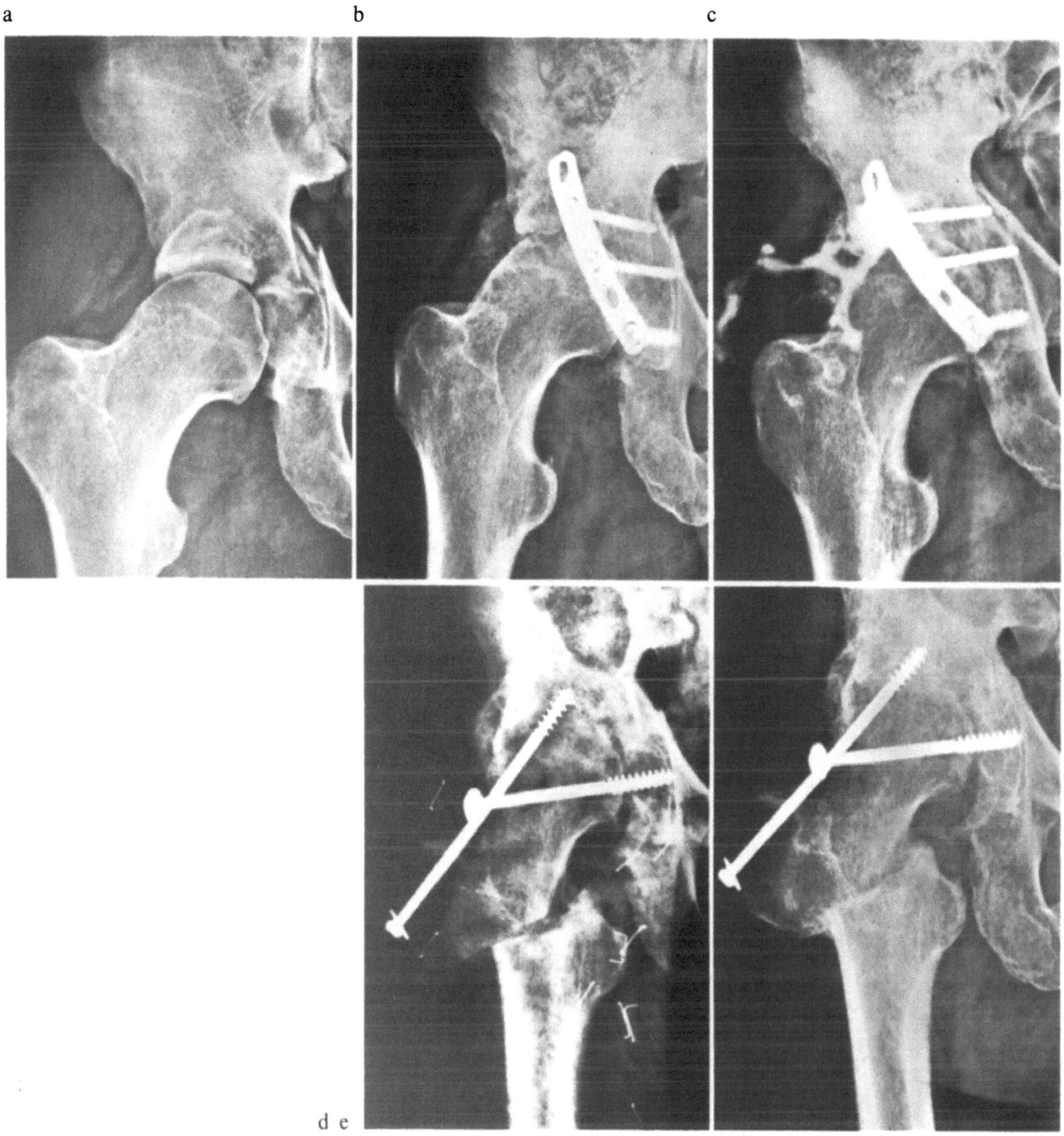

Fig. 170. *Type IV HA with PO in an old tuberculous hip*. I. S., ♀, aged 45 years, No. 161 143.

a) Severe destruction of the hip joint following juvenile tuberculosis of the joint.

b) At operation.

c) Two months following HA. Because of ınadequate internal fixation an exception was made and a hip spica was applied for 6 weeks.

d) Five months following HA. Bone union with good leg position

a b c

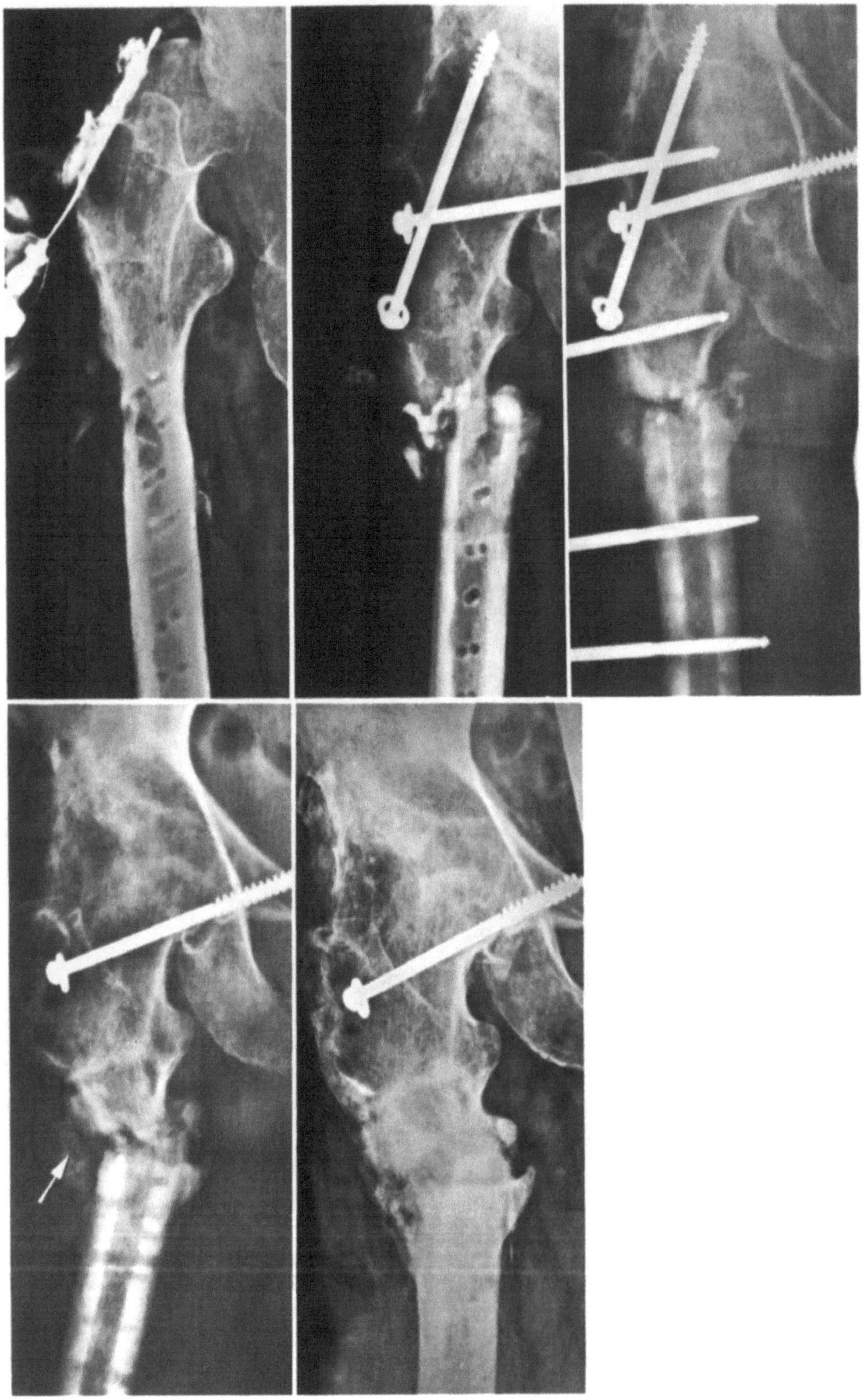

d e

a b c d e

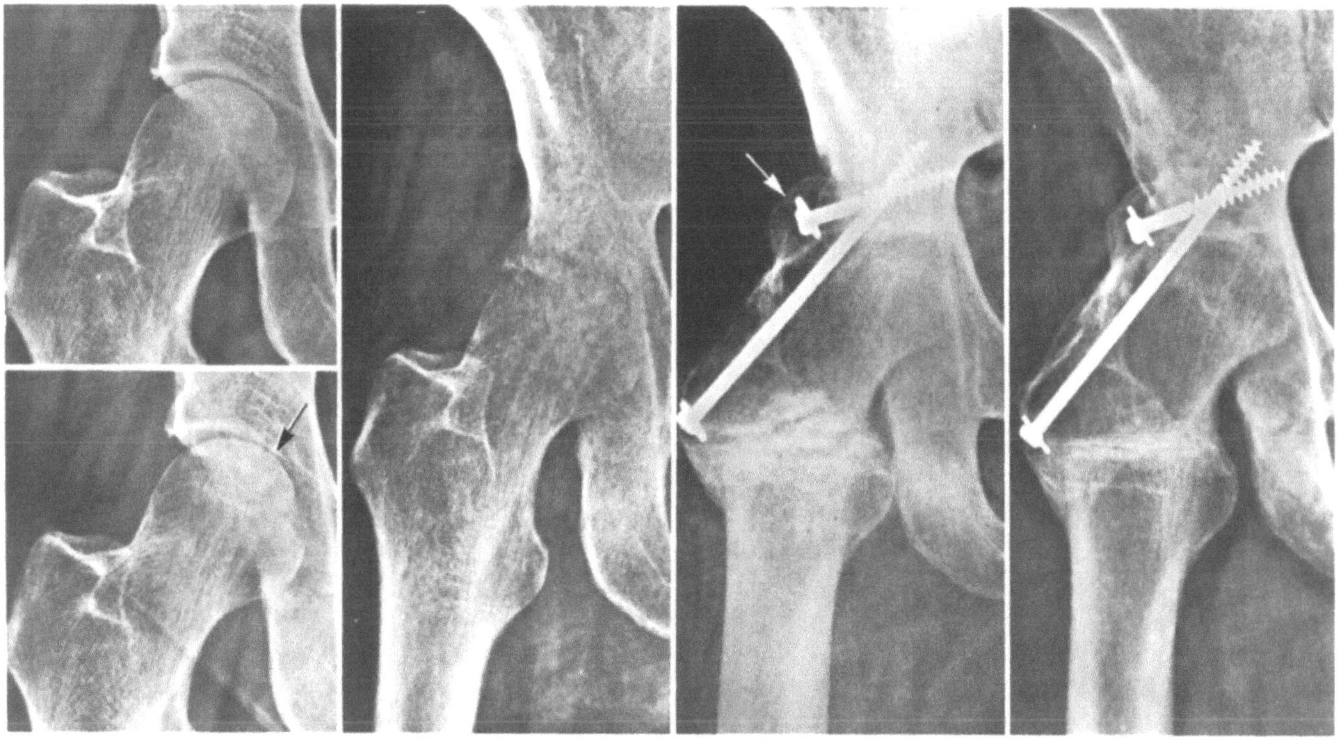

Fig. 173. *HA with minimal internal fixation in a staphylococcal hip infection secondary to sepsis.* H. H., ♀, aged 39 years, No. 102958.

a) One month following admission to hospital for a facial furuncle which developed into sepsis. Incipient sepsis of the hip not yet radiologically visible.

b) Six weeks later. Medial narrowing of the joint space. Bone structure slightly blurred on comparison with (a).

c) Four weeks later. Severe destruction of the hip joint; joint space almost obliterated.

d) Three months after arthrodesis of the hip which was infected with Staphylococcus. The iliofemoral graft is clearly visible. The HA has already united. The IO is still visible but partially united.

e) Eleven months after operation. Osteotomy and HA united. Ideal leg position with 1 cm leg shortening. Patient complaint-free and working full time as housewife

Fig. 172. *HA in a case of staphylococcal hip infection.* B. W., ♂, aged 44 years, No. 142697.

a) Femoral head completely dislocated. Staphylococcal hip infection with osteitis following internal fixation of a compound comminuted subtrochanteric fracture with an angled blade plate

b) Ten weeks following HA with minimal internal fixation and IO. Bones are united with good leg position. Infected refracture secondary to subtrochanteric osteitis. Treated by cancellous bone plasty and application of external compression clamps. Eight months later, failure to heal; formation of infected subtrochanteric pseudarthrosis.

c) Two months following further cancellous bone plasty and renewed application of external compression clamps. Callus formation but absence of bone union.

d) Two months later. PA still present. Removal of the external compression clamps and the loose distal screw. Freshening of the bone and "tension band" cancellous bone plasty on the lateral side.

e) Seven months later. PA healed. Leg capable of full weight bearing. No complaints

a b c

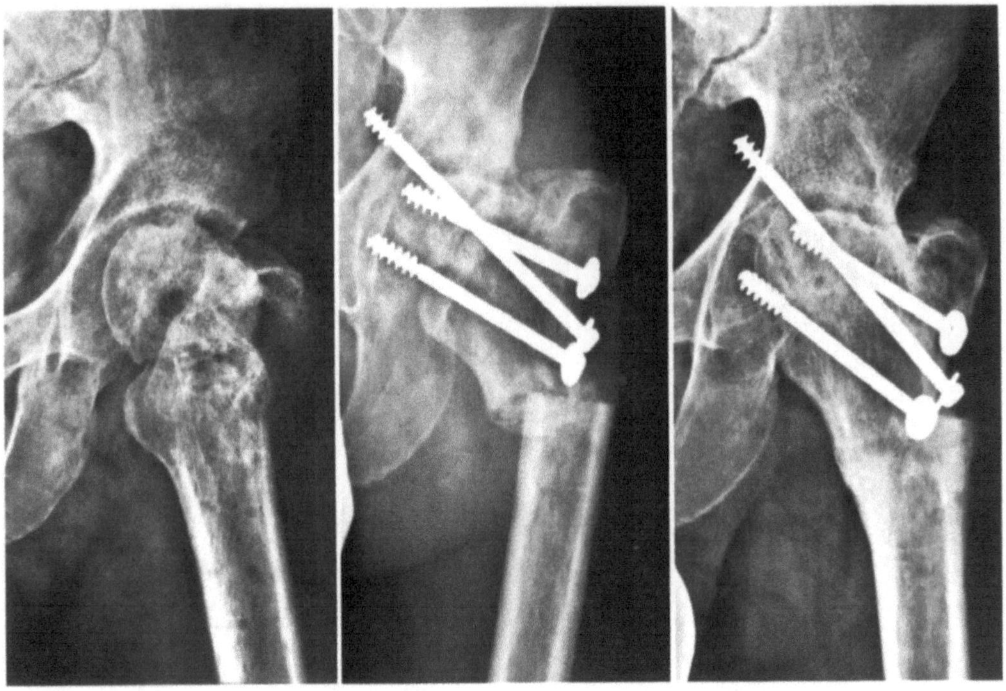

Fig. 174. *Screw arthrodesis of an infected PA of the femoral neck.* V. R., ♂, aged 32 years, No. 144100.

a) Infected PA and necrosis of the femoral head following internal fixation of a medial fracture of the femoral neck with an angled plate.

b) HA with screw fixation and subtrochanteric osteotomy.

c) Fourteen months later. HA united. Patient complaint-free

a b c d

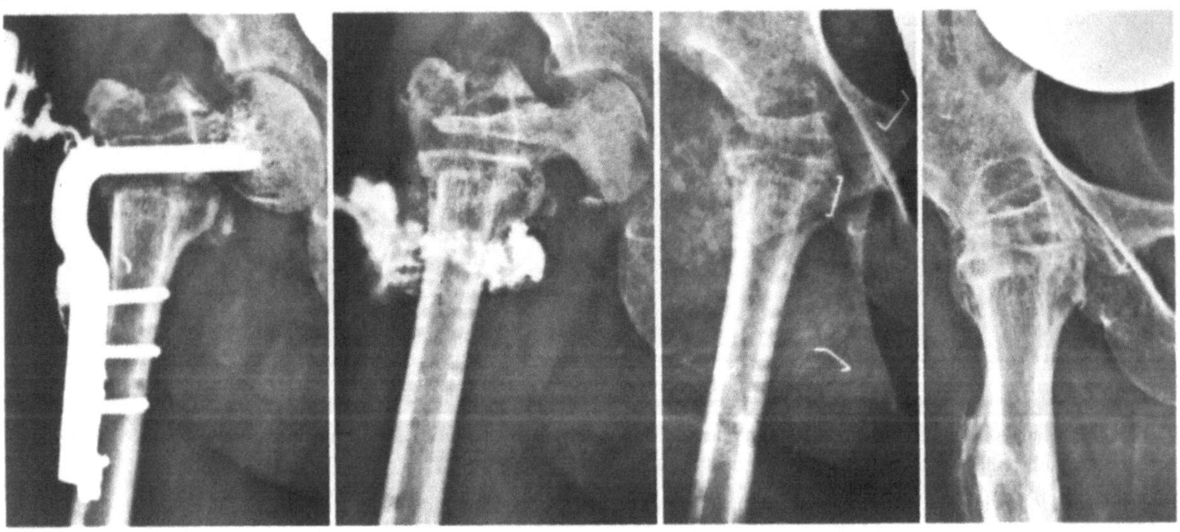

Fig. 175. *Freshening arthrodesis of a hip which had become septic following treatment of CDH by IO.* M. R., ♀, aged 29 years, No. 106025.

a) Fistula secondary to IO has been filled with contrast medium as far as the blade of the plate.

b) Repeat filling of the fistula 1 month following implant removal. Large abcess cavity. Drainage of the abcess.

c) Freshening arthrodesis 2 months later with renewed perfusion drainage. Cast applied with the leg in abduction. Two months later subtrochanteric corrective femoral osteotomy and cancellous bone plasty.

d) Follow-up 2 years later. Arthrodesis united with 8° abduction. Patient complaint-free and working full time

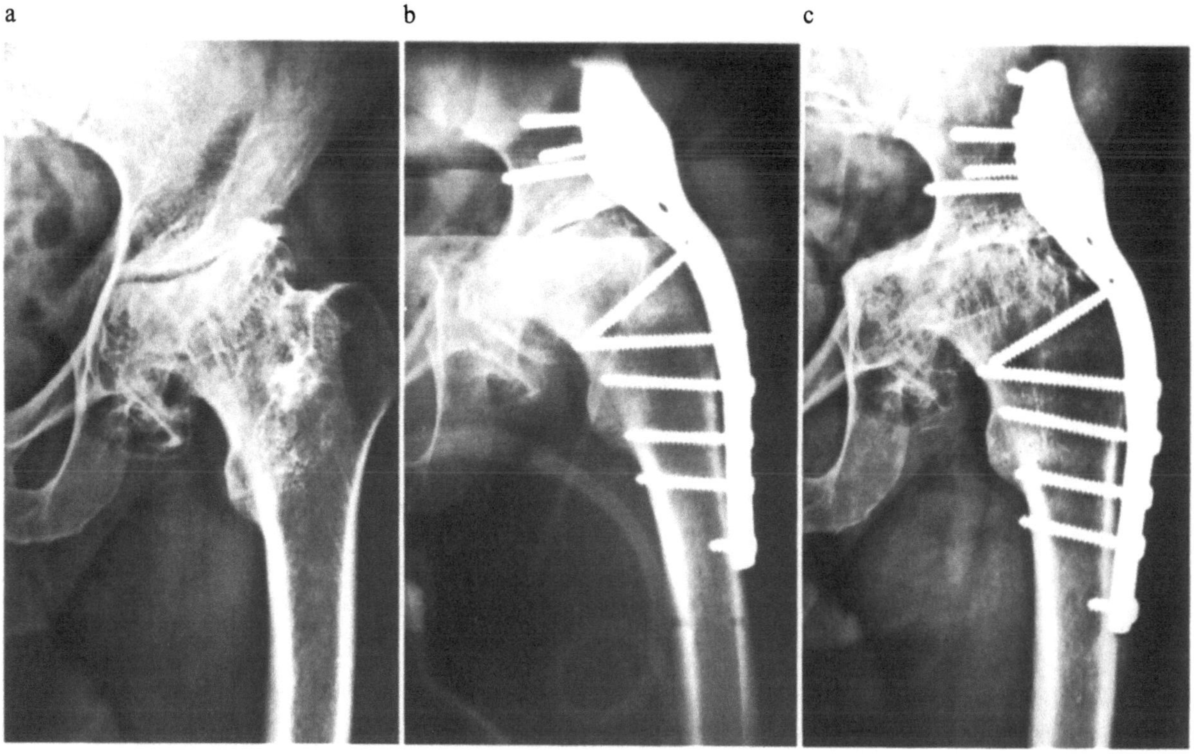

Fig. 176. *Type IV HA PO following partial necrosis of the femoral head.* S. R., ♂, aged 52 years, No. 145092.

a) Severe arthrosis of the hip. Necrotic femoral head largely resorbed.

b) HA with cobra-head plate. Osteotomy sloping somewhat. Because of the shape of the acetabulum and femoral head bone resection was kept to a minimum in order to prevent increased shortening.

c) Nine months later. HA united with ideal leg position. No difference in leg length

5 Hip Arthrodesis for Necrosis of the Femoral Head

5.1 Introduction

We differentiate between:
a) Idiopathic head necrosis
b) Head necrosis subsequent to orthopaedic operations
c) Post-traumatic head necrosis

Despite the differences in etiology, all femoral head necroses present the same problem in respect to HA. The reason is the more or less extensive disintegration of the head in the weight-bearing area which is always present.

5.2 Idiopathic Head Necrosis

5.2.1 Head Necrosis Alone

In advanced necrosis in which resorption has already occurred (evidenced radiologically by sclerosis) with resulting adaptation of the contact surfaces, the situation is advantageous for HA. Such cases are rare (Fig. 176).

5.2.2 Head Necrosis with Subluxation of the Femoral Head

More often subluxation occurs with rapidly worsening and severely painful degenerative changes which cause the patient to consult the doctor at an early stage. A totally necrotic area results which has to be resected at operation. The resulting leg shortening must, if possible, be taken account of in the choice of operative procedure (valgus correction of the proximal femur is required) (Figs. 177, 178).

a b c

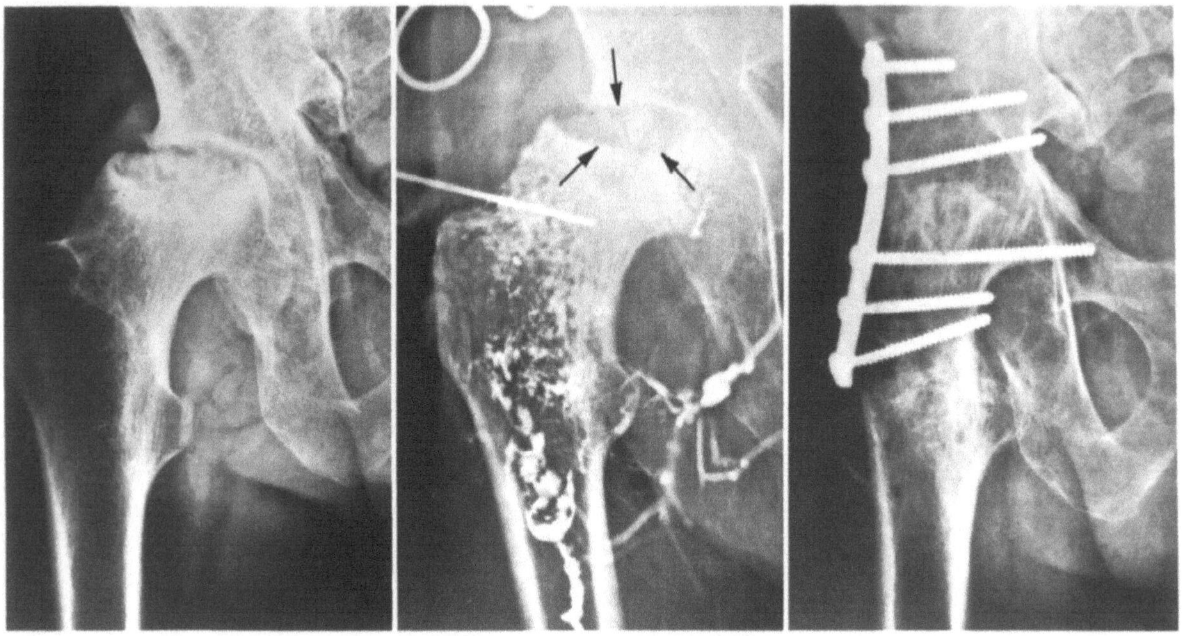

Fig. 177. *Type II HA in a case of idiopathic necrosis of femoral head.* Z. A., ♂, aged 55 years, No. 115077.

a) Arthrosis of the hip with idiopathic necrosis and subluxation of the femoral head.

b) Venography. Good return flow from the still-vitalised head segment. Marked demarcation of the necrosis.

c) Eleven months after HA. Arthrodesis united. Slight adduction (9°). Correction of 2.5 cm functional leg shortening by raising heel of shoe

a b c

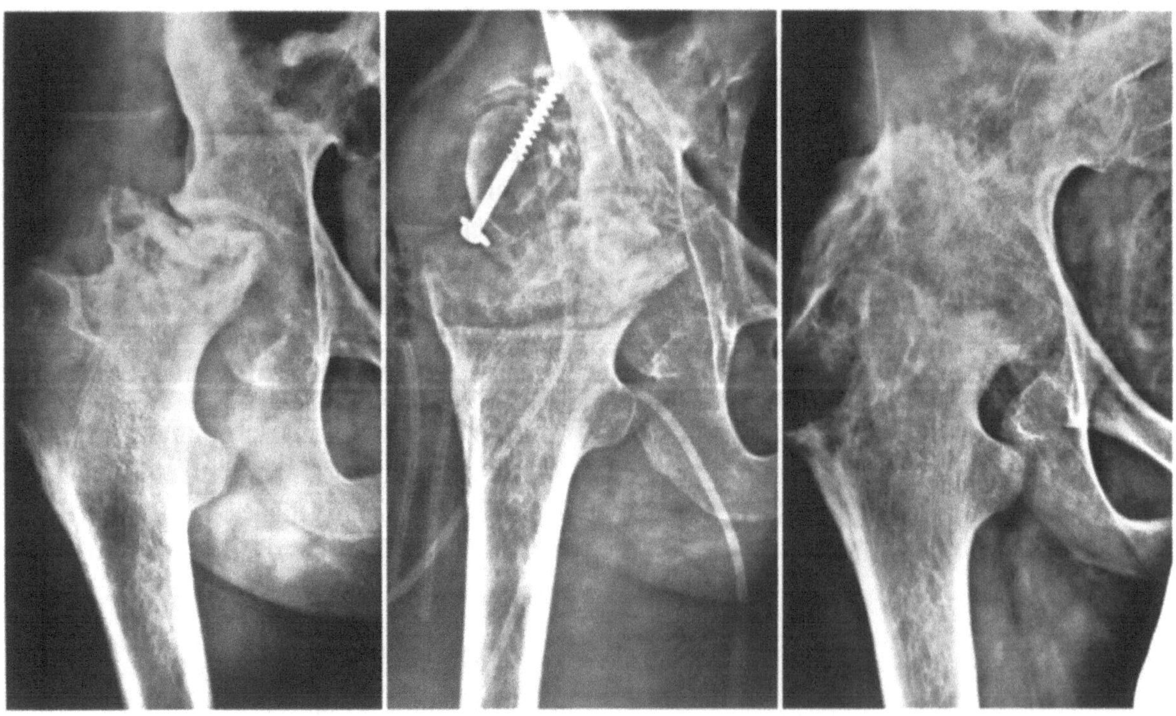

a b c

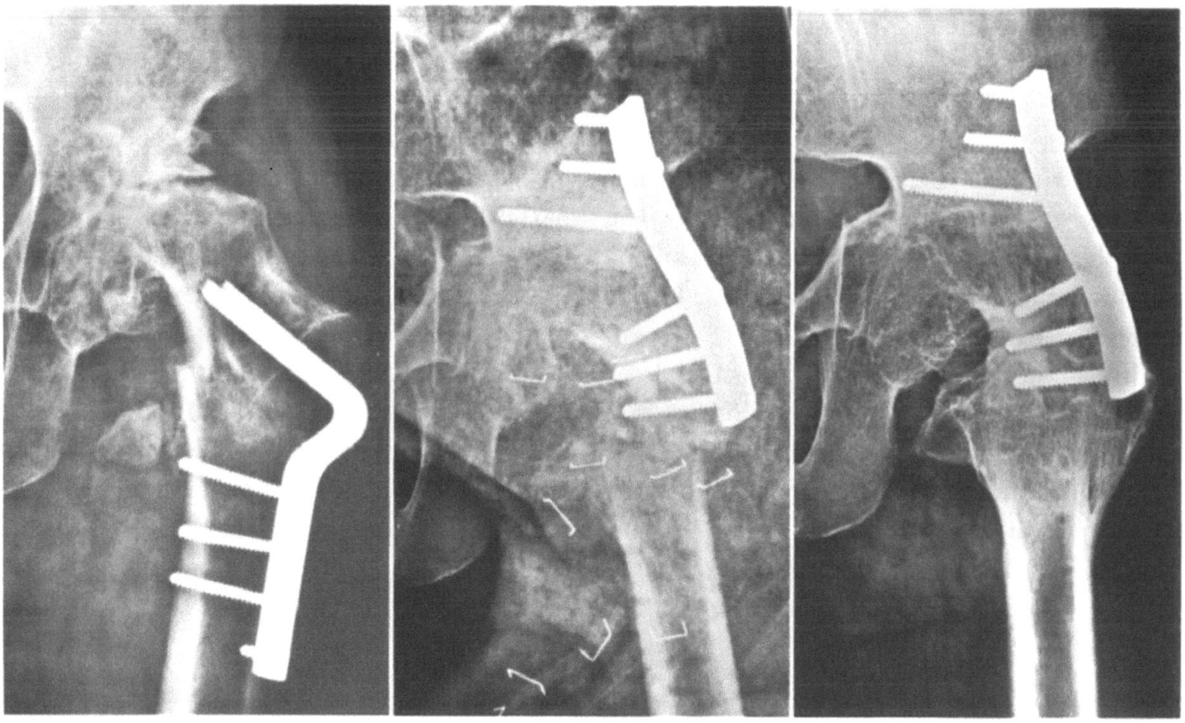

Fig. 179. *Type II HA in a case of NHF following IO*. W. K., ♂, aged 58 years, No. 92238.

a) Four months following IO. Marked NHF.

b) Type II HA in a cast.

c) Twenty-eight months later. HA united with good leg position. Correction of 3.5 cm leg shortening with orthopaedic shoe. Trouble-free gait without cane

←

Fig. 178. *Type I HA in idiopathic NHF*. M. A., ♂, aged 22 years, No. 88276.

a) Very painful arthrosis of hip with idiopathic necrosis and subluxation of the femoral head.

b) Type I HA with high IO. Large iliofemoral bridge graft.

c) Result 46 months following HA. Ideal union

5.3 Femoral Head Necroses Subsequent to Orthopedic Operations

These frequently occur if the indication is unsuitable or the technique was inadequate. The complication results from interruption of the blood circulation in the femoral head. In our series, such cases have followed IO for hip arthrosis and following old Type I arthrodeses in which the osteotomy was performed too high up. In all such cases the vascular supply to the femoral neck and head was partially interrupted by damage to individual nutrient vessels. The latter are, with the exception of the artery to the head of the femur, found at the trochanteric base of the femoral neck. Branches of the medial circumflex artery of the femur which pass along the dorsal aspect of the femoral neck supply the mediodorsal and lateral part of the femoral neck and pass into the bone at the junction of head and neck. The ascending branch of the lateral circumflex artery of the femur passes ventrally; it only supplies the ventral and superior parts of the femoral neck but does not supply the head. Thus, during orthopaedic procedures, the dorsal vessels which are so important in supplying the femoral head should be carefully protected (Figs. 179 – 182).

Fig. 181. *Cobra-head plate arthrodesis in a case of arthrosis of the hip and partial NHF following IO*. M. A., ♀, aged 57 years, No. 66894.

a) Twelve months following IO for arthrosis of the hip. Flattening and partial NHF.

b) Three years after Type IV HA. The arthrodesis is united with good leg position and 2.5 cm leg shortening

a b c

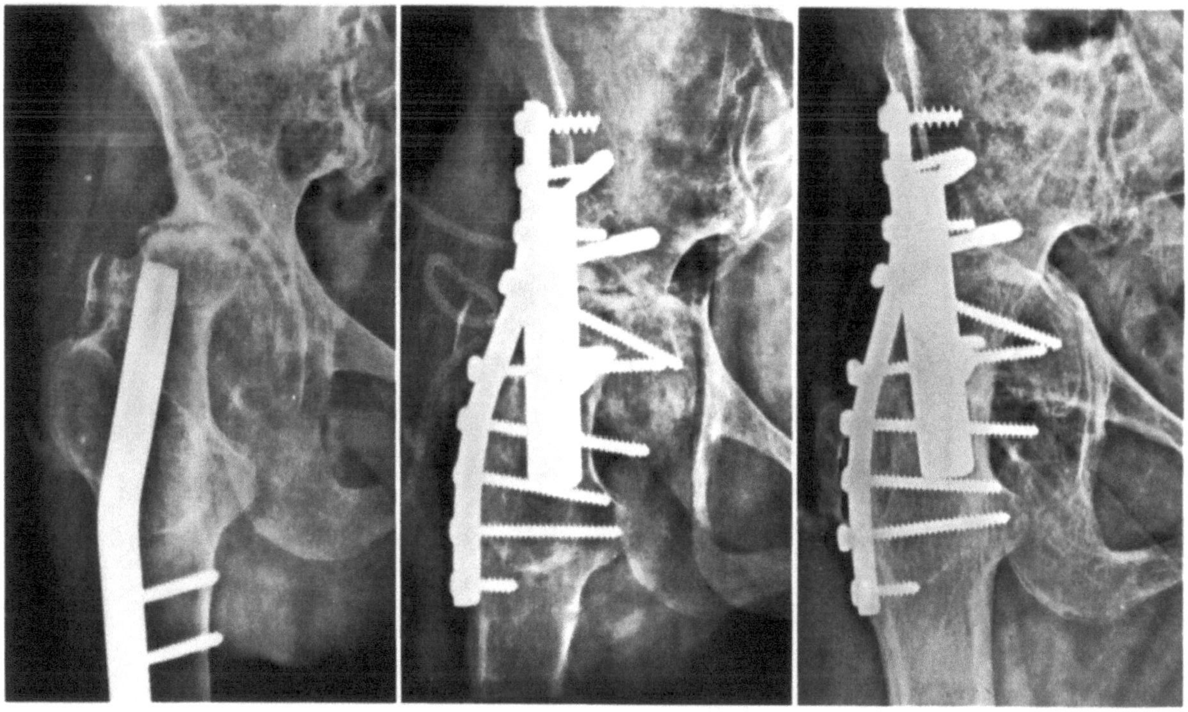

Fig. 180. *Type III HA in a case of partial NHF following IO*. M. M., ♀, aged 64 years, No. 71 118.

a) Partial NHF 2 years after IO performed for arthrosis of the hip.

b) Double-plate arthrodesis with PO.

c) Follow-up 7 years later. Arthrodesis united with good leg position and 3.5 cm leg shortening. Good subjective result with no complaints

a b

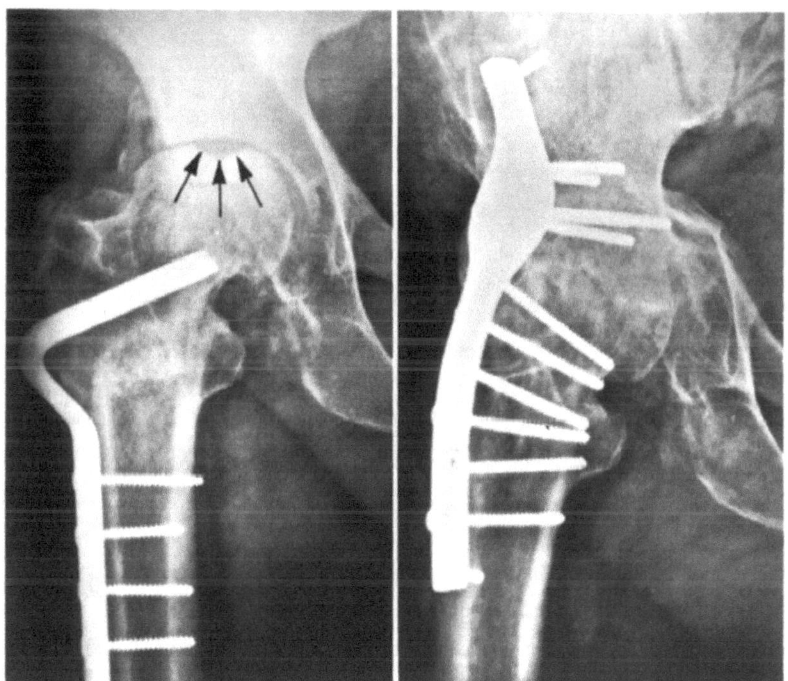

a b c

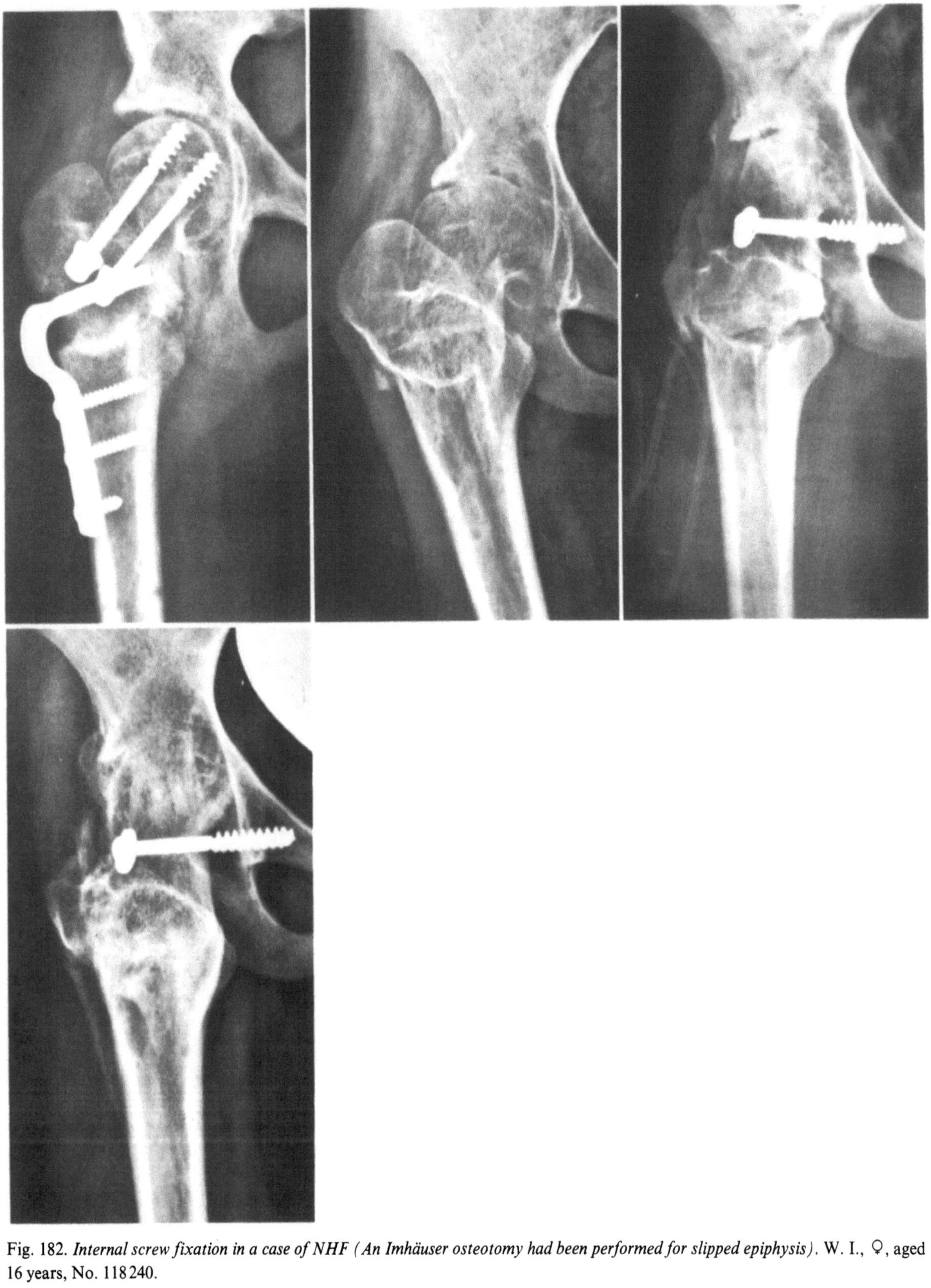

Fig. 182. *Internal screw fixation in a case of NHF (An Imhäuser osteotomy had been performed for slipped epiphysis).* W. I., ♀, aged 16 years, No. 118240.

a) One month following Imhauser osteotomy.

b) Deformation of the femoral head. Clinically almost complete ankylosis.

c) Screw arthrodesis (the proximal femur is brought into the vertical position; transverse IO).

d) Fourteen months later. Ideal arthrodesis. With 0.5 cm functional leg shortening.

e f g

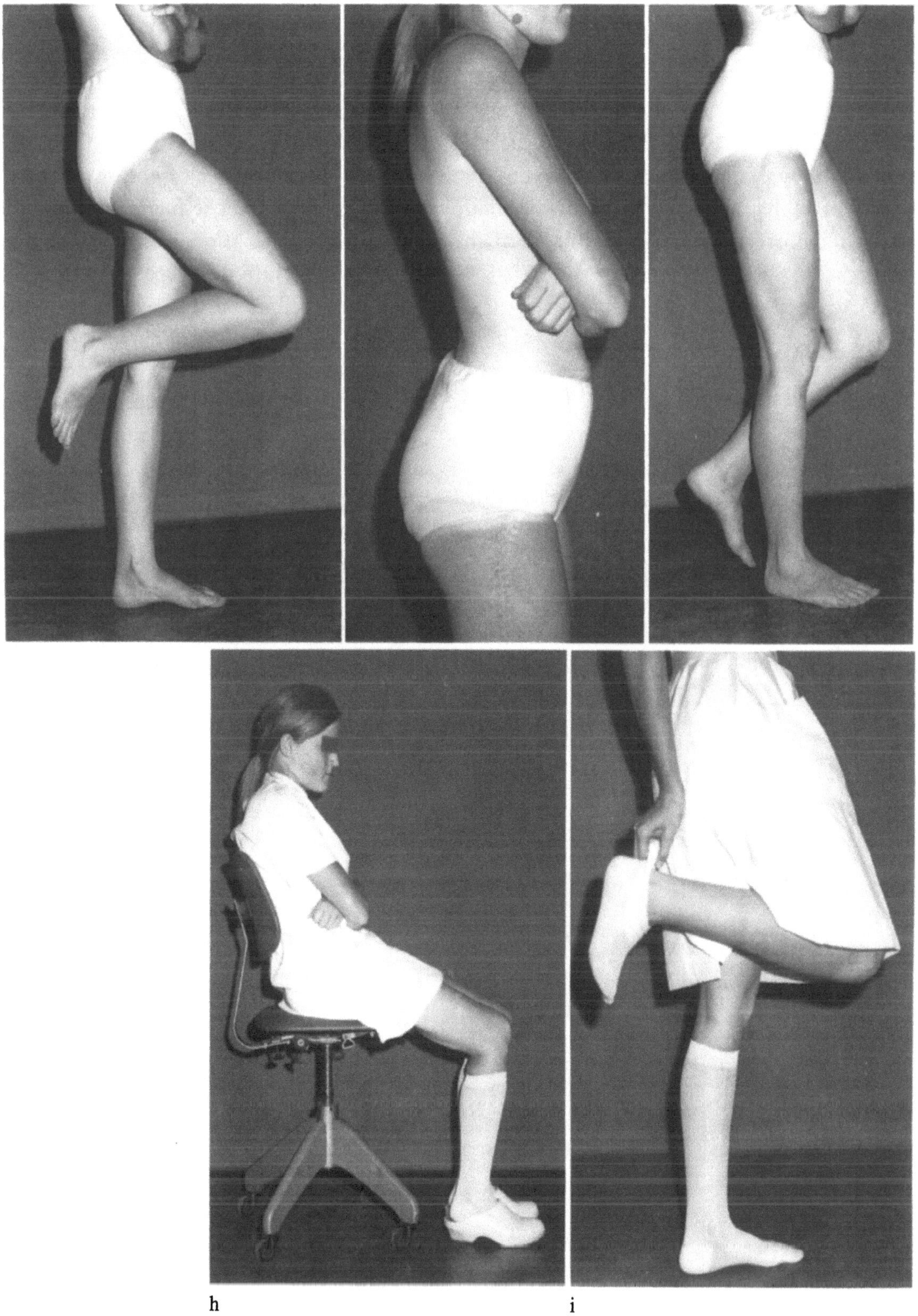

h i

Fig. 182e – i) Flexible LS allows sitting and gait of normal appearance. Socks can be pulled on easily since knee joint is freely mobile

5.4 Post-traumatic Necrosis of the Head of the Femur

Our series includes NHF following successful bone union of a femoral head fracture, following PA of such fractures and following inade quate or incorrect operative treatment of the fractures.

5.4.1 United Fracture

Statistics show that NHF results in 30% – 40% of femoral neck fractures as a direct result of the trauma or (sometimes additionally) as a consequence of the operation.

Frequently the necrosis is circumscribed and lies in the weight-bearing area but it may also include the whole head, corresponding to the area supplied by the vessel or vessels damaged. The prognosis in femoral neck fracture has not significantly improved despite more precise knowledge of the blood supply and new operative procedures. Although nowadays bone union of a femoral neck fracture almost always results from correct reduction, impaction and rigid internal fixation, disintegration of the head as a result of necrosis of the femoral neck may still occur 2 – 5 years following the fracture or even later.

An early sign of necrosis is loss of head sphericity. In fortunate cases, revitalisation and restructuring of the head may still occur at this stage. The final result is "head shrinkage."

However, if necrosis continues and is accompanied by weight bearing, the head disintegrates. In such cases prosthetic replacement is indicated in older patients and HA in younger patients (Fig. 183 – 189).

Fig. 183. *Type II HA in a case of post-traumatic arthrosis of the hip*. N. D., ♂, aged 28 years, No. 10637.

a) NHF with almost complete ankylosis of the hip 5 years after nailing (Smith-Petersen) of a fracture of the femoral neck.

b) HA with PO following resection of the necrotic superior part of the femoral head.

c) One year following operation. HA united with ideal leg position. With 1 cm leg shortening

a b c

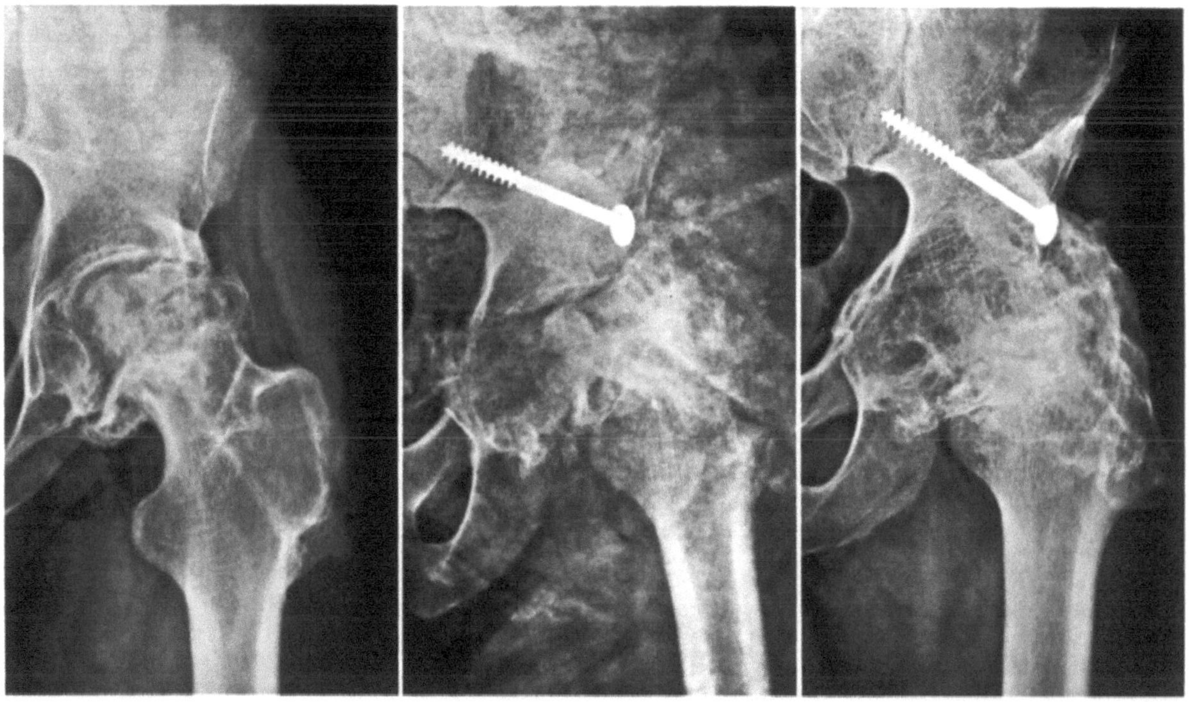

Fig. 184. *Type I HA following post-traumatic NHF.* E. K., ♂, aged 38 years, No. 75976.

a) NHF 13 years following nailing of a fracture of the femoral neck.

b) Immediately following arthrodesis. A cast has been applied.

c) Twenty-three months later. Perfect healing with 2.5 cm leg shortening

a b c

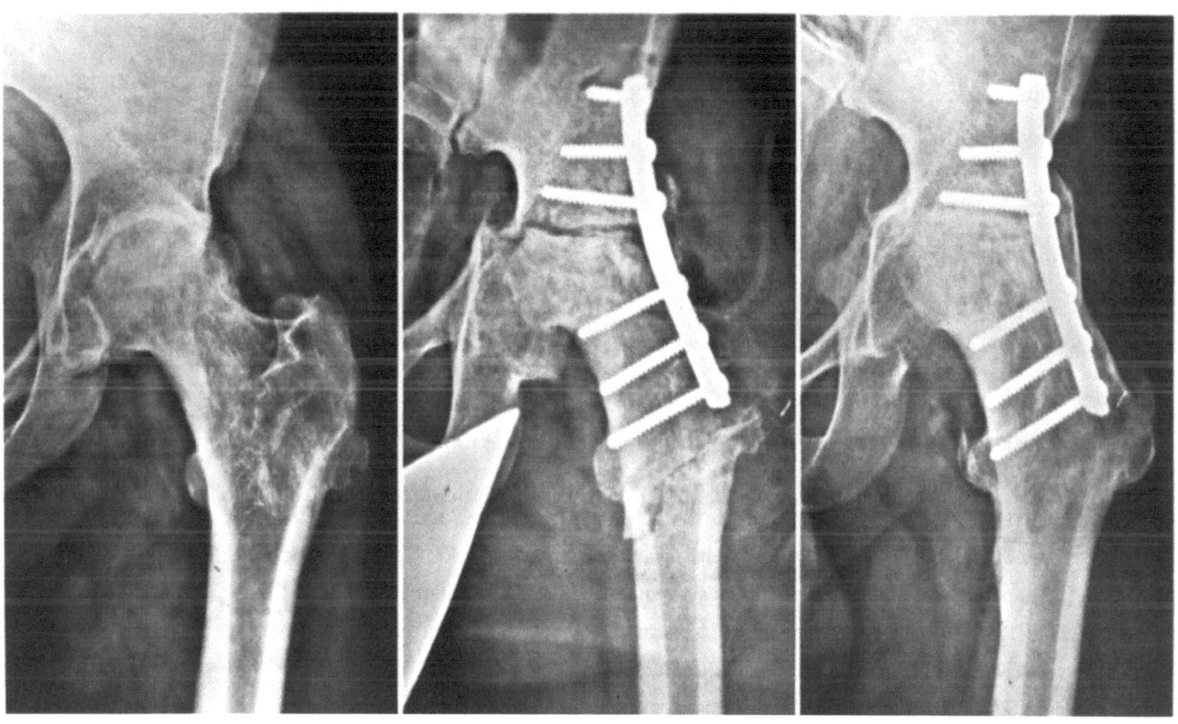

a b

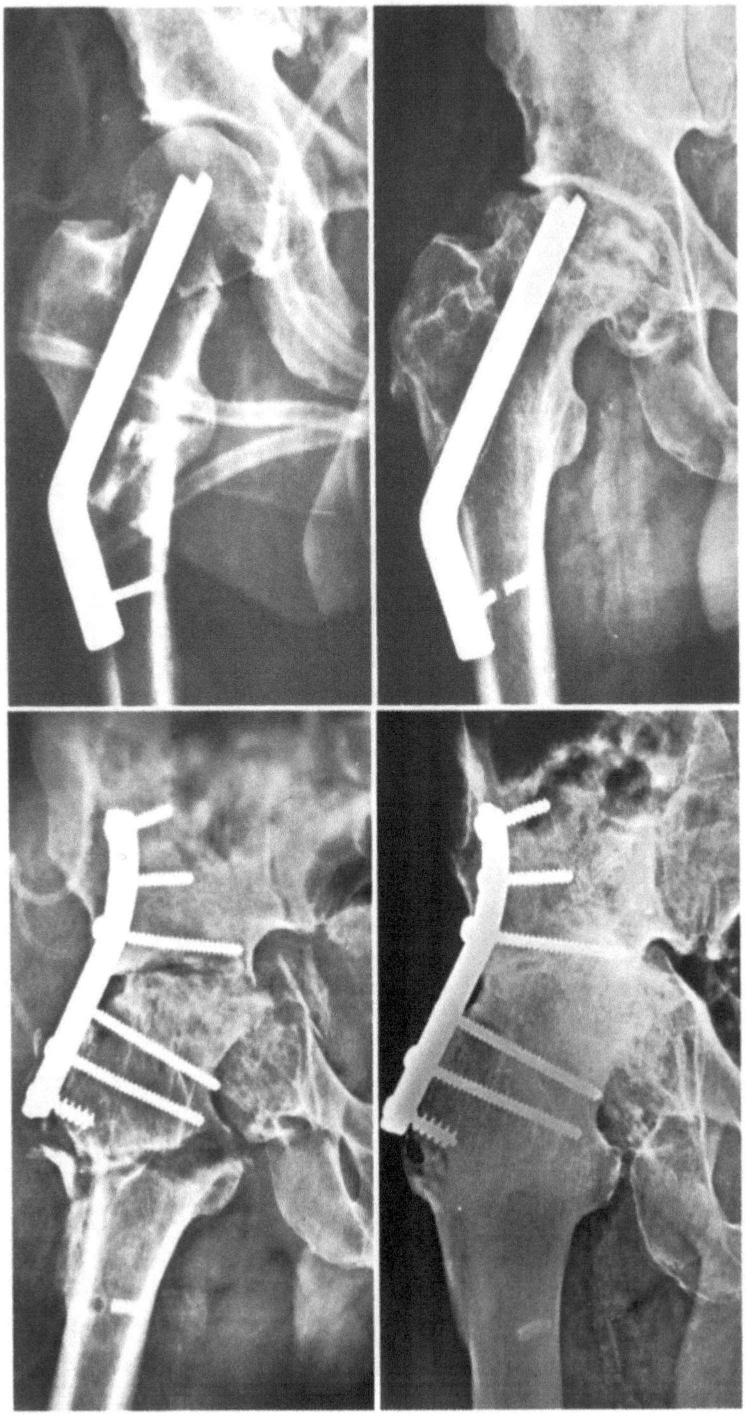

c d

Fig. 185. *Type II HA in a case of NHF following nailing of a femoral neck fracture*. M. J., ♂, aged 52 years, No. 68489.

a) Internal fixation of the month-old fracture of the medial femoral neck with restoration of neck angle.

b) Five years later. Radiotranslucency around the nail is a sign of loosening. Screw fracture and NHF.

c) Type II HA following PO and partial resection of the femoral head.

d) Five years later. HA and osteotomy united with ideal leg position and 3.5 cm leg shortening

a b c

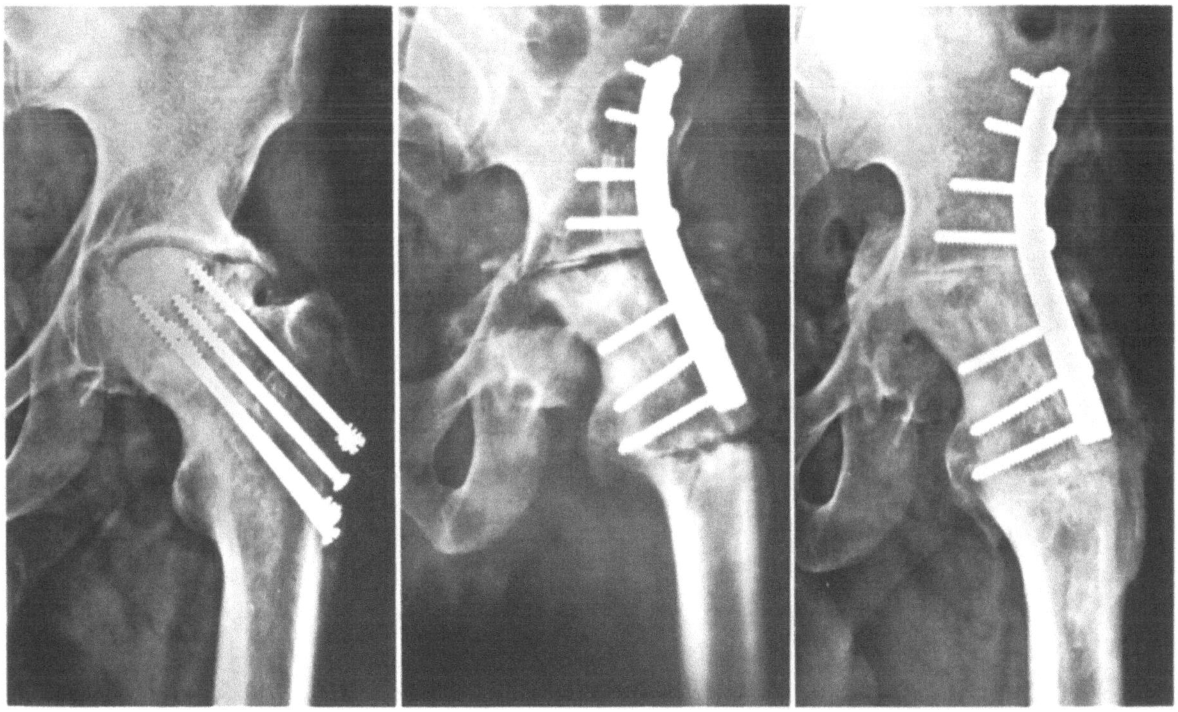

Fig. 186. *Type II HA in a case of NHF following screw fixation of a femoral neck fracture.* F. L., ♂, aged 42 years, No. 91401.

a) Five years after screw fixation. NHF.

b) Nineteen days following Type II HA. The necrotic femoral head has been largely resected.

c) Nine months later. HA and osteotomy united with ideal leg position. Limp-free gait; patient has returned to full-time work as labourer

a b

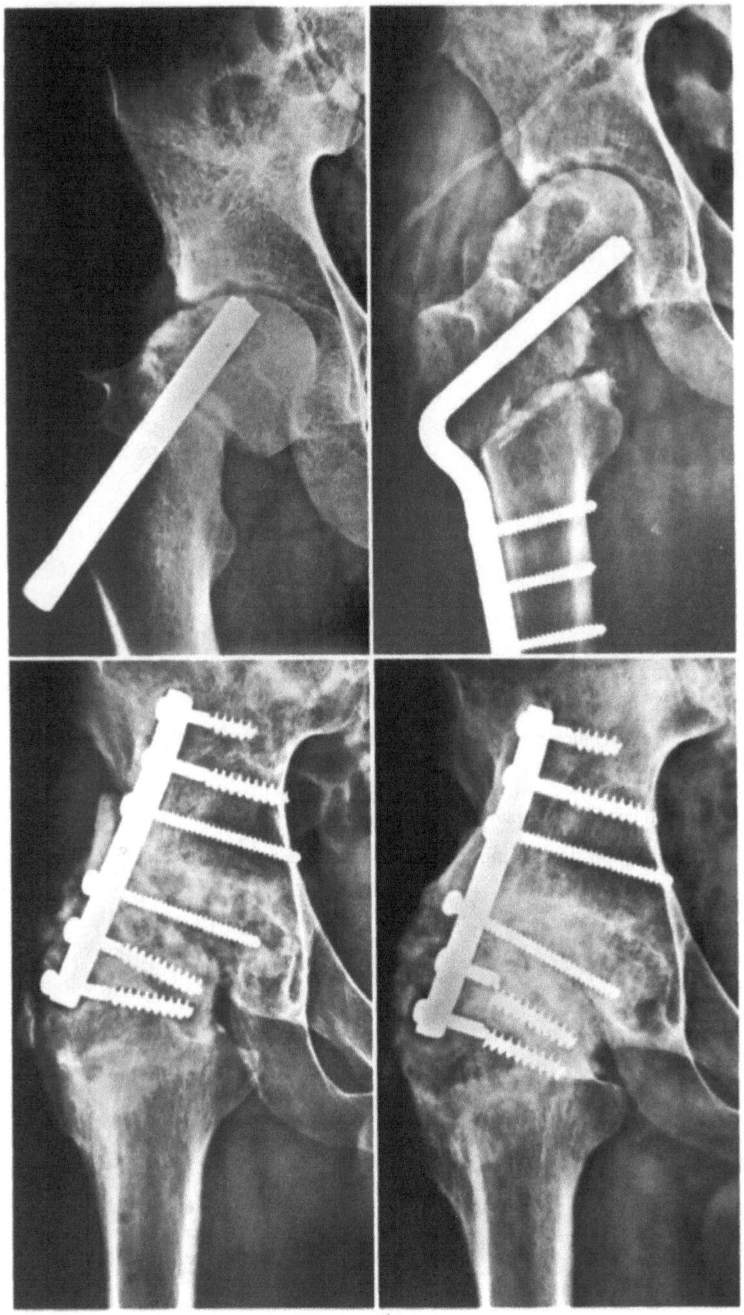

c d

Fig. 187. *Type II HA following PA and NHF.* H. F., ♂, aged 22 years, No. 81516

a) Seven months after nailing of a fatigue fracture of the femoral neck.

b) Transposition osteotomy for PA of the femoral neck. The loss of head sphericity is a sign of necrosis in the weight-bearing zone.

c) One year following Type II HA for extremely painful NHF. Incomplete union of the osteotomy. HA clinically united. The radiotranslucency around the plate and the heads of the screws indicates implant loosening which is a sign of inadequate rigidity.

d) Result $6^1/_2$ years following HA. Loosening and fracture of the distal screws. HA clinically and radiologically united. Good subjective result

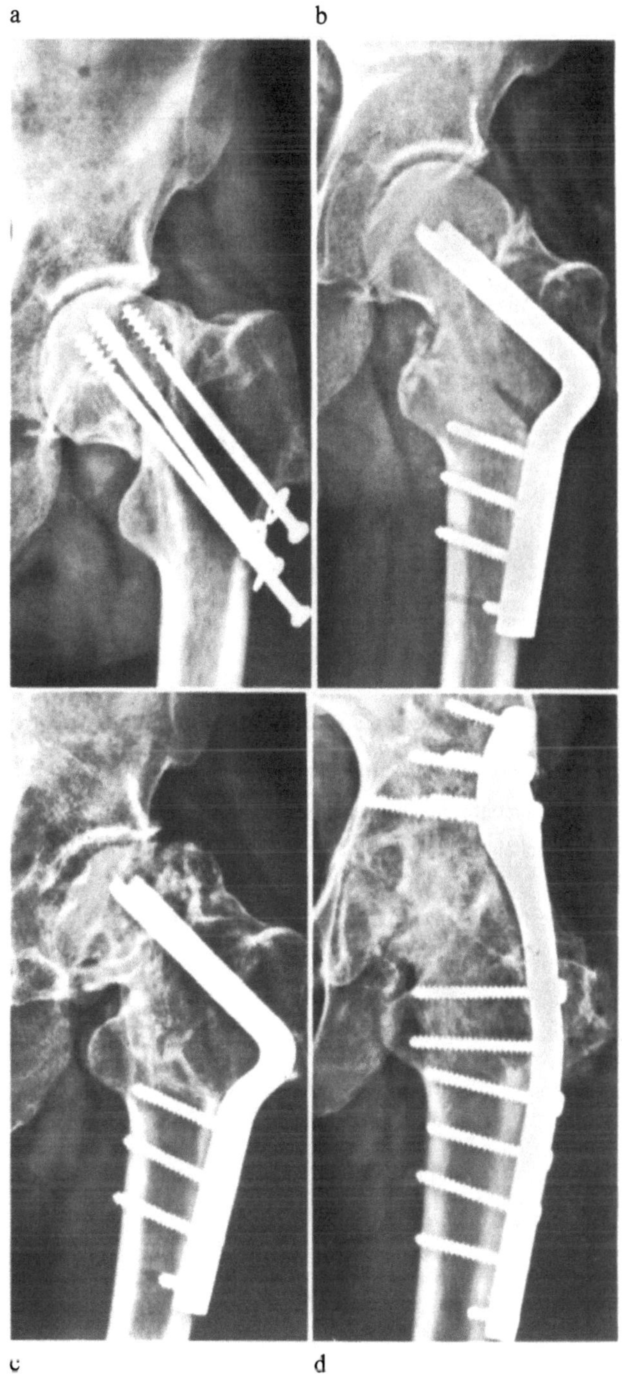

Fig. 188. *Type IV HA in a case of NHF.* A. J.-C., ♂, aged 39 years, No. 105248.

a) PA 10 months after screw fixation of a medial femoral neck fracture.

b) Transposition osteotomy with 30° valgus correction.

c) Two years later. PA united but NHF apparent.

d) Twenty-six months following cobra-head plate arthrodesis without PO. United with ideal leg position

a b c

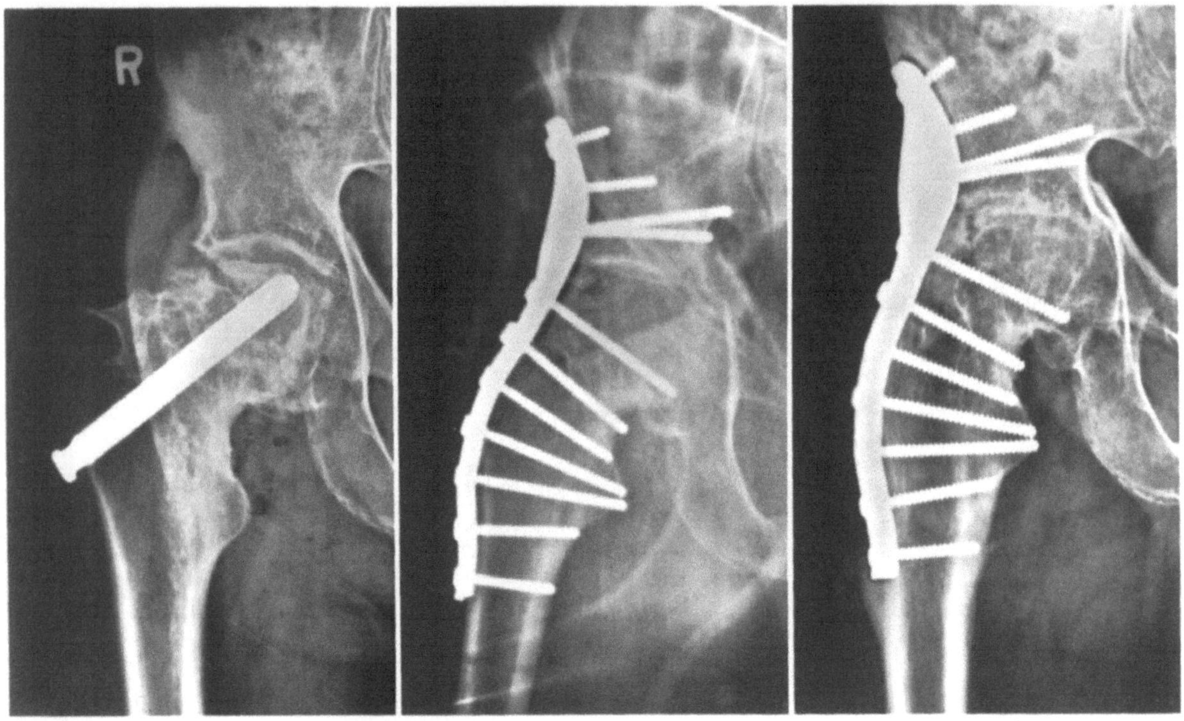

Fig. 189. *Cobra-head plate arthrodesis for painful ankylosis following NHF.* S. E., ♂, aged 60 years, No. 102422.

a) Eighteen months following nailing of the femoral neck. NHF.

b) Immediately following cobra-head plate arthrodesis with PO (following resection of the completely necrotic medial femoral head).

c) Two years following HA. United with good leg position. Good subjective result

a b c

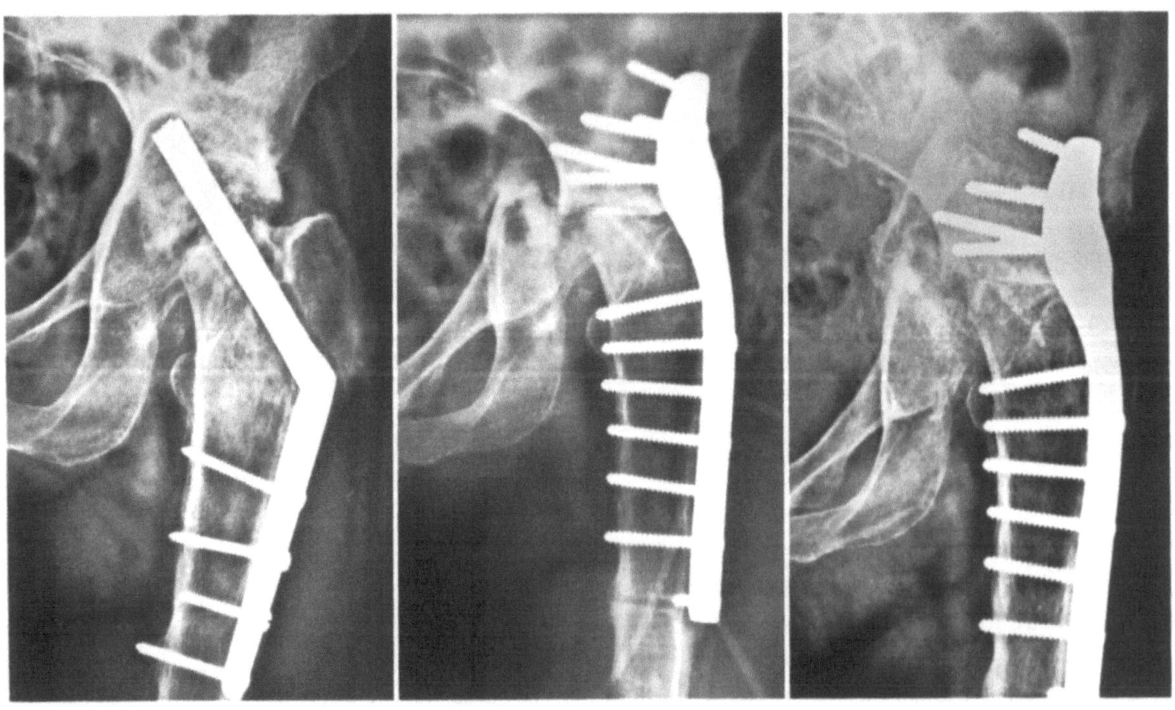

a b c d

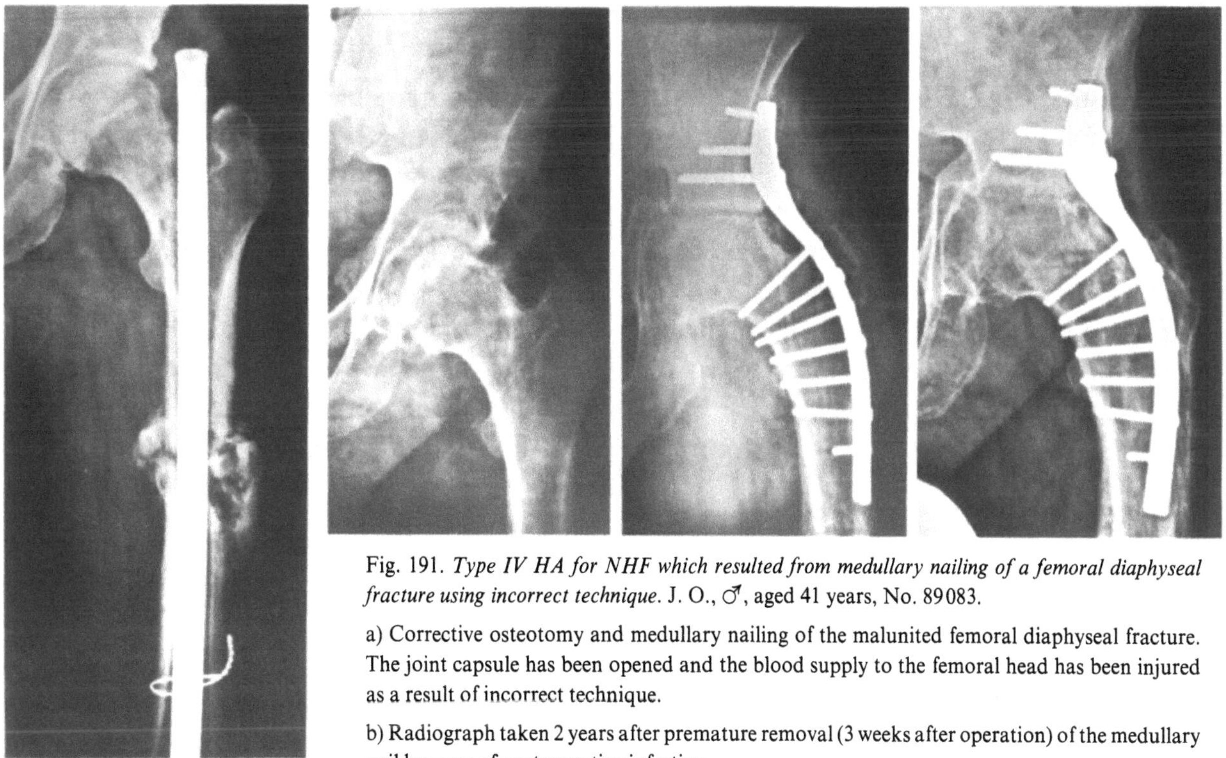

Fig. 191. *Type IV HA for NHF which resulted from medullary nailing of a femoral diaphyseal fracture using incorrect technique*. J. O., ♂, aged 41 years, No. 89083.

a) Corrective osteotomy and medullary nailing of the malunited femoral diaphyseal fracture. The joint capsule has been opened and the blood supply to the femoral head has been injured as a result of incorrect technique.

b) Radiograph taken 2 years after premature removal (3 weeks after operation) of the medullary nail because of postoperative infection.

c) Immediately following HA with rigid internal fixation and PO.

d) Radiograph 38 months following operation. HA united with ideal leg position

5.4.2 Pseudarthrosis Following Femoral Neck Fracture

Head necrosis is not infrequently accompanied by PA of the femoral neck. The more medial the fracture, the greater the chances of PA occurring. The frequency of PA following medial femoral neck fractures depends on whether the treatment was operative (average PA frequency = 14.6% in 4916 operations) or nonoperative (average PA frequency = 36.7% in 708 cases). The PA frequency also depends on whether the fracture was dislocated or not (only four PA in 318 nondislocated fractures) (Nigst, Banks).

The circumstances are ideal for HA is cases where a partially necrotic and partially revitalised head is incorporated into the acetabulum. An economical wedge resection of the PA is performed and complemented by rigid cobra-head plate fixation (Fig. 190).

5.4.3 Hip Arthrodesis as a Result of Inadequate or Incorrect Operative Technique

Although medullary nailing may be regarded as a conventional internal fixation method we still see NHF as a result of incorrect technique. Particularly introduction of the guide

Fig. 190. *Type IV HA for PA of the femoral neck and partial NHF*. B. M., ♂, aged 49 years, No. 152062.

a) PA 6 months following internal fixation of a medial fracture of the femoral neck. The partially necrotic and partially revitalised femoral head is incorporated into the acetabulum.

b) HA with cobra-head plate following resection of a 1 cm-thick bone disc right through the PA and the pelvis.

c) Four months after HA. PA and HA united. Ideal leg position and 1.5 cm leg shortening rod from the distal end in a proximal direction instead of from the tip of the trochanter causes the joint to be opened on driving in the nail and the joint capsule is partially torn. This causes damage to the vessels supplying the weight-bearing area of the head. Damage to the vessels or postoperative infection cause NHF or joint infection. In order to prevent this complication, the ASIF recommends downward open nailing with precise reduction of the fracture under direct vision (Fig. 191).

6 Hip Arthrodeses in Girdlestone Hip and Similar Conditions

6.1 Introduction

The femoral head resection first described by GIRDLESTONE in 1924 is a mutilating operation with severe permanent disadvantages. The original wide range of indications (hip arthrosis, rheumatoid arthritis, tuberculitic and nontuberculitic hip infection) is now limited to TP failure and infected fractures of the femoral neck.

The main indication for GH nowadays is the infected prosthesis in which no improvement can be expected by perfusion drainage or TP replacement.

The permanent disadvantages are the considerable degree of leg shortening and reduced hip stability. Follow-up of 30 GH patients in our clinic showed the result to be unsatisfactory in almost a quarter (poor hip stability; average maximum duration of walking 45 min; mean leg shortening of 4 cm; muscle insufficiency). For this reason, HA is certainly to be preferred to resection of the femoral head if the former is feasible.

Arthrodesis of a GH is one of the problem operations in orthopaedic surgery. Loss of the femoral head and femoral neck causes considerable leg shortening. If GH followed removal of a cemented TP, the bone in the proximal femoral diaphysis is biologically inferior (inadequate trochanteric cancellous bone). Furthermore, there is always the possibility of quiescent infection.

For these reasons the biological and biomechanical environment is disadvatageous to HA. The situation is better following prosthetic replacement without cement since there is less bone destruction in the proximal femur.

In our series we differentiate between:

a) GH
b) GH-like conditions

6.2 Girdlestone Hips

We have performed HA in the following situations:

a) Subsequent to prosthetic replacement
b) In GH without infection
c) In GH with clinically eradicated infection

6.2.1 Subsequent to Prosthetic Replacement

In these cases, HA is technically possible either immediately following removal of the prothesis or, if the latter has already been removed, for the treatment of painful instability of the hip.

Fig. 193. *Type III HA following Judet prosthesis implanted for arthrosis of the hip*. M. M., ♀, aged 58 years, No. 93166.

a) Thirteen years following implantation of the prosthesis. Up to a year ago the patient had had no problems.

b) HA with rigid internal fixation with double plate following PO.

c) Six weeks later. Incipient bone union. Patient walking with canes (50% weight bearing). Standing on one leg possible without pain

a b c

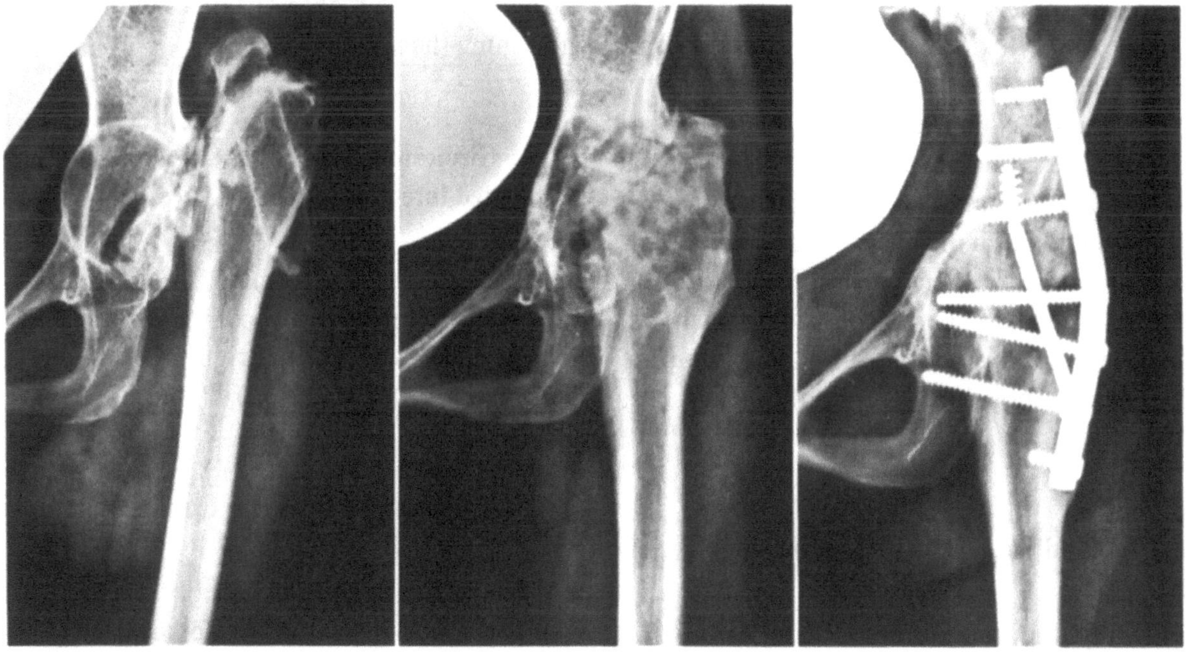

Fig. 192. *Type II HA following Judet prosthesis (CDH)*. B. E., ♀, aged 29 years, No. 74068.

a) Eight months following implantation of a Judet prosthesis the prosthesis had to be removed because it had fractured and dislocated.

b) Five years following impaction of the trochanter in the acetabulum. Painful but mobile hip (65 – 0 – 0°, 10 – 0 – 10°, 0 – 0°) with formation of a secondary joint between the acetabulum and the trochanter.

c) Three years following HA. United with good leg position. Only sensitivity to weather change remains

a b c

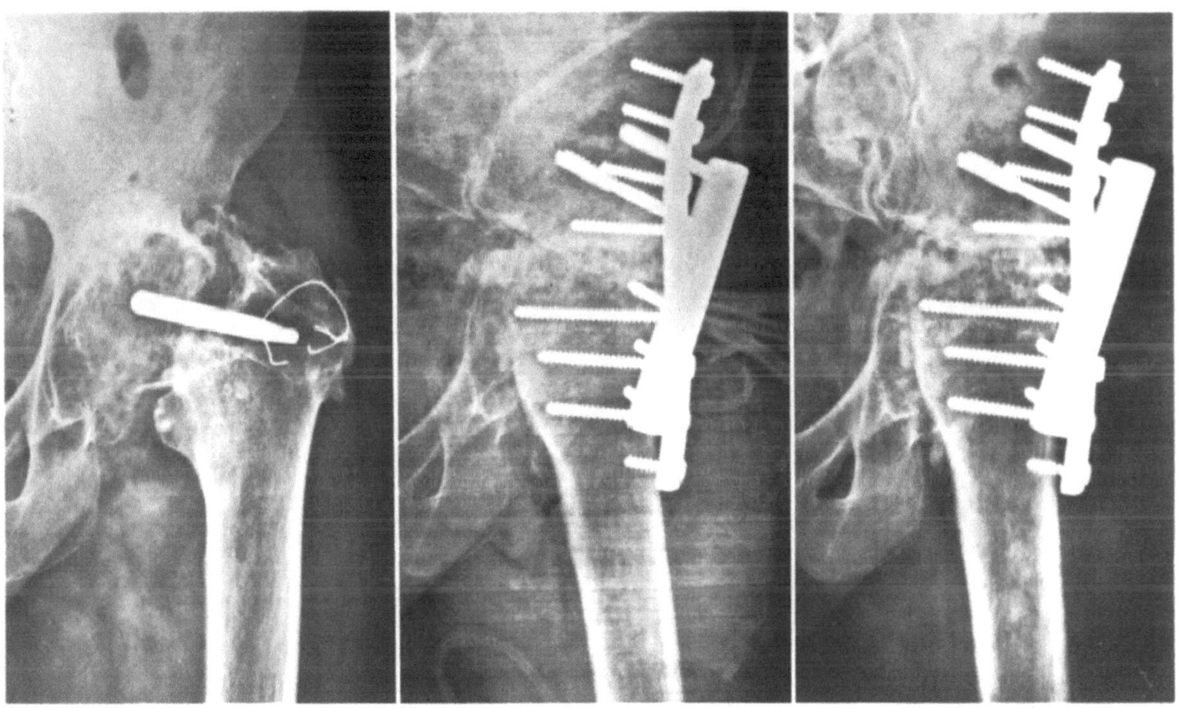

In our three cases of this type, reoperation was necessary twice because of instability and PA of the first HA.

Since the healing tendency is markedly reduced, the internal plate fixation must be very rigid. Cancellous bone plasty must be performed simultaneously to accelerate healing and fill the bone defect. Medialisation following PO improves contact between the surfaces and application of the plate with the leg correctly positioned is simplified (Figs. 192, 193).

6.2.2 Girdlestone Hip without Infection

Basically the same rules obtain as in HA following removal of an endoprosthesis.

In special cases where a viable head is incorporated into the acetabulum (such as is possible in the presence of femoral neck PA) decortication of the sloping contact surfaces and internal plate fixation suffices.

This technique makes HA possible without shortening the leg (Fig. 194).

6.2.3 Girdlestone Hip Following Clinically Eradicated Infection

In these cases, HA with minimal internal fixation is to be preferred. Following Tb of the hip, however, HA with normal rigid internal plate fixation is allowed (Fig. 195).

6.3 Girdlestone-Hip-Like Conditions

HA is indicated and technically feasible in young patients in whom the femoral head is either resorbed or totally necrotic (post-traumatic cases). In these cases, the necrotic bone of the femoral head and possibly that of the femoral neck is resected. HA with the usual internal compression fixation follows (Figs. 196 – 199).

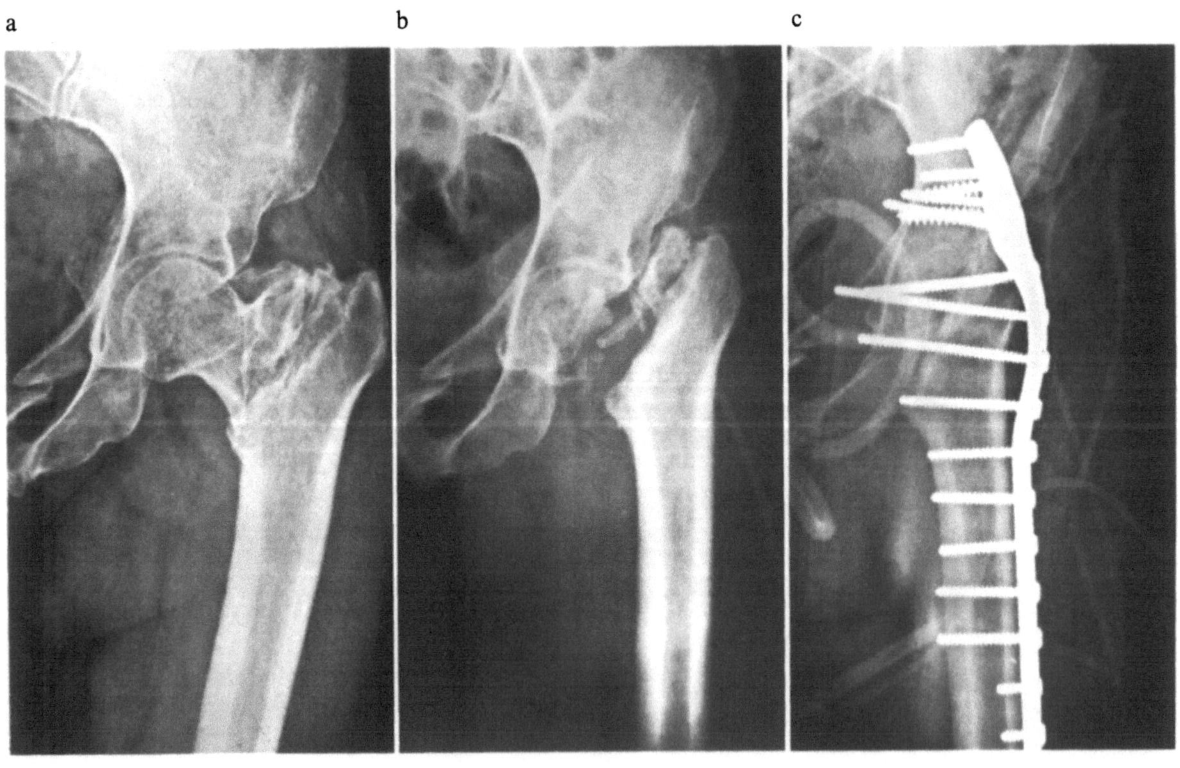

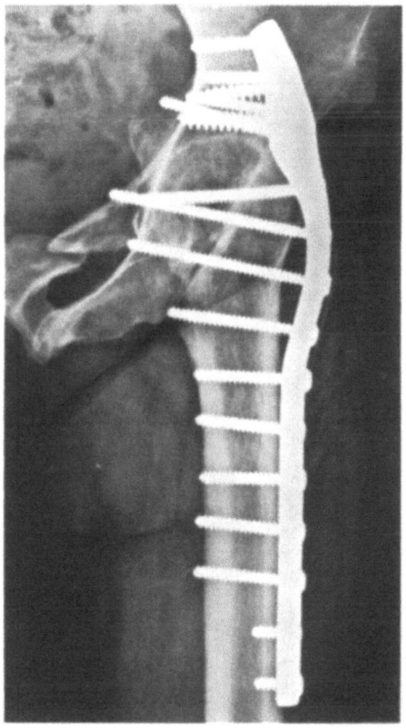

e

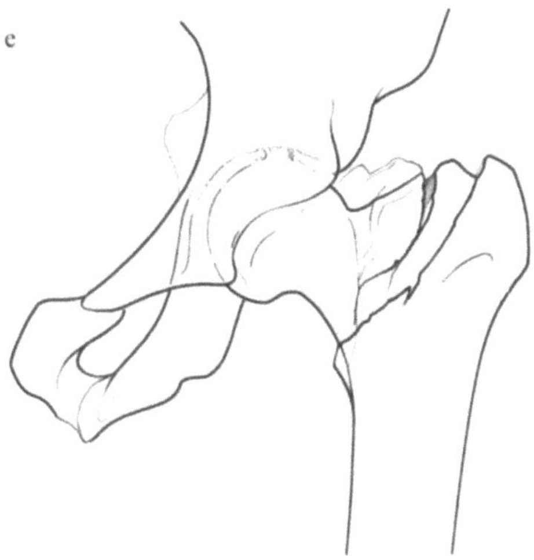

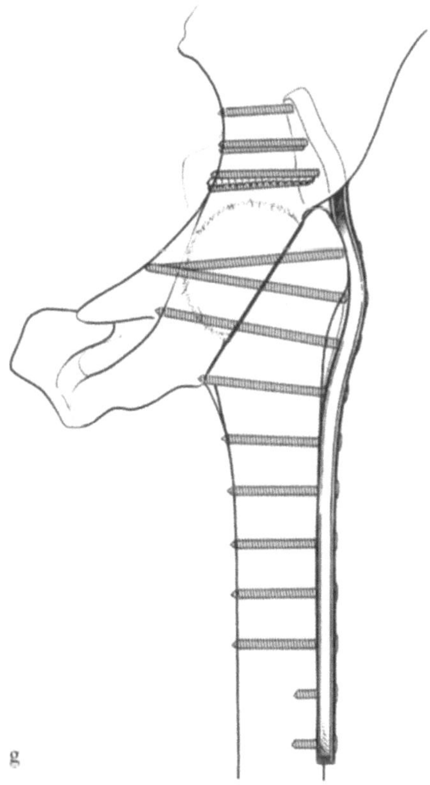

g

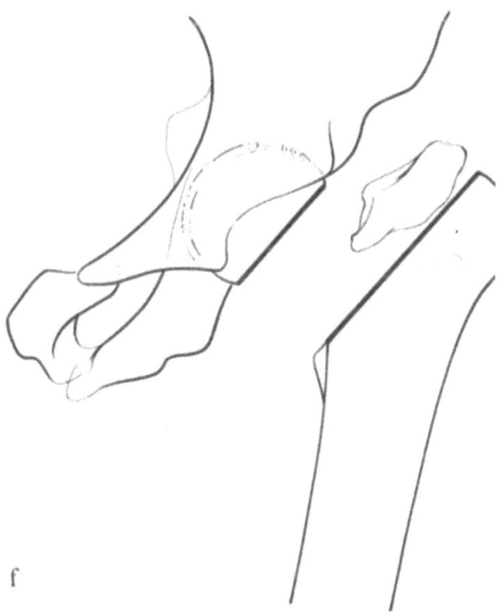

f

◀ Fig. 194. *Type IV HA following resection of the femoral head.* B. J., ♀, aged 46 years, No. 150431.

a) One year following fracture of both pubic rami on both sides. PA of a conservatively treated intratrochanteric femoral fracture with tilting of the head in varus.

b) First stage: resection of the femoral head. The planned transposition osteotomy was impossible since the viable femoral head had been walled into the acetabulum.

c) Second stage: cobra-head plate arthrodesis 2 weeks later.

d) Four months later. The HA is united. Painless gait without cane. Return to full-time work.

e – g) Diagrammatic representation of a – c.

e) Femoral head walled in. PA.

f) Viable head left in acetabulum. Osteotomy at level of PA.

g) Ideal contact between femoral head and proximal end of femur. Perfect stability with the cobra-head plate.

a b c

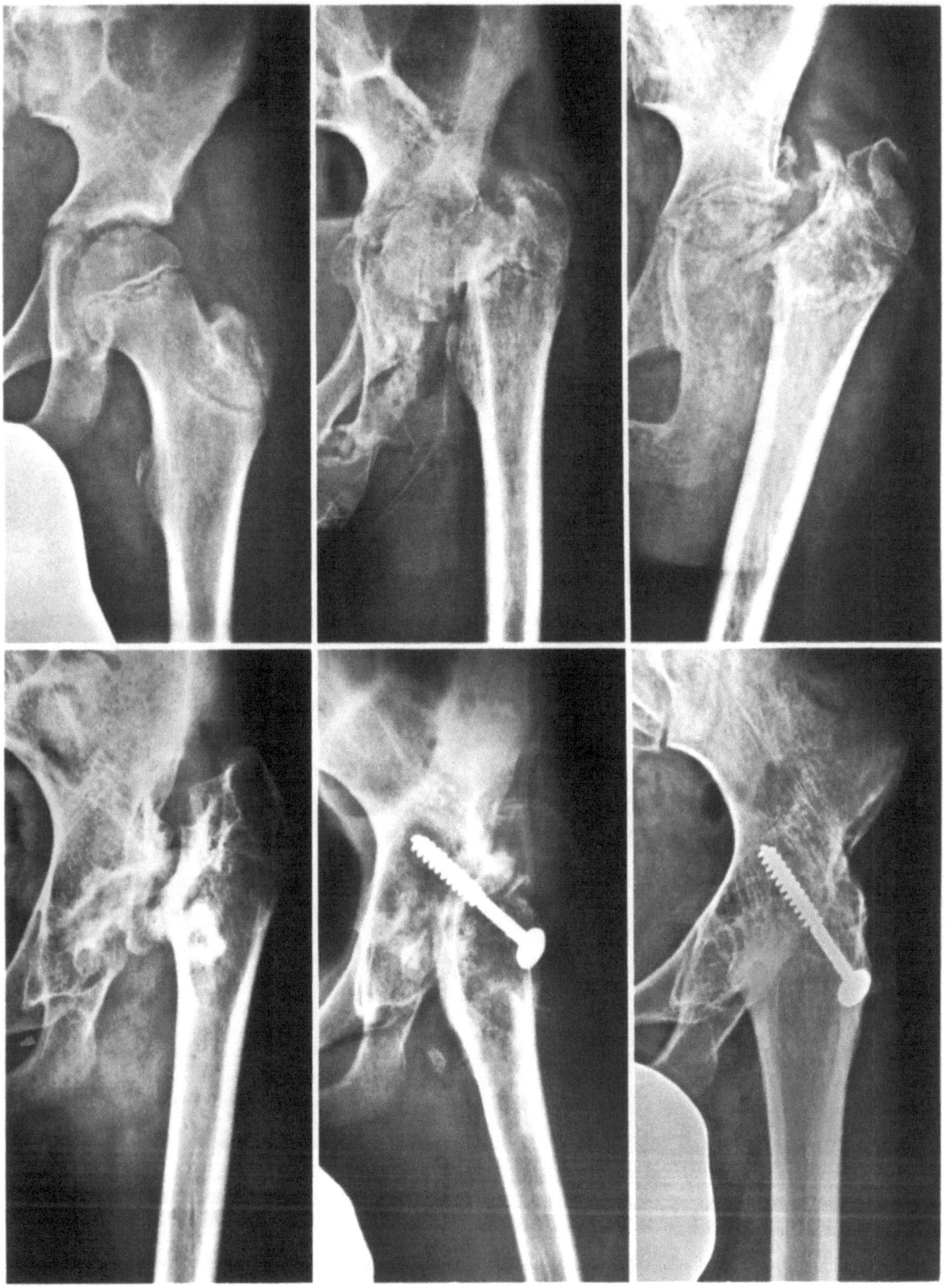

d e f

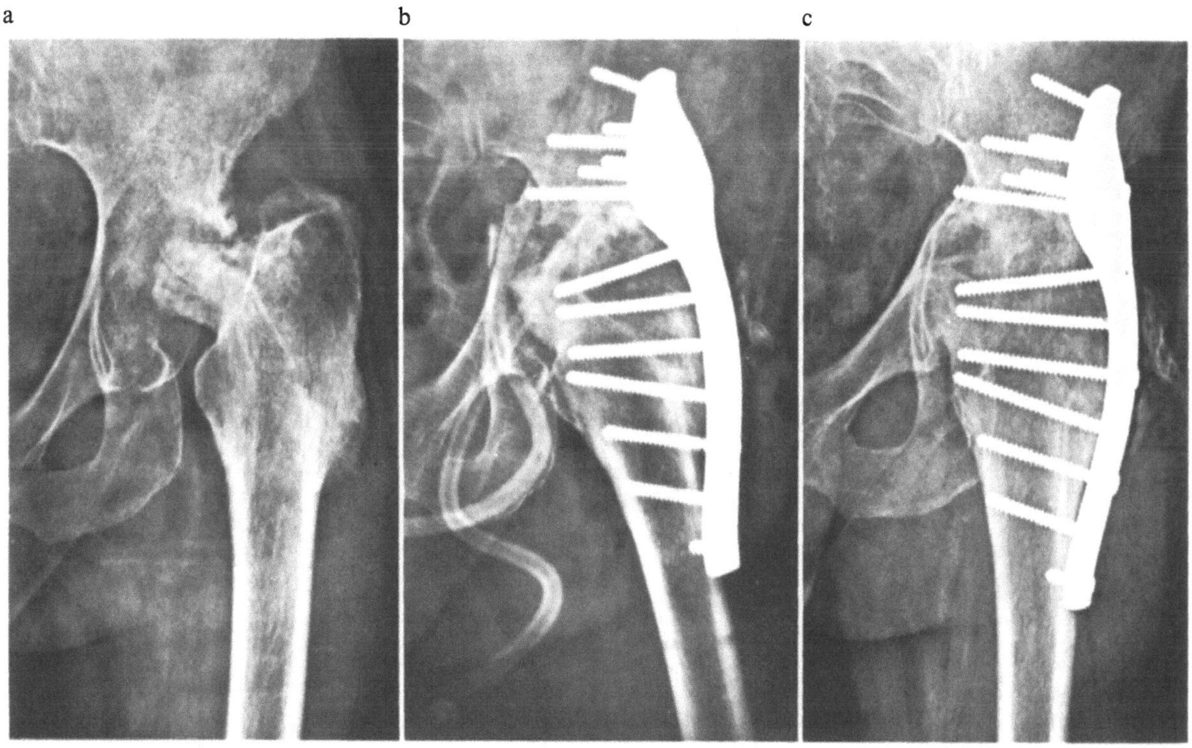

Fig. 196. *Cobra-head plate arthrodesis for NHF following nailing of a femoral neck fracture.* H. B., ♀, aged 64 years, No. 98864.

a) Twenty-eight months after nailing of the femoral neck fracture (nail removed 1 year after insertion) there is NHF and ankylosis of the joint in flexion, adduction and external rotation.

b) Following excision of the NHF and resection of the femoral neck, PO is performed with a moderate degree of medial displacement and is followed by cobra-head plate arthrodesis.

c) Ten months later. HA objectively and subjectively ideal

←

Fig. 195. *Arthrodesis of a Girdlestone hip.* M. Ch., ♂, aged 15 years, No. 99268.

a) Incipient septic arthritis not yet radiologically visible.

b) Nine weeks later following drug therapy.

c) A further 4 months later. Necrosis in the region of the femoral epiphysis with spontaneous fracture of the femoral neck and extensive joint destruction.

d) Two years after removal of the necrotic femoral neck and head. 6 cm leg shortening.

e) HA and hip spica following preparatory supracondylar traction with Steinmann pins and adductorotomy.

f) Twenty-nine months after HA. The latter is united in 10° adduction

a b

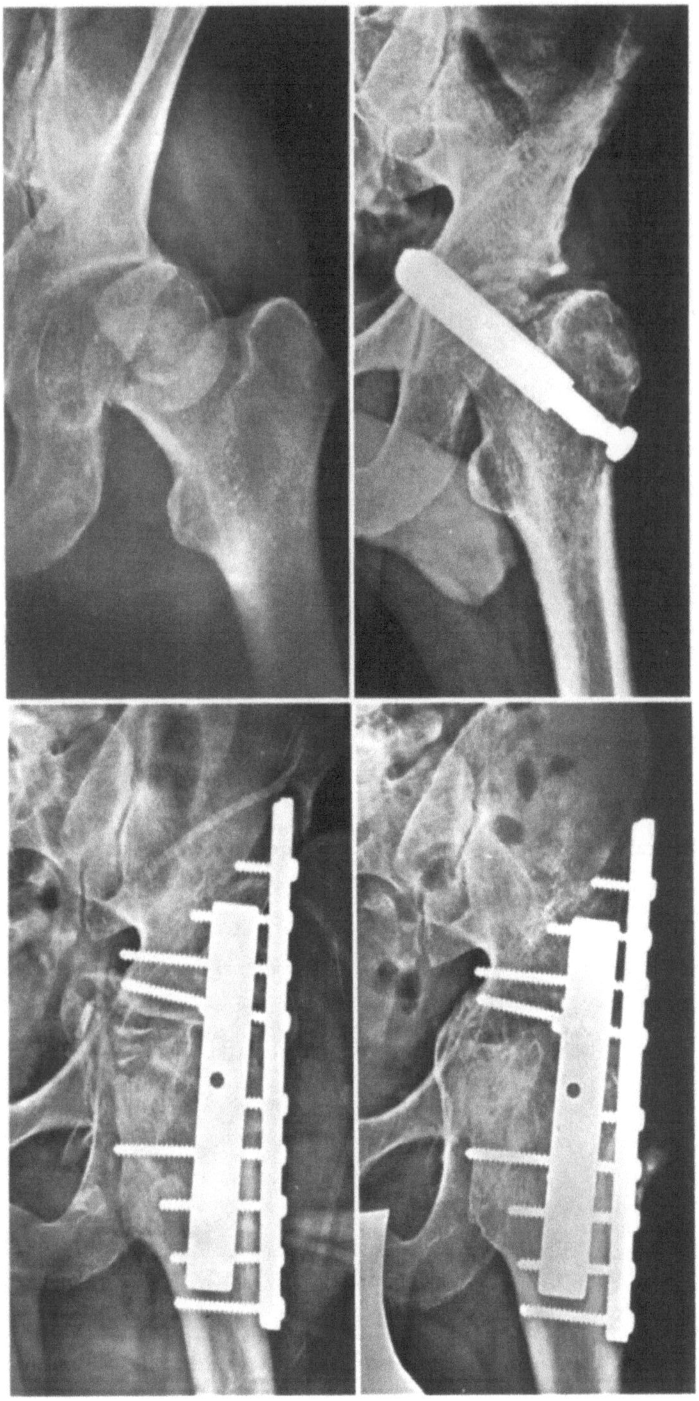

c d

Fig. 197. *Type III HA for PA following attempted HA with trifin nail in another hospital.* J. H., ♂, aged 35 years, No. 73416.

a) Ten days after accident.

b) Unstable HA with trifin nail.

c) HA with rigid internal fixation and PO.

d) Twenty-five months later. HA and PA healed

a b c

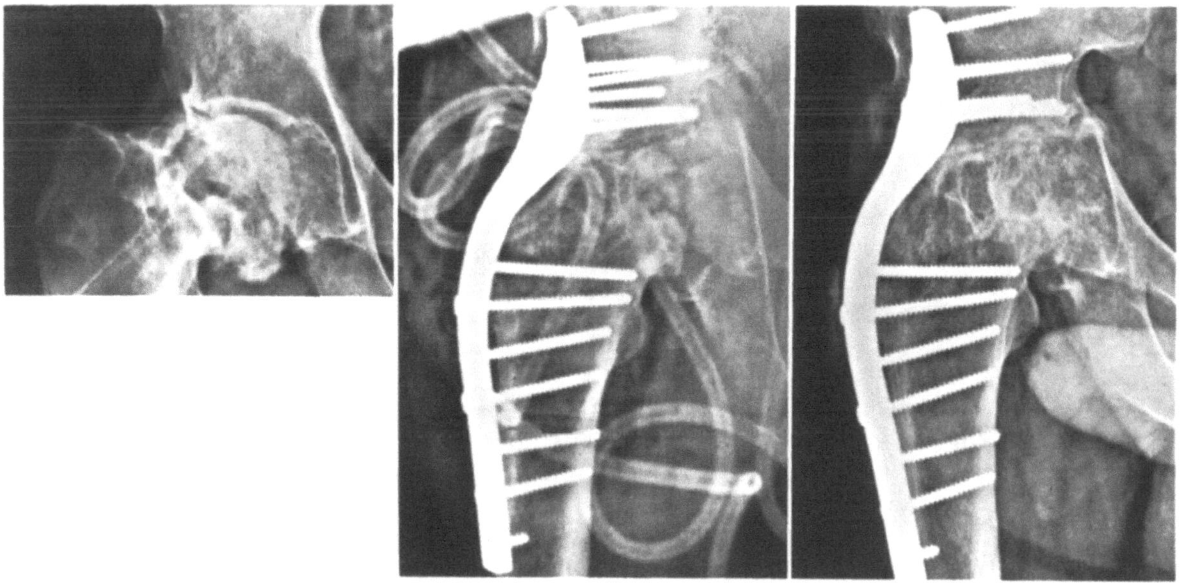

Fig. 198. *Type IV HA in a case of NHF secondary to nailing of a femoral neck fracture*. R. J., ♂, aged 50 years, No. 106819.

a) Four years following nailing of the femoral neck fracture (2 years after implant removal). PA and NHF visible.

b) Cobra-head plate arthrodesis with PO. The completely devitalised femoral head was resected.

c) Ten months after HA. Clinically and radiologically united arthrodesis with 2 cm leg shortening. Patient has returned to full-time work as innkeeper

a b c

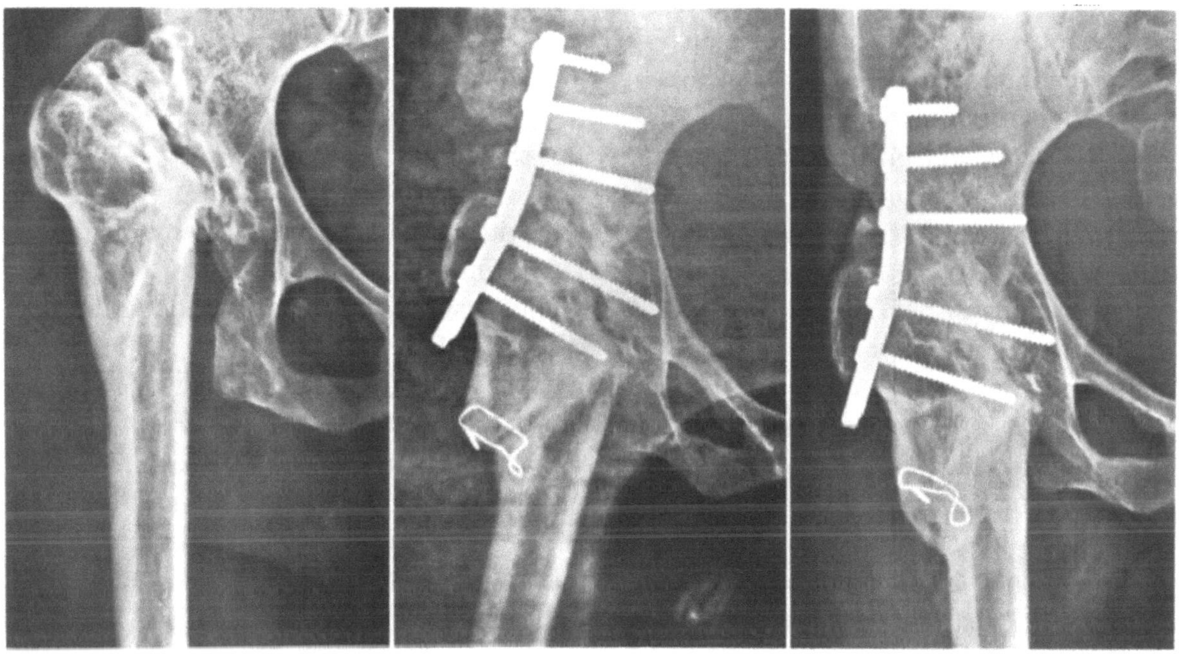

Fig. 199. *Type II HA following infantile hip sepsis*. W. M., ♀, aged 48 years, No. 136438.

a) Very high trochanter with completely deformed hip joint. Pseudoacetabulum. Loss of femoral head and femoral neck, and *9 cm* leg shortening.

b) Two months following Type II HA (still in cast). Cerclage wiring to prevent displacement of the osteotomy.

c) Twenty months following HA. Bone union with good leg position. Still 6 cm leg shortening (corrected with orthopaedic shoe). Patient complaint-free and working full time in a post office

III. Hip Arthrodesis and Total Prosthesis

1 Introduction

Of the three most frequent hip operations (IO, HA and TP), TP has become the commonest in the last 7 years. Some orthopaedic and general surgeons were, or still are, of the opinion that TP is now the operation of choice for all forms of hip arthrosis and have rejected IO almost completely and HA totally. TP certainly has many advantages (freedom from pain, very good range of motion, no difficulties with adaptation, simple postoperative management), but the experience of approximately 10 years to date is inadequate and the increasing occurrence of problems to which solutions have not yet been found (loosening of anchorage, signs of wear, secondary trophic changes) is such that wholesale acceptance of the technique and rejection of other techniques is not yet justifiable. Early or late TP infections usually have more serious consequences than those occurring following IO or HA (Boitzy and Zimmermann; Charnley and Eftekhar). Continuing improvement in the design of artificial joints, simplification of operative techniques and measures to prevent infection (prophylactic vaccination, sterile operating boxes) justify the hopes that the problems may one day be solved but until then, caution should be exercised in the choice of indications. A certain optimism is justified, but euphoria is not.

The situation was well summarised by the still-valid statement of Hanslik and Friedebold: "Prognoses as to the duration of adequacy of function are valid for precisely as long as the duration of past experience."

It is always possible that the TP will later be partially replaced by another biomechanically better operation since, as Hackenbroch emphasised in 1959: "arthrodesis and arthroplasty are only replacements; they offer apparent healing, a sanatio per defectum."

HA and TP represent the two extremes in surgical treatment of hip disease. Sometimes, if both hips are affected one side is arthrodesed and the other is replaced with a joint prosthesis. Until now little has been published on the problems and results of combined TP-HA. We have therefore followed up all our cases and the results are reported in the first part of this chapter.

IO still has its place and will survive the present widespread movement towards TP (Müller). It has the advantage that a second operation is usually possible without considerable difficulty if the IO fails or if postoperative complications result. However, reoperation is more and more frequently considered following HA and TP. Thus it is now possible to replace an HA by a TP in cases where increasing age of the patient is accompanied by intolerable back complaints or increasing knee stiffness. The limits, difficulties and results of replacement of an HA by a TP are discussed in the second part.

Systematic follow-up of all patients in whom a TP has been implanted has shown that 4 – 5 years following the operation, a further operation was indicated or had been carried out in approximately 30% of cases (SCHNEIDER: 35% reoperated in a first series of 109 patients from September 1961 – 31st December 1967 and 5.9% in a second series of 1572 patients from 1st January 1968 – 31st May 1973: HUGGLER, 10% – 30%). With increasing frequency cups, shafts or whole prostheses have been replaced, usually with success as far as one can judge. Nevertheless we are chary about performing primary implant replacement in a case of infected TP since in our opinion the risk of renewed infection is too great despite the use of perfusion and suction drainage, gentamycin-containing bone cement and antibiotics. We still prefer a staged procedure, i.e., preliminary removal of the TP and bone cement followed by perfusion and suction drainage and then, 6 – 12 months later, implantation of a new TP if there are no signs of local or generalised infection.

If the latter is impossible, however, there are only two main surgical possibilities available, namely GH and HA. HA is certainly preferable to GH if feasible since it offers more hip stability, less leg shortening and less muscle insufficiency. In our series we have only a few cases of prosthetic replacement (Judet or Thompson prostheses, TP) following HA. The last part of this chapter deals with this latter problematical procedure.

2 Hip Arthrodesis Combined with Total Prosthesis on the Opposite Side

2.1 Statement of Problem

In cases of bilateral hip disease, particularly in young working patients, the question is frequently raised as to whether an HA on the side with the more limited range of movement should be combined with a TP on the opposite side. The detrimental effects of a HA on the contralateral TP are always being mentioned. One might theoretically expect increased prosthesis wear since the stress on the prosthesis is increased by the total transfer of rotatory motion from the arthrodesed side. With this in mind we followed up all our patients clinically and radiologically but were unable to confirm the latter supposition on comparing our findings to those obtained in other TP patients. Furthermore, we found no difference in range of movement of the TP hip between patients with a HA on the opposite side and patients with unilateral or bilateral TP. In the presence of severe bilateral hip joint changes, bilateral TP should be limited to patients over 60 years of age. Severe degenerative change in the lumbosacral region which frequently occurs at this age is also a contraindication to HA. Again, in the opinion of many authors (WITT et al; GOEB, DEBEYRE et al; WALCHER) bilateral TP is preferable to combination of HA with TP, even in some exceptional cases of rheumatic disease in younger patients, e.g., progressive chronic rheumatoid arthritis or ankylosing spondylitis. This is supported by our follow-up findings: in the rheumatoid hips we found none of the complications which are known to occur following TP for other indications. There were no cases of cup loosening (even after 6 – 7 years) and patients remained free from pain over periods of years with good mobility and unchanged walking ability as well as increase of the bone density around the cemented cup (SEGMÜLLER).

In other cases we prefer to combine HA with TP if IO is no longer possible.

Basically, we first perform HA on the more severely affected side. This is for a number of reasons:

a) HA creates a pain-free rigid hip with permanent function. The psychological attitude of the patient to the arthrodesis is important. The freedom from pain and ability to bear weight compensates greatly for the loss of movement.
b) We prefer a period of partial weight bearing of approximately 2 months following implantation of a TP and this is facilitated

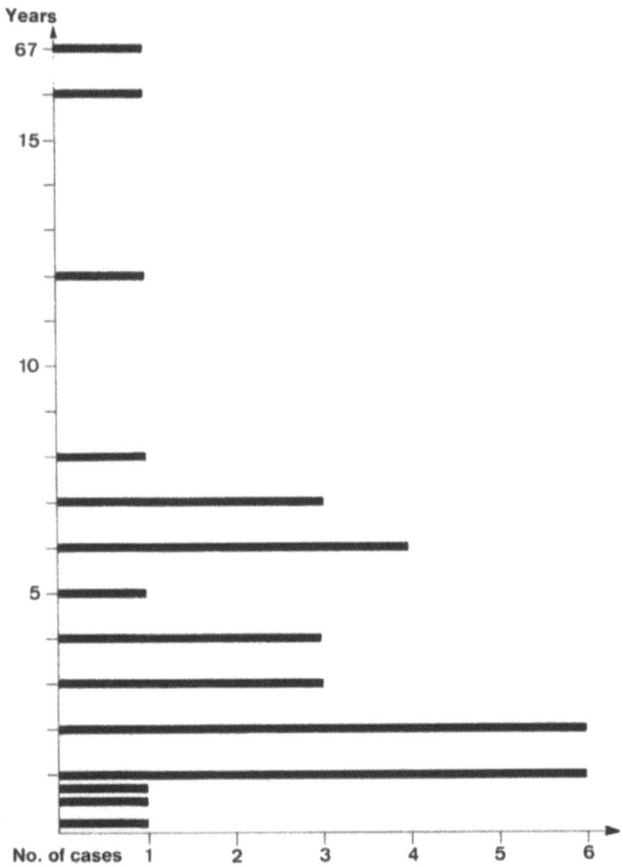

Fig. 200. Time interval between TP and HA

if the opposite hip is arthrodesed and capable of full weight bearing.

c) Equalisation of leg length or the slight shortening (1 cm) desired on the arthrodesed side is technically easier to carry out on implantation of the TP.

d) If TP complications occur, full weight bearing on the arthrodesed hip is possible. This permanent security is not a feature of IO or, for the time being, of TP.

Exceptions occur in which TP may be performed first. These are the cases of severe bilateral ankylosis. It is interesting that implantation of a TP in such cases frequently reduces pain on the opposite side since the TP side has a greater range of movement and bears weight, thus reducing the load on the opposite side.

2.2 Case Material

Between 1965 and 1972 at the Cantonal Hospital in St. Gall, TP was performed on one side and HA on the opposite side in 33 patients. In 29 cases the first operation was HA and in four cases TP. The time interval between HA and TP ranged from 1 month to 67 years with a mean of $5^1/_2$ years (Fig. 200).

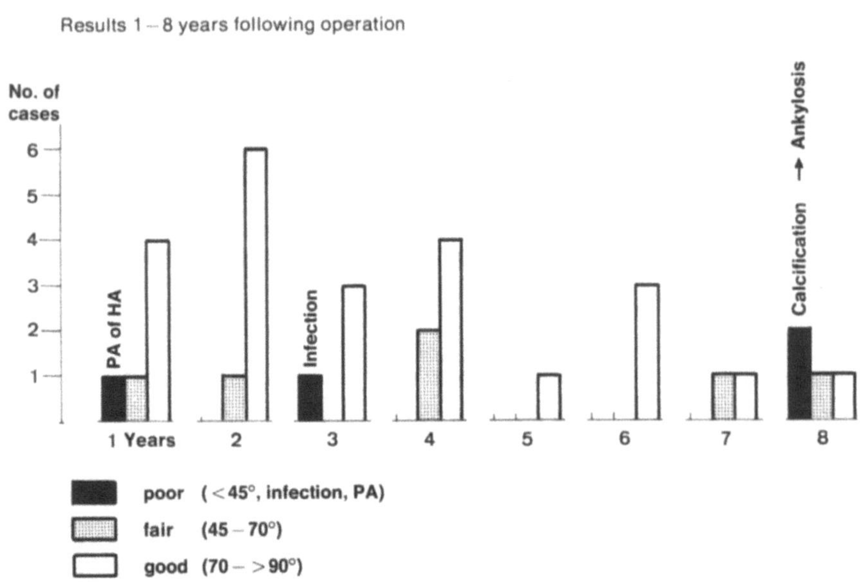

Fig. 201. Results of combining TP with HA
Results 1 – 8 years following operation

2.3 Results

The results were examined 1 – 8 years following the last operation in 13 female and 20 male patients. The results were good (range of hip movement on the TP side was 70° to more than 90°) in 23 patients; six were satisfactory (45° – 70°) and four were poor (Fig. 201). In addition to the failures detailed (one HA pseudarthrosis, one infection following TP which necessitated GH, one complete ankylosis and one partial ankylosis as a result of calcification around the prosthesis) three cases of prosthetic loosening occurred. In one such case the cup was replaced 2 years following TP and in another case, TP was performed 4 years following the original TP. Both patients are now complaint free. The third case only shows radiological signs of loosening 4 years following TP; clinically and subjectively, the patient is problem-free. This frequency of loosening (9%) is actually considerably below that which we have observed on systematically following up our TP cases. However, the comparison is not completely valid since there are insufficient cases in our series (33 cases) to allow statistical conclusions to be reached.

2.4 Case Material

(Figs. 202 – 210)

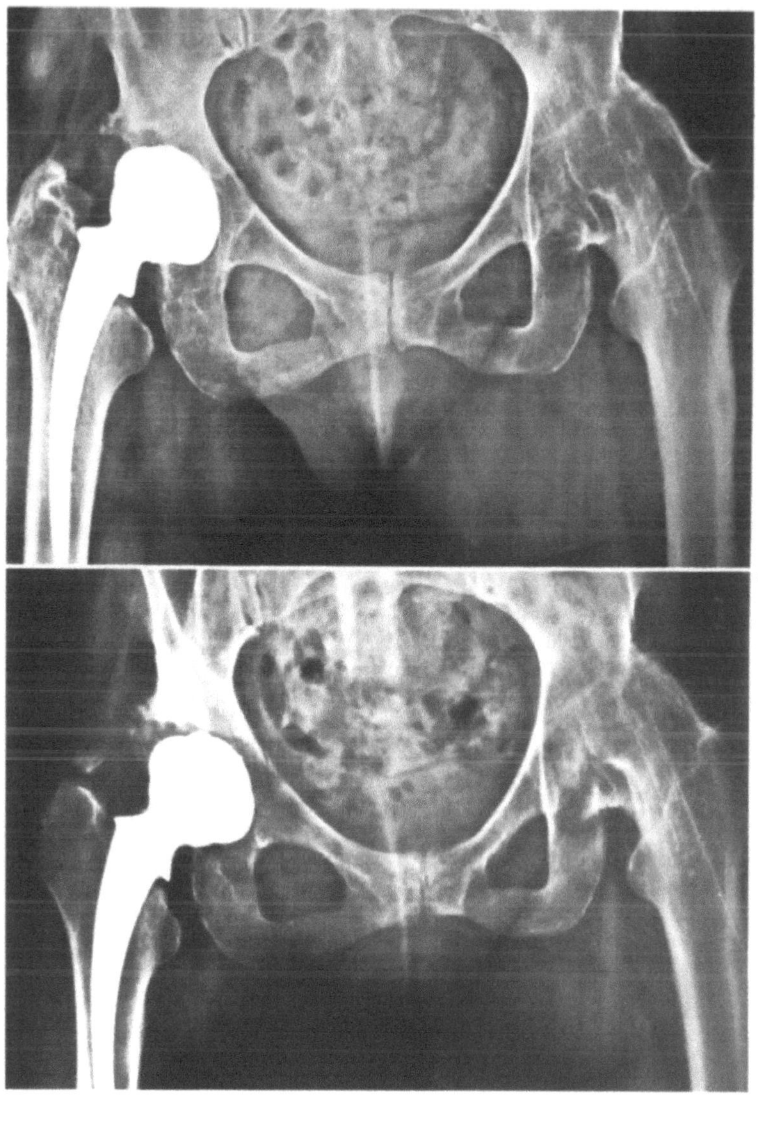

a

b

Fig. 202. *HA and TP in a case of bilateral hip arthrosis.* B. M., ♀, aged 52 years, No. 108050.

a) One month following TP planned 10 years following HA.

b) Six years later. The patient is complaint-free. Trendelenburg weakly positive. Flexion/extension 40 – 0 – – 0°

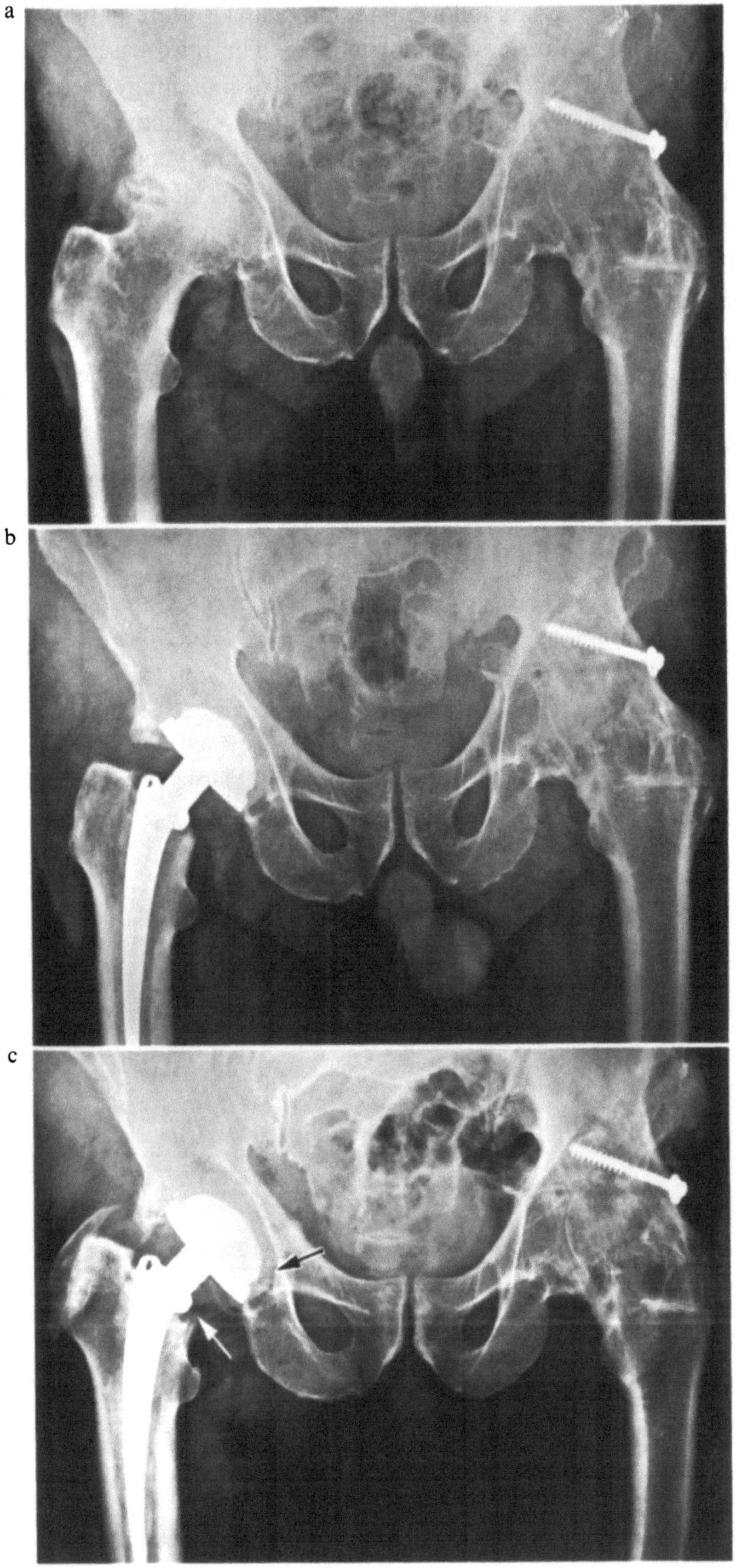

Fig. 203. *HA and TP in a case of bilateral hip arthrosis*. R. E., ♂, aged 65 years, No. 73813.

a) Eight years following Type I HA. Bone union with ideal leg position. Severe arthrosis of the opposite hip.

b) One month after TP.

c) Forty months later. Complaint-free. With 15 cm abduction of leg. Flexion/ extension 80–0–0°. Radiograph shows incipient translucency around the weight-bearing zone and slight bone resorption at the calcar. Patient working full time as forester

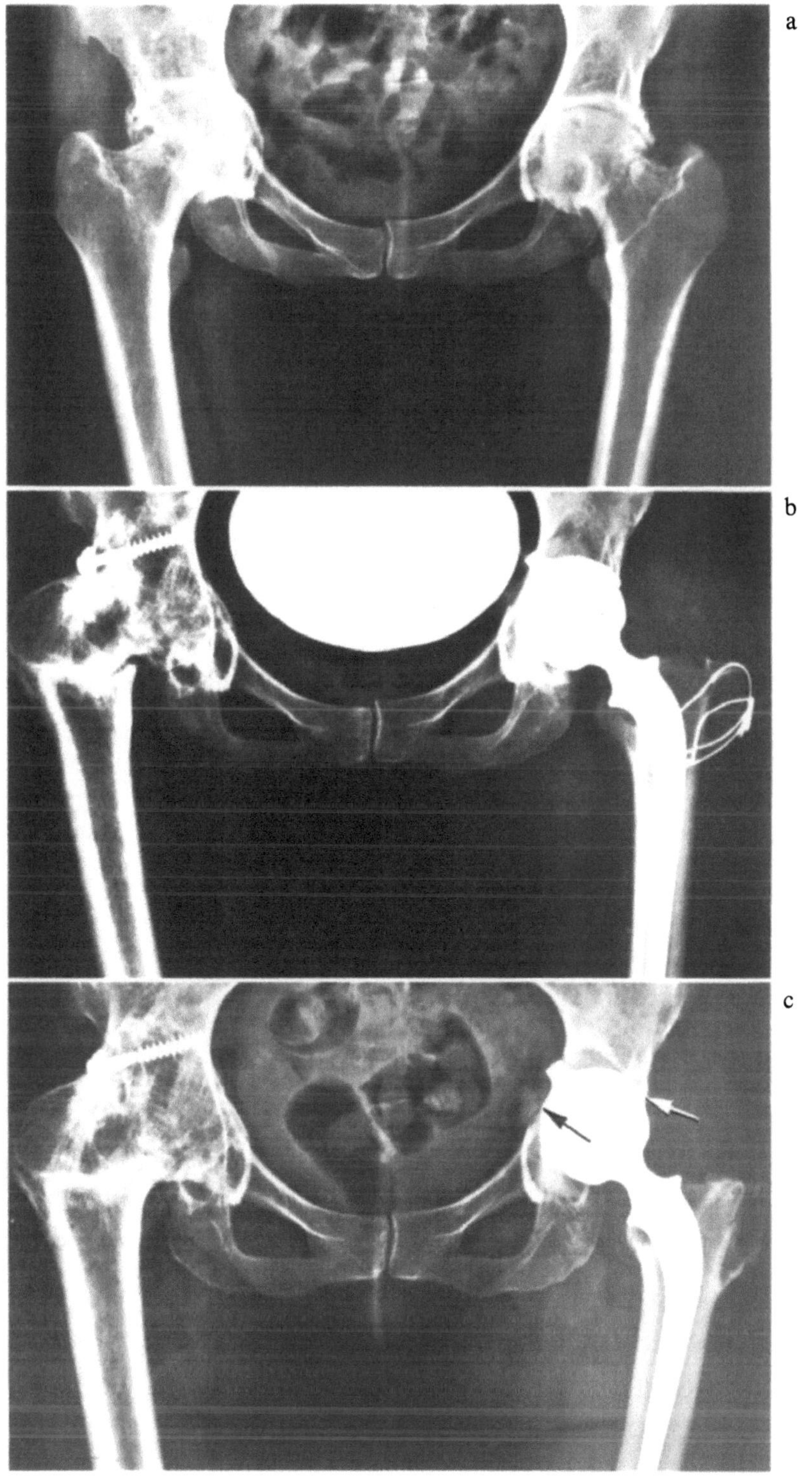

Fig. 204. *Combination of HA and TP in a case of bilateral hip arthrosis with acetabular protrusion.* I. S., ♀, aged 42 years, No. 96300.

a) Before operation.

b) Eight months following HA, 1 month following TP.

c) Follow-up 7 years later. Ideal result with 65 cm leg abduction. Flexion/extension 80–0–0°. Acetabulum somewhat medially displaced but no other signs of loosening. Patient working full time. The cerclage wire was removed because of trochanteric bursitis

a

b

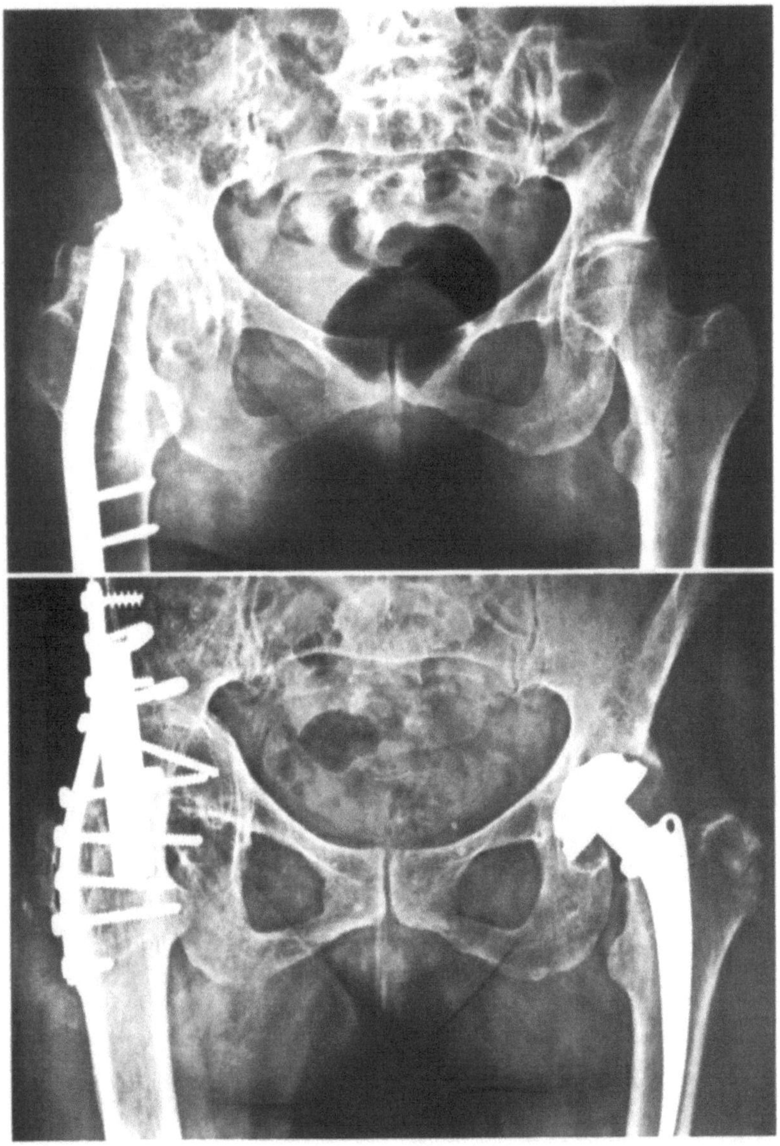

Fig. 205. *Combination of HA and TP (bilateral arthrosis; NHF following IO on the right side)*. N. N., ♀, aged 64 years, No. 71118.

a) Before operation.

b) Seven years following HA and 16 months after TP. Arthrodesis united with good leg position. Flexion/extension 80 – 0 – 0°

a

b

c

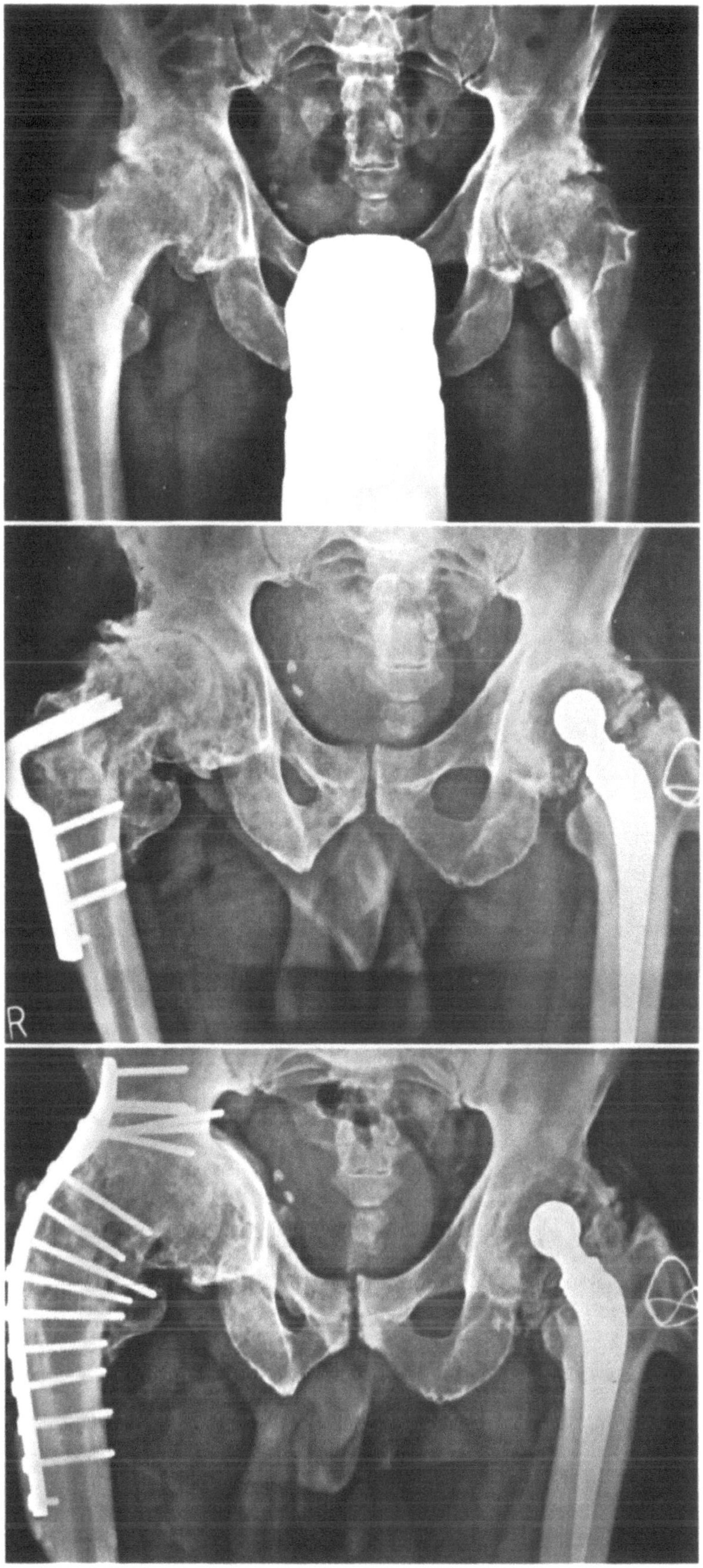

Fig. 206. *Combination of HA and TP in a case of very severe bilateral hip arthrosis.* W. J., ♂, aged 50 years, No. 85483.

a) Before operation.

b) Four years after IO and 3 years after TP. Considerable problems on the right side.

c) Four and a half years after HA and 8 years after TP. No complaints on the arthrodesed side. Flexion/extension 65–0–0°, with 45 cm leg abduction despite extensive calcification of gluteus medius. Patient farming full time

a
b
c

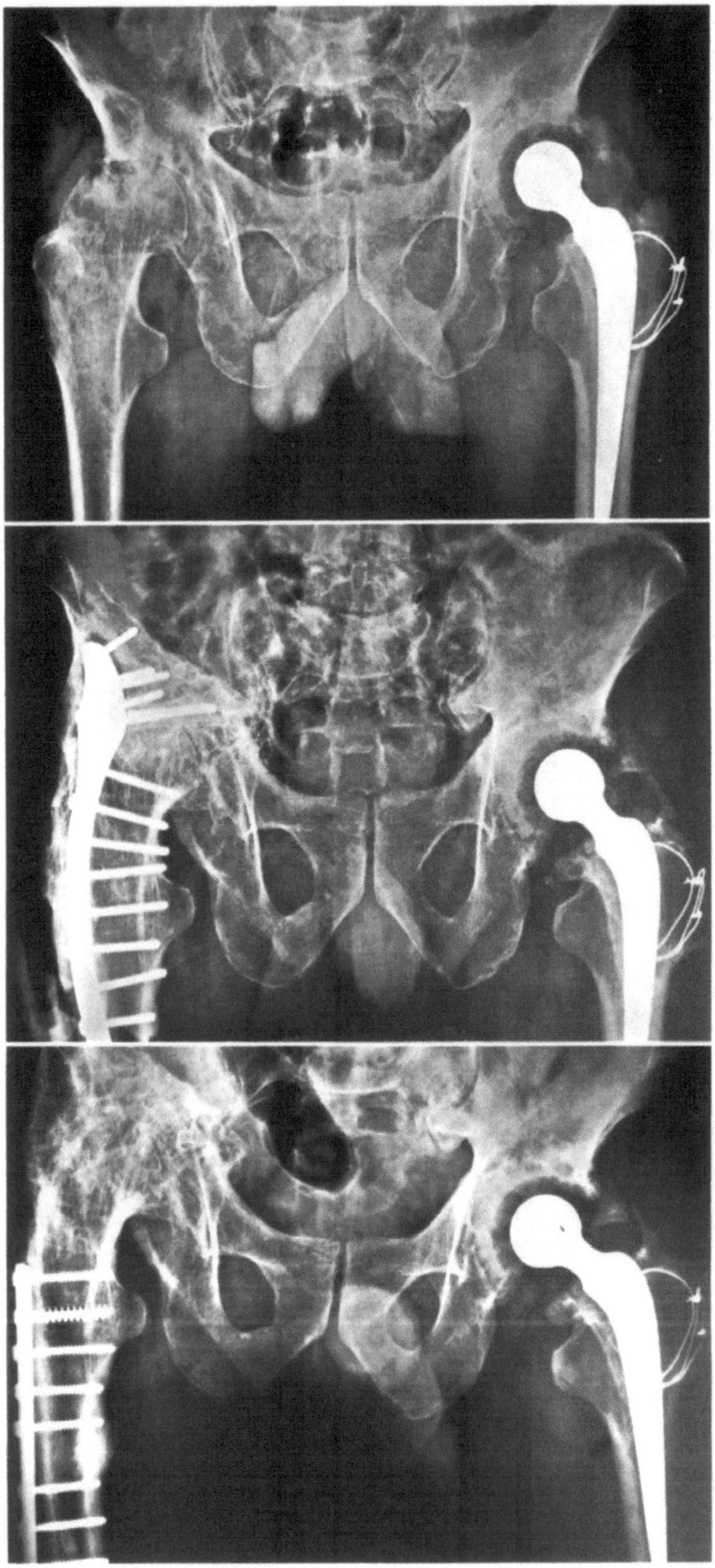

Fig. 207. *Combination of HA and TP in a case of bilateral hip arthrosis.* M. J., ♂, aged 57 years, No. 115300.

a) Five months after TP.

b) Three and a half years after Type IV HA and $4^1/_2$ years after TP. Fracture of the femoral diaphysis at the distal end of the cobra-head plate following severe fall.

c) Eleven months later the fracture is united and the TP is still in good condition. Flexion/extension 75 – 0 – 0°. Slight calcification of gluteus medius. Works full time as labourer

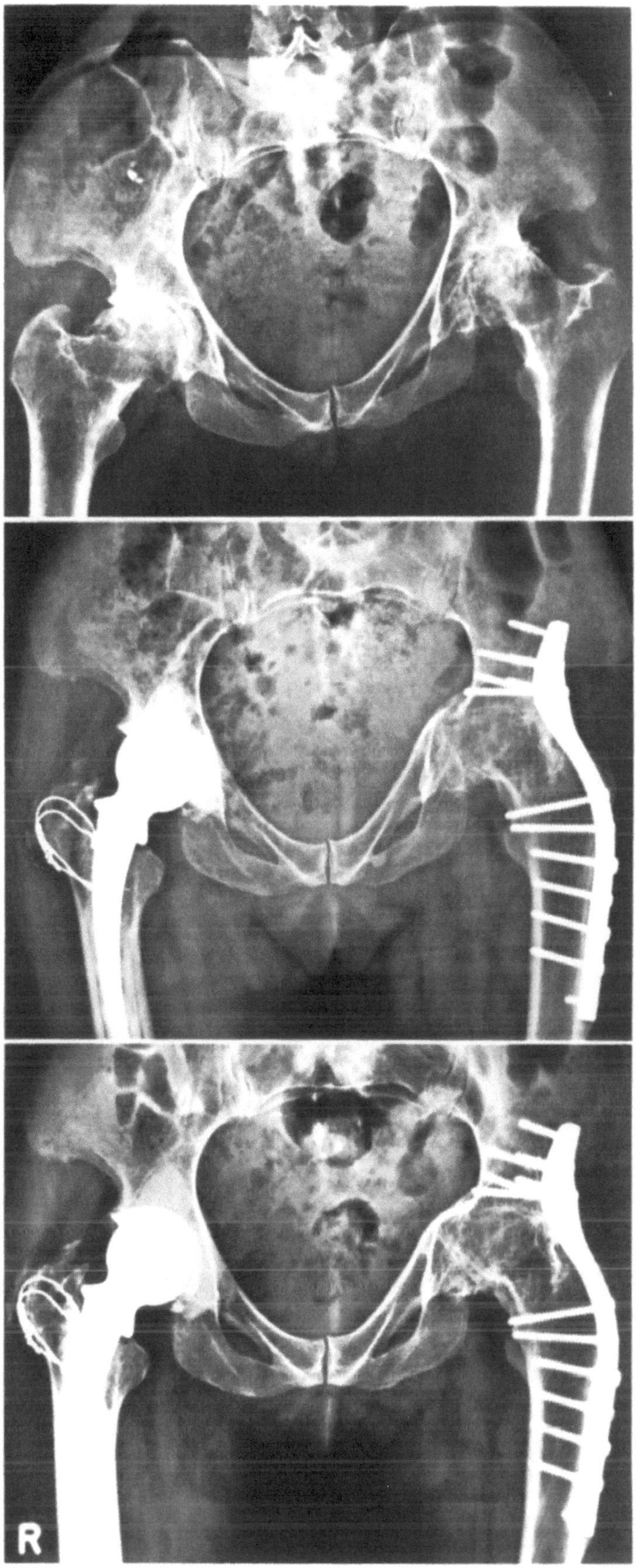

a

b

c

Fig. 208. *Combination of HA and TP in a case of bilateral arthrosis of the hip and coxa vara.* F. F., ♀, aged 62 years, No. 102546.

a) Before operation.

b) One year after HA and 5 months after TP.

c) Four years later. 50 cm leg abduction. Flexion/extension 70 – 0 – 0°. No signs of loosening. Patient complaint-free

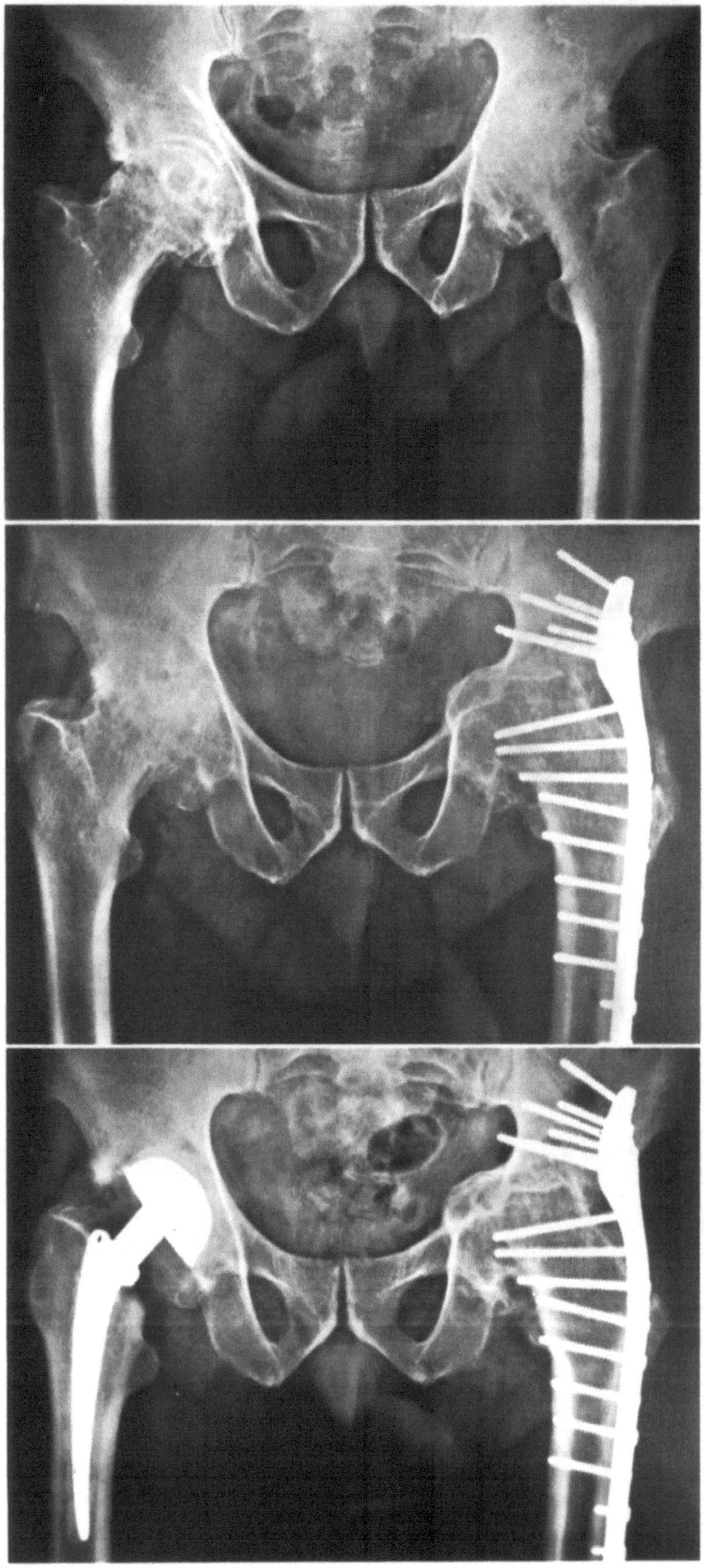

a

b

c

Fig. 209. *HA and TP in a case of very severe bilateral hip arthrosis.* N. O., ♂, aged 64 years, No. 112817.

a) Before operation.

b) Three years after cobra-head plate arthrodesis and PO. No problems on the arthrodesed side but marked worsening on the opposite side.

c) Fifteen months after TP. Flexion/extension 70 – 0 – 0°. With 35 cm leg abduction. Still works as engineer

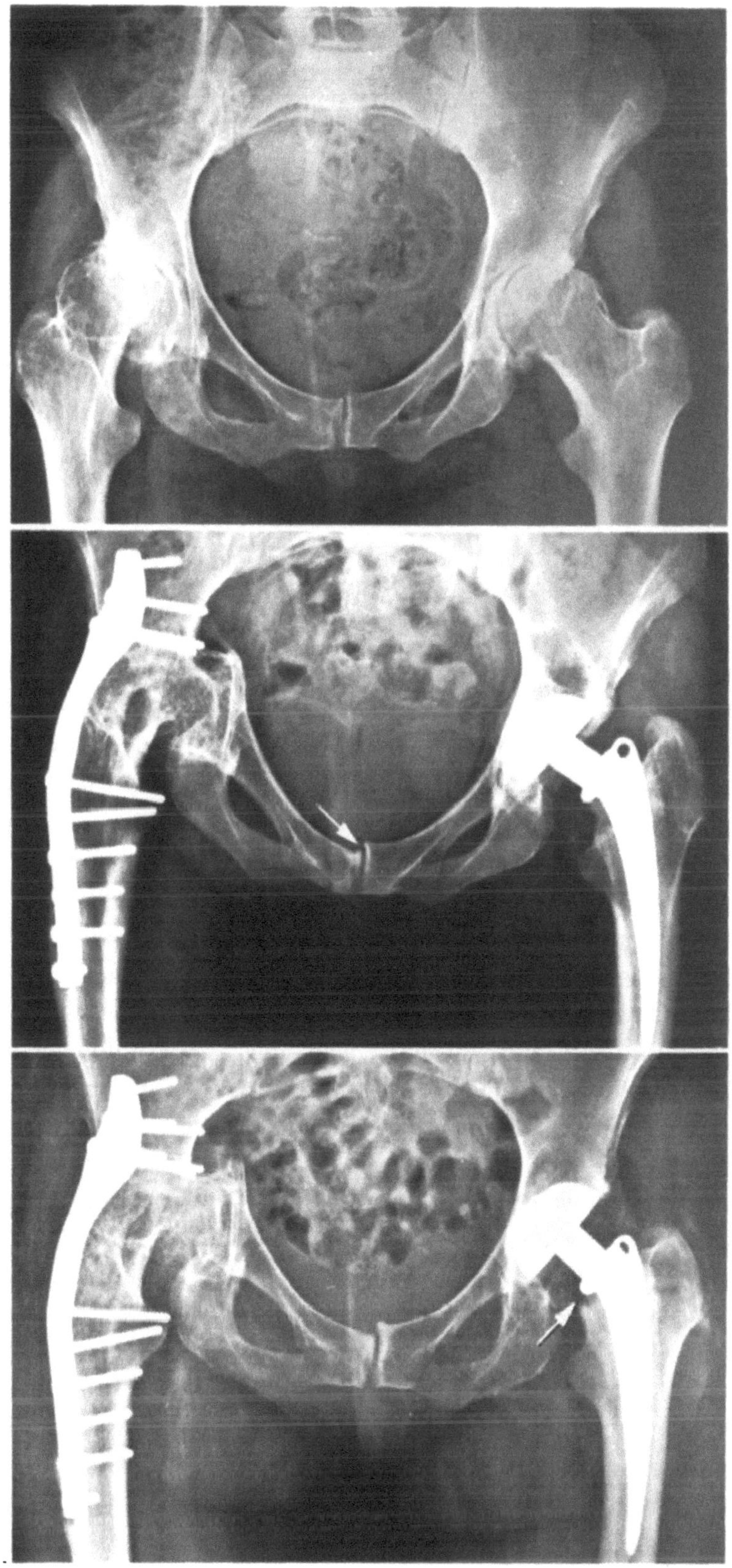

Fig. 210. *HA and TP in a case of bilateral hip arthrosis following bilateral acetabular dysplaysia.* C. E., ♀, aged 49 years, No. 91077.

a) Before operation.

b) One year after HA and 3 weeks after TP. Note the slight subluxation of the symphysis.

c) Three years later. Perfect result. Flexion/extension 100 – 0 – 0°. No complaints whatsoever. Slight bone resorption at the calcar

3 Total Prosthesis Following Hip Arthrodesis

3.1 Introduction

TP has become so popular and its advantages are so obvious that patients whose hips have been arthrodesed frequently feel frustrated. It is therefore understandable that many HA patients ask whether the HA could be converted into a TP. This was confirmed by answers to our questions put to the patients. It is interesting that the majority of patients did not desire a TP because of pain but because of their appearance on sitting and walking. An approximately normal range of hip movement is therefore of primary importance to the patient and also to the doctor.

The situation is completely different in cases where considerable symptomatic problems arise in the neighbouring joints, particularly in the ipsilateral knee joint, the contralateral hip and the lumbar spine, or if pain occurs in the arthrodesed hip, usually as a result of PA. In such cases a TP is expected to bring not only an improved range of movement but also freedom from pain and possibly also correction of deformity or difference in leg length. The problems associated with this difficult operation will now be discussed and this will be followed by a statement of our policy in respect of the indications.

In St. Gall we only found a few cases of TP following hip ankylosis. These were younger patients with total stiffening of the hip resulting from ankylosing spondylitis. However, these cases cannot be used as examples of replacement of an HA by a TP. MÜLLER in Berne and GERTSCH in Grosshochstetten have larger series of cases. They have generously offered us all their case material (case histories and radiographs) for evaluation. From the data presented the reader may get an idea of the possibilities and limitations of such operations.

3.2 Statement of Problem

3.2.1 Changes in the Musculature Following Hip Arthrodesis

For years there has been disagreement about the functional state of the musculature following HA. Despite extensive electromyographic investigation of the hip musculature (FRIEDEBOLD, TÖNNIS, BAUMANN and BEHR; BURCKHARDT) differences in opinion continue to exist. It is undisputed and can always be clinically observed that HA leads to so-called disuse atrophy. BAUMANN and BEHR investigated M. gluteus medius, the adductors and the iliopsoas electromyographically in 42 patients 3 months – 8 years following HA. The results show only relatively slight disuse atrophy in these muscles without signs of degeneration, which is due to continuation of muscle activity. Following HA, the musculature loses its dynamic function but isometric contraction in response to static-dynamic requirements remains. Years following HA, a normal pattern of innervation was found in the muscles mentioned above both on standing and on walking. The leg shortening which is frequently present following HA leads to relaxation of the hip muscles. Following HA the latter exert considerable pressure which promotes bone union and also function as a supporting corset for the skeletal system (PAUWELS).

M. gluteus medius and M. gluteus minimus should always remain intact to increase the stability of the arthrodesed hip. According to FRIEDEBOLD, the disuse atrophy may lead to degenerative changes despite the nerve remaining intact and this may cause irreversible deterioration of function.

We are of the opinion that severe degenerative muscle changes of this nature are only seen in special cases, e.g., accompanying painful unstable arthrodesis or extensive scarring of the hip muscles. Clinical experience has shown that in cases like these, the range of movement with a prosthesis remains markedly limited. Friedebold has made the interesting observation that the electrical activity in the gluteal muscles 6 months after carrying out HA is almost as strong as that on the side of the hip plasty which was performed at almost the same time.

Blaimont has reported a case in which M. gluteus medius recovered its original static and dynamic function following implantation of a total prosthesis in a hip which had been arthrodesed for 40 years. Follow-up of our patients who had received a TP following HA has shown that in all cases the *abductors have recovered their ability to maintain pelvic equilibrium.*

3.2.2 Technical Difficulties at Operation

These are created by the previous procedure. There are frequently severe anatomical changes. Muscle insertions and the greater trochanter are missing and extensive scarring renders good exposure difficult. Rüter and Ganz have called attention to specific problems: if leg lengthening of more than 3 cm is required to counteract a considerable reduction in true leg length, the insertion of M. iliopsoas has to be sacrificed; earlier HA combined with osteotomies or deformities may make unusual positioning of the femoral prosthetic component (retrotorsion, increased antetorsion) necessary; PA of the PO makes reinforcement of the bone cement with K-wires and screws or even a medial internal plate fixation necessary. Furthermore, if the remnant of the proximal femur no longer contains cancellous bone, anchorage of the femoral prosthetic component may create considerable problems.

The increased risk of postoperative infection should not be underestimated since the local powers of resistance are weakened (scarring, marked tendency to bleeding).

Kölbel and Weigert recommend that the prosthesis cup be cemented in place far medially in order to prevent or reduce Trendelenburg gait which occurs as a result of interference with active joint control.

3.3 Indications

It follows from what has been said that the conversion of an HA into a TP is a serious operation. It is irresponsible to risk performing this operation in order to satisfy a patient's demands for restoration of joint movement if that patient is otherwise complaint-free.

Conversely, the procedure is undoubtedly indicated in the following cases:

a) Severe complaints arising in neighbouring joints, particularly knee or lumbar spine problems.
b) Failure of the arthrodesis within the hip itself. Prosthetic replacement may be indicated in place of rearthrodesis, particularly in those cases where one would nowadays have implanted a TP instead of performing arthrodesis.

3.4 Case Material

The cases listed in Table 33 were made available to us by Professor Müller (cases 1–11) and Dr. Gertsch (cases 12–17). The two last cases are from our clinic; in the last case (case 19) bilateral hip ankylosis secondary to ankylosing spondylitis was the indication for bilateral TP.

The original indications for HA were: five cases of congenital dysplasia; seven hip arthroses; one hip arthrosis secondary to rheumatoid arthritis; three post-traumatic hip arthroses; two post-traumatic NHF. The hips of the last patient with ankylosing spondylitis were completely ankylosed on both sides and bilateral gonarthrosis was also present.

The indications for TP were: lumbar spinal complaints (five cases); ipsilateral knee problems (one case); contralateral knee problems (one case); ten cases of PA of the HA with lumbar spinal pain in five of these cases, pain in the opposite hip in two cases and in the ipsilateral knee joint in one case. In one case, the back complaints were caused by abduction deformity with an apparent increase in leg length of 2.5 cm on the arthrodesed side.

The time interval between HA and TP ranged from 1–22 years with a mean of 8.4 years.

3.5 Results

The period of observation following TP implantation ranged from 3 months–8 years with a mean of 2 years, 3 months. All patients are

Table 33. TP following HA (11 cases from Berne, 6 cases from Grosshöchstetten, 2 cases from St. Gall)

Initials, sex and year of birth	Primary hip disease	Age at HA	Interval HA–TP (years)	Complaints	Follow-up period after TP (months)	Course
1. E. F., ♀, 1946	CDH	19	5	LS	24	No complications, complaint-free
2. R. A., ♀ 1932	CDH	19	20	LS (+opposite. hip)	6	No complications, complaint-free
3. C. V., ♀, 1927	CDH	22	22	Knee+LS	12	No complications, complaint-free
4. U. D., ♀, 1924	CDH	41	$3^1/_2$	PA	36	Loosening of cup, complaint-free after 2 × replacement of TP
5. S. H., ♀, 1907	CDH	41	19	PA	60	Dislocation of TP; replacement of TP 1 year later; complaint-free
6. W. E., ♀, 1909	Hip arthrosis	56	4	PA (+opposite hip)	36	No complications complaint-free
7. G. D., ♀, 1907	Hip arthrosis	60	1	PA (+LS)	42	No complications complaint-free
8. B. E., ♀, 1902	Hip arthrosis	64	4	PA (+LS+opposite hip)	24	Loosening of prosthesis shaft; replacement of TP 2 years later
9. K. E., ♂, 1935	Post-traumatic hip arthrosis	22	14	PA (+knee)	6	No complications, complaint-free
10. H. A., ♀, 1907	Post-traumatic hip arthrosis	58	$3^1/_2$	PA (+LS)	36	No complications, complaint-free
11. B. A., ♂, 1899	Post-traumatic NHF	62	2	PA (+LS)	96	Teflon wear. TP replacement 6 years later. Complaint-free.
12. R. F., ♂, 1923	Hip arthrosis	44	4	LS	30	No complications, complaint-free.
13. S. M., ♀, 1917	Hip arthrosis	40	13	PA (+LS)	36	No complications, complaint-free
14. G. E., ♂, 1926	Hip arthrosis	42	5	Abduction deformity, increased apparent leg length (LS)	4	Hematoma. Still slight lumbar spinal trouble.
15. B. M., ♂, 1908	Rheumatoid arthritis	53	12	Knee, LS	3	No complications, complaint-free
16. N. H., ♂, 1905	Post-traumatic hip arthrosis	63	5	PA implant fracture	6	Hematoma; complaint-free.
17. H. C., ♀, 1939	Post-traumatic NHF	27	7	LS, knee	6	No complications, complaint-free
18. G. H., ♀, 1918	Hip arthrosis	52	7	PA (+knee)	60	No complications, complaint-free
19. B. B., ♂, 1940	Ankylosing spondylitis	–	–	Bilateral complete hip and knee ankyloses.	18	No complications, complaint-free

complaint-free and very satisfied with their range of hip motion. However, it should be noted that in three cases (cases 5, 8 and 11) the TP had to be replaced once (TP dislocation, loosening, Teflon wear) and in one case (case 4) two TP replacements have been necessitated by loosening of the cup.

The postoperative course was usually uneventful. In only two cases did a haematoma occur; one case was managed conservatively and the other required operative revision.

No infections have occurred to date. Furthermore, despite detrimental local factors (scar tissue, reduced blood perfusion, extensive bone resection) no calcifications have occurred.

Flexion was worse than is normally the case with a TP but nevertheless in all cases followed up it was at least 50°. It was particularly limited in cases where the insertion of the abductors was absent before operation (usually following resection of the greater trochanter). With the exception of one case the Trendelenburg sign was always negative.

In all cases, restoration of hip mobility led to significant or total relief of back complaints. Knee complaints were less frequently affected (severe arthrotic knee joint changes which were present before operation).

3.6 Case Material

(Figs. 211–217).

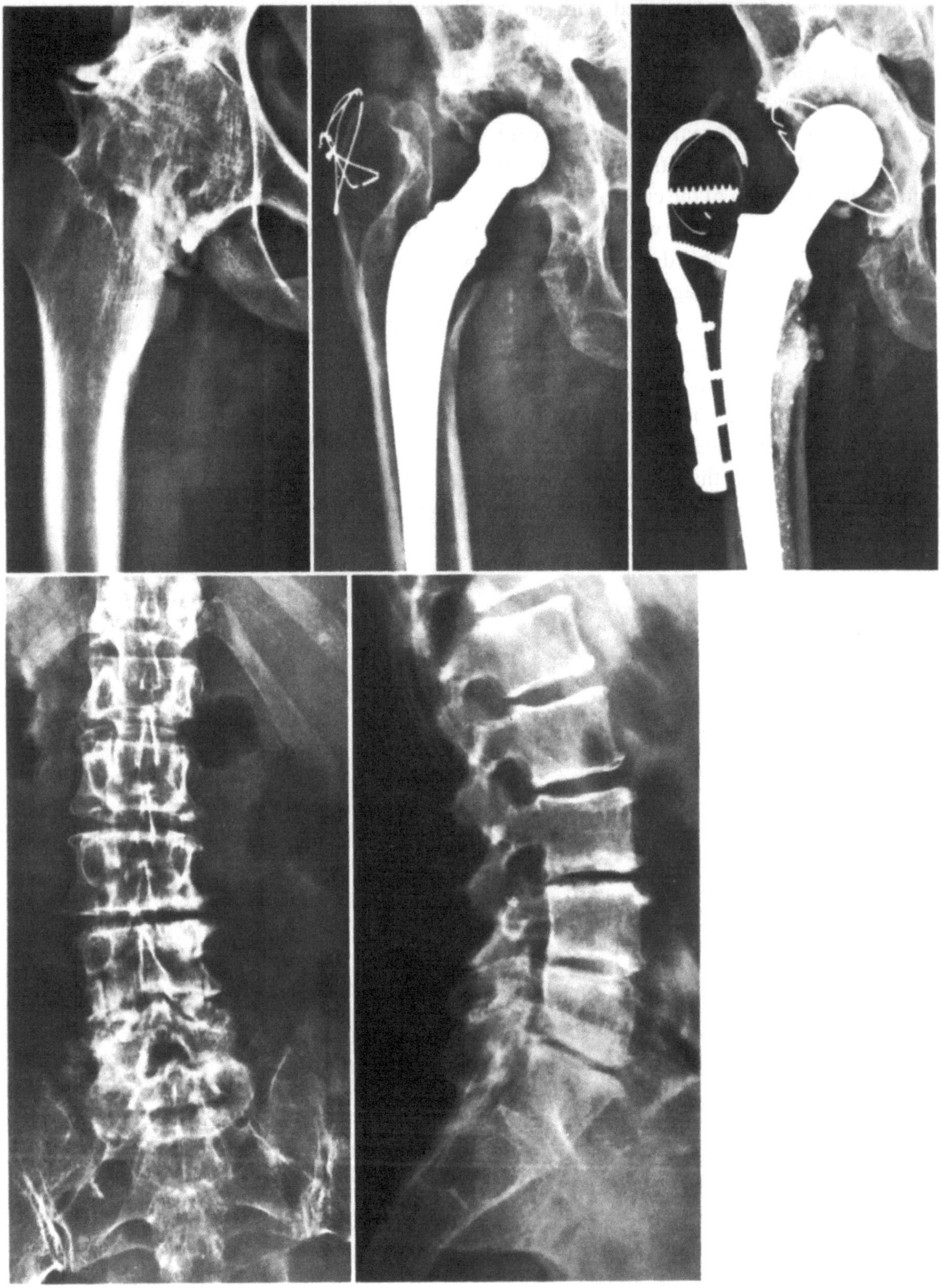

Figs. 211 – 217. TP following HA

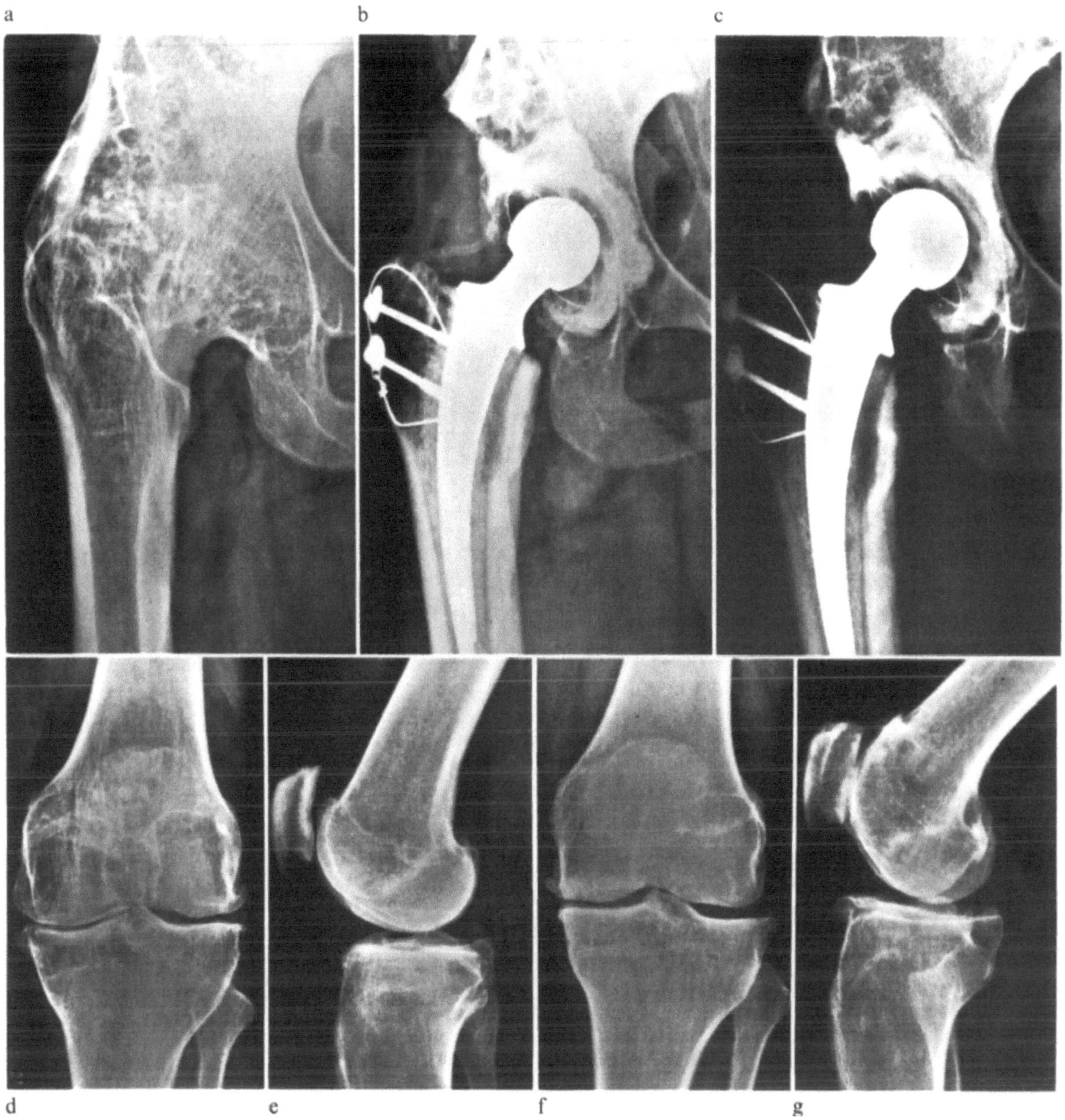

Fig. 211. *Replacement of prosthesis because of loosening (TP performed for hip ankylosis secondary to tuberculosis).* D. E., ♀, aged 66 years, D. E. 06 708 283.

a) Forty years after operation on the Tb hip. Complete ankylosis. The suspected PA was not found at operation.

b) Eight years after TP. Loosening of the prosthesis with severe bone resorption at the calcar.

c) Three months following TP replacement. Patient complaint-free. Function: 90 – 0 – 0°.

d and e) Extensive degenerative changes in the LS

Fig. 212. *TP following HA for knee complaint.* C. V., ♀, aged 44 years, No. BE 6712/71.

a) Seventeen years following HA which had united in 40° flexion, 45° external rotation and 20° abduction. Severe knee complaints.

b) TP on day of operation.

c) Two years and 3 months later. TP intact. Arthrotic knee pain still present (varus knee).

d and e) Knee joints before TP operation.

f and g) Two years later the arthrotic changes have not worsened. The medial joint space seems to have increased but this could be an artefact due to the angle at which X-ray was taken

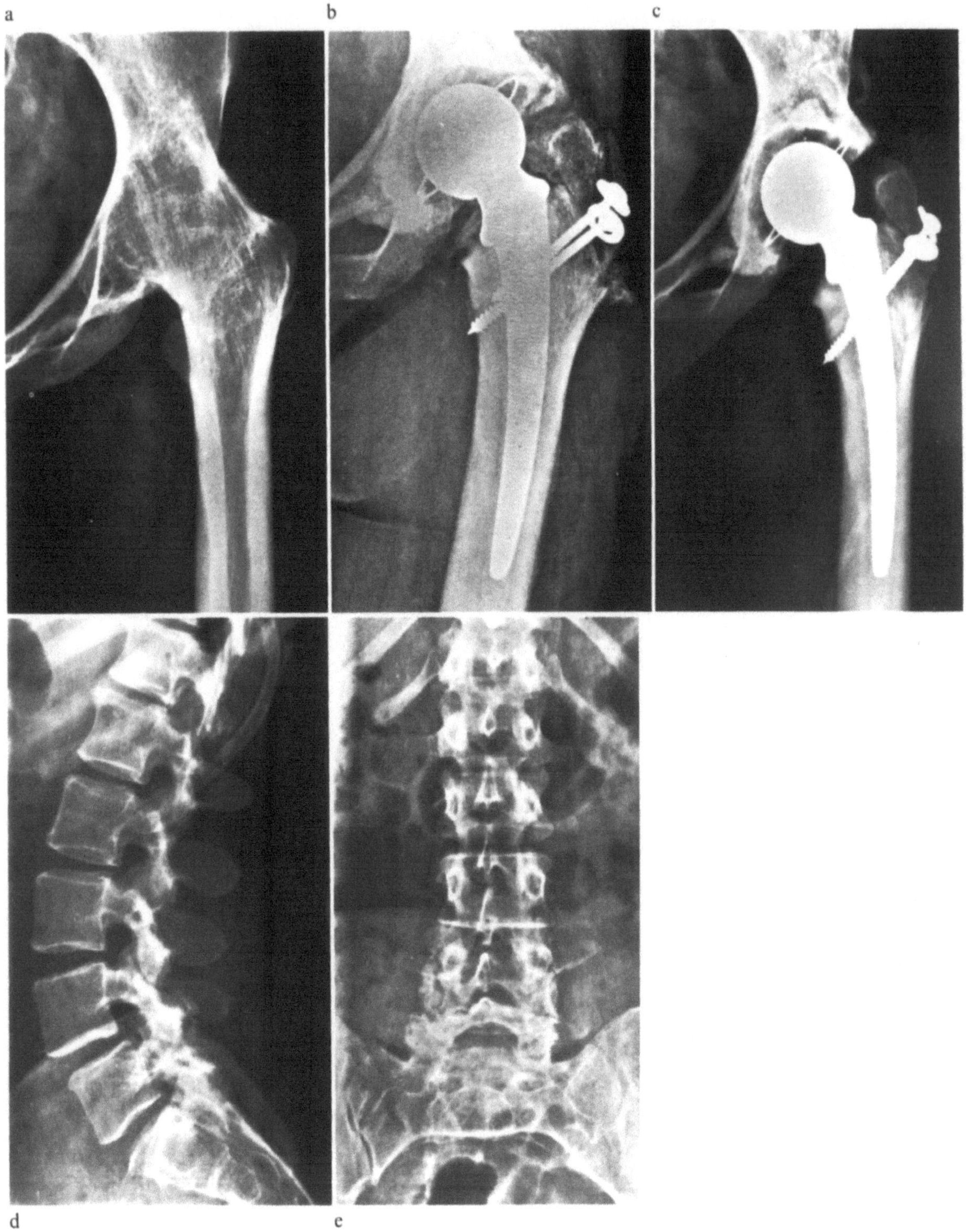

Fig. 213. *TP following HA for lumbar pain.* C. R., ♀, aged 41 years, No. BE 7981/73.

a) Before operation. HA secondary to Tb hip infection with 40° fixed flexion deformity.

b) TP on day of operation.

c) Three months later. Patient compaint-free. Flexion/extension 90 – 0 – 0°.

d) Despite the considerable subjective complaints there are no signs of important degenerative changes in the LS

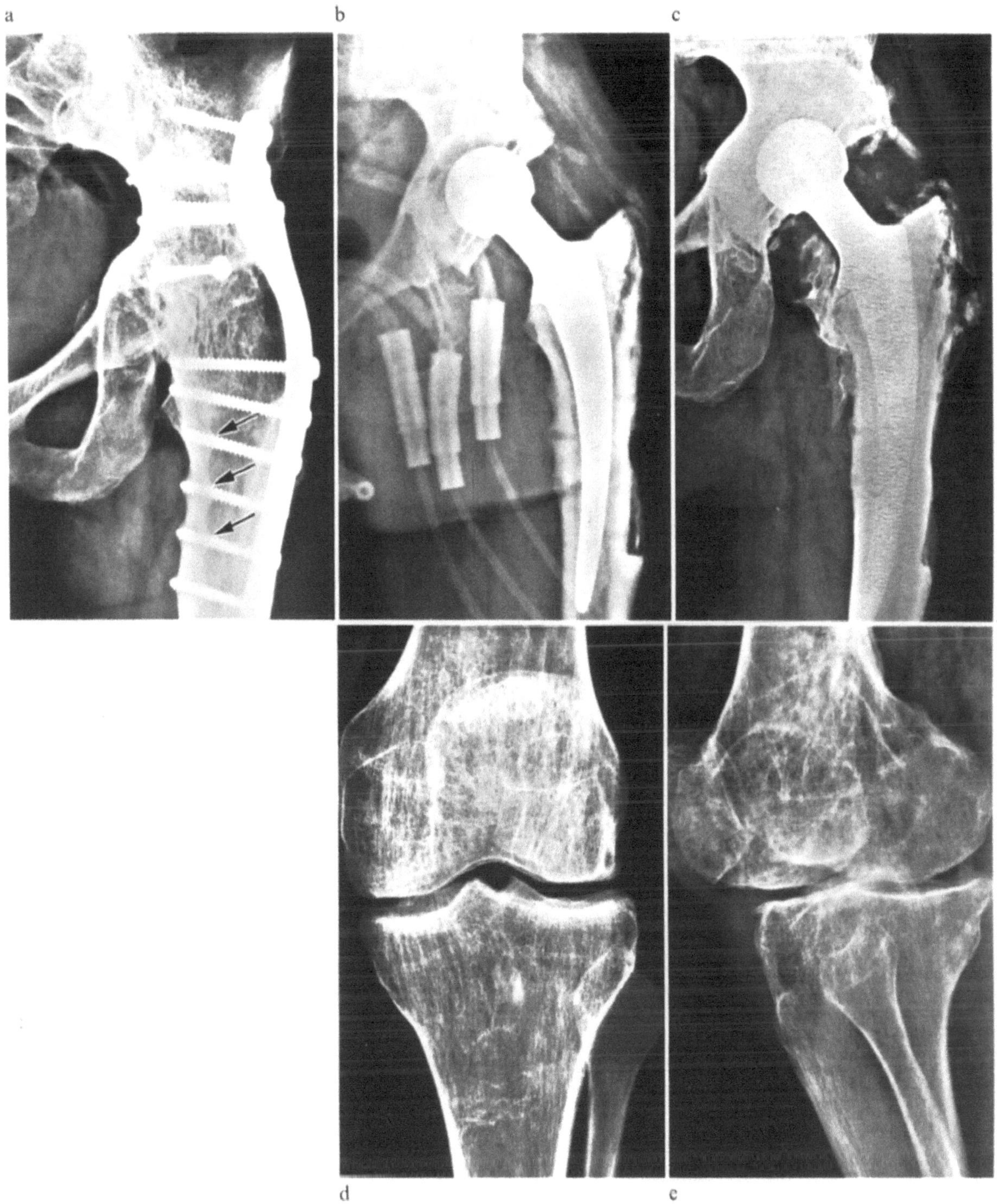

Fig. 214. *TP following HA for severe knee complaints*. H. C., ♀, aged 34 years, No. GH 1276.

a) Seven years following cobra-head plate arthrodesis for post-traumatic NHF. Note the thickening of the cortex around the screws.

b) TP on day of operation.

c) Four months later. 8 cm leg abduction. Flexion/extension 90 – 0 – 0°. Patient complaint-free.

d and e) Post-traumatic arthrosis of the knee. Function still good (80 – 0°)

a b

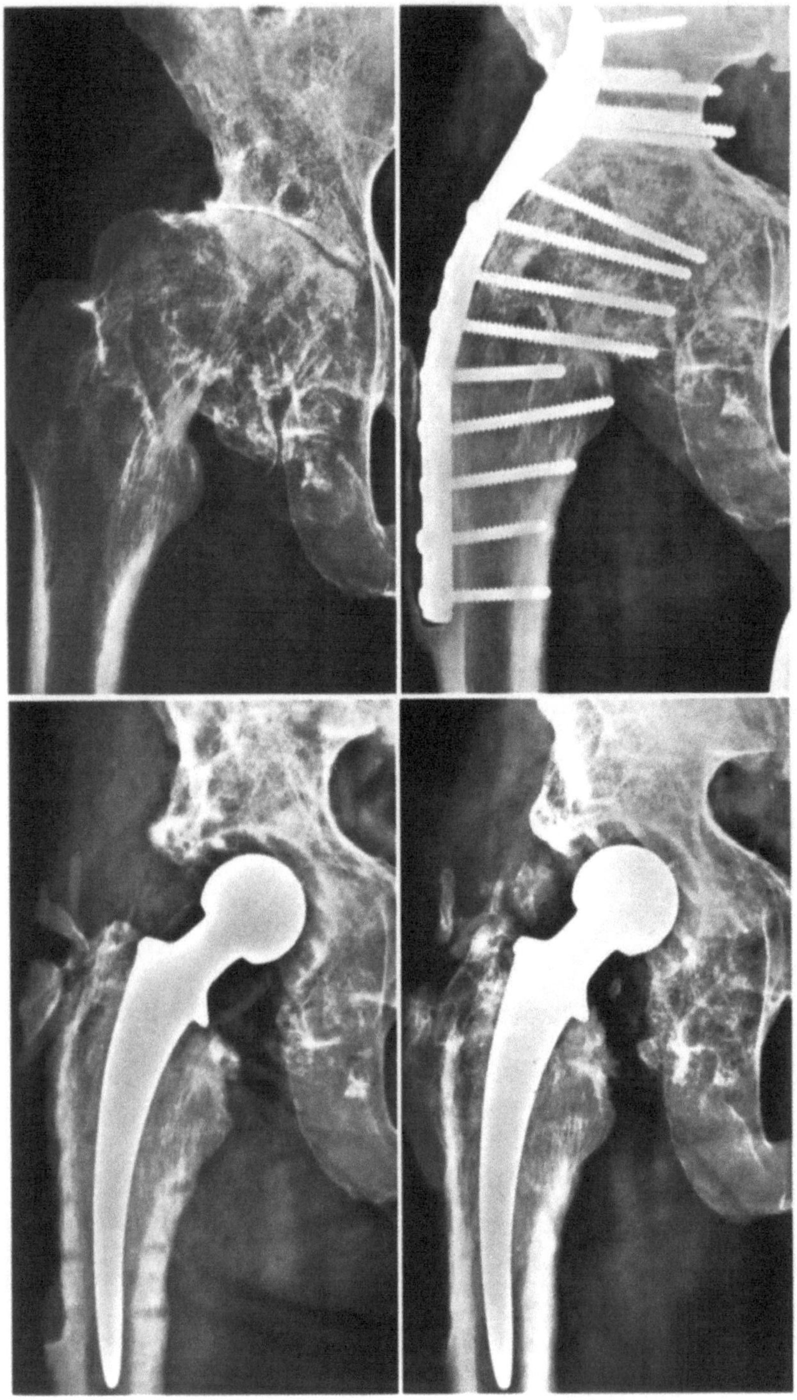

c d

Fig. 215. *TP performed subsequent to HA for lumbar pain and pain in the opposite hip*. R. F., ♂, aged 48 years, GH 1002.

a) Severe arthrosis of the hip.

b) Five years after HA. Worsening of the back complaints. Arthrodesis otherwise successful.

c) TP on day of operation.

d) Twenty eight months later. Very successful TP. Leg abduction 80 cm. Flexion/extension 65 – 0 – 0°. No further back complaints

a b c

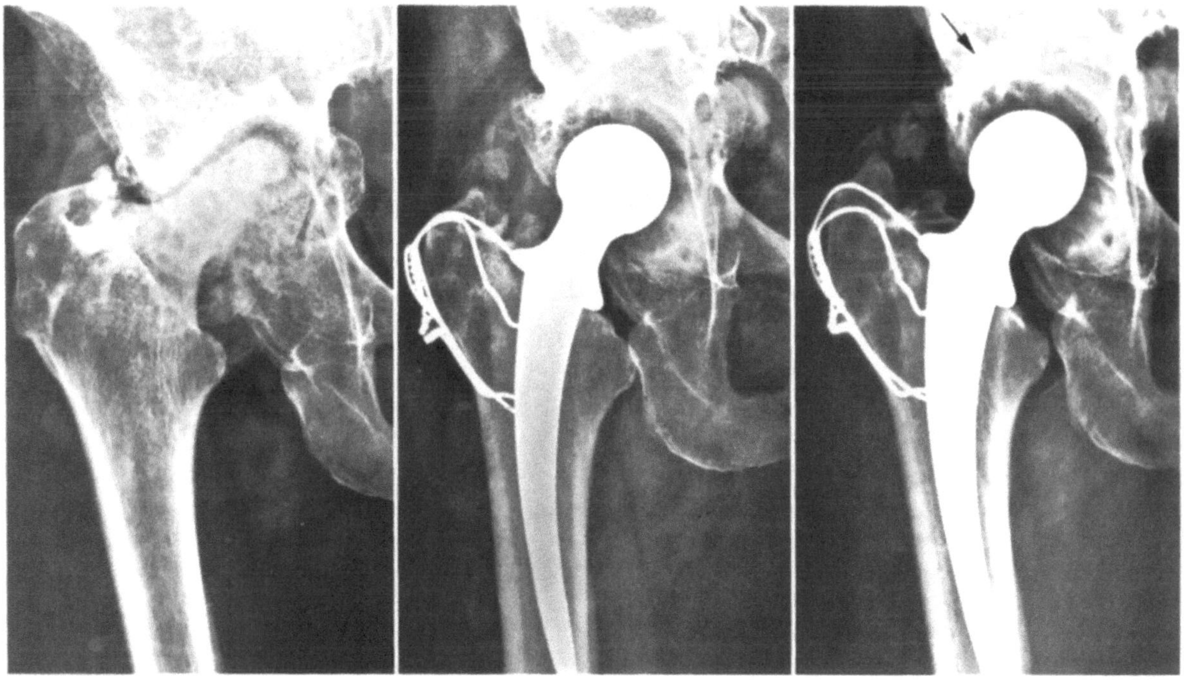

Fig. 216. *TP following attempted arthrodesis and PA in a case of hip arthrosis.* G. E., ♀, aged 50 years, No. 117946.

a) HA pseudarthrosis. Lack of rigidity clinically evident. Hardly able to stand on one leg.

b) Four months after TP.

c) Forty months after TP. 80 cm leg abduction. Flexion/extension 90 – 0 – 0°. Considerable cortical increment visible on comparison with radiograph (b). No subjective problems

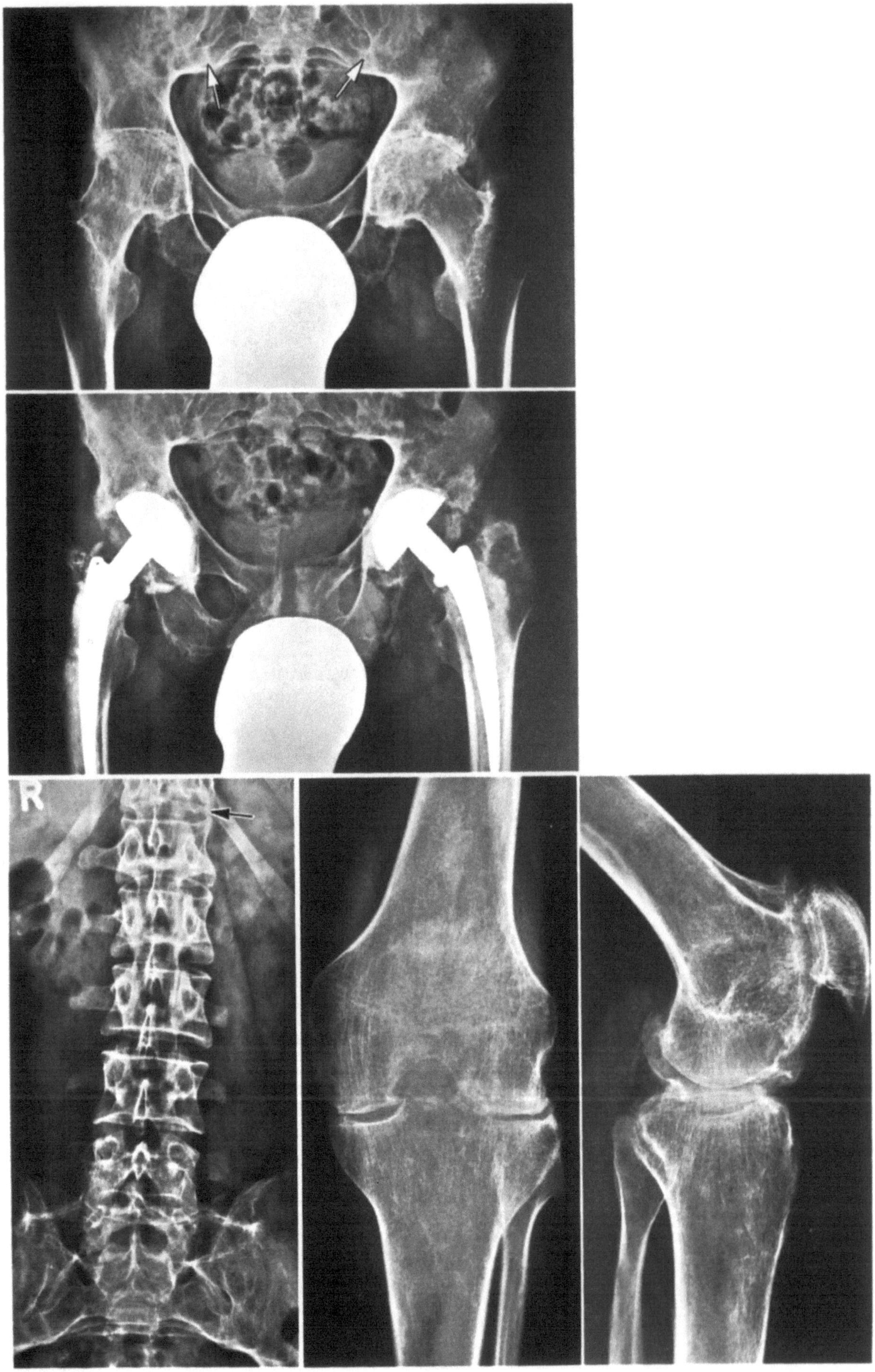
a
b
R
c
d
e

4 Hip Arthrodesis Following Total Prosthesis

4.1 Introduction

Whereas a lot has been published on the usually excellent early results following implantation of a TP, little has been written about the long-term results and complications. Up until now the problems associated with wear of, and body tolerance of, the plastic materials, loosening of the anchorage, secondary trophic changes in the bone and periarticular joint calcification remain partially or totally unsolved. Fortunately, reoperation in such cases, particularly replacement of the cup, shaft or of the whole prosthesis, is usually successful even if difficult. This is not the case when TP implantation is followed at an early or late stage by infection. From 1967–31 July 1972, 44 infections (total 3.5%) occurred following 1234 TP in our clinic. Although the infection rate following TP of the hip joint could be reduced from 6.8% (1967) to 0.9% (1973) as a result of systematic prophylactic immunisation with staphylococcal antigen and prevention of wound contamination by strict asepsis in a sterile operating box, the infected TP is still the complication most feared by us. If perfusion drainage or replacement of the TP fails there are only two possibilities remaining following removal of the implant and of the bone cement. These are the GH resection and arthrodesis of the hip. If the latter operation is possible it is preferable to the Girdlestone procedure with its unsatisfactory result, particularly in active working patients whose general condition is good.

Fig. 217. *TP in a case of bilateral ankylosis secondary to ankylosing spondylitis and bilateral arthrosis of the knee in a young patient.* B. R., ♂, aged 32 years, No. 157624.

a) Before operation. Typical bilateral sacroiliac joint changes.

b) One and six months, respectively, following TP operation. Hips giving no more trouble. Abduction 65 cm. Flexion/extension (right) 50–0–0°, (left) 75–0–0°.

c) Suggestion of bone union at the thoracolumbar junction.

d and e) Severe arthrosis of the knee and femoropatellar joint

4.2 Statement of Problem

Basically one must differentiate between HA following partial prosthetic replacement and HA following TP.

4.2.1 Hip Arthrodesis Following Partial Prosthetic Replacement

These were already discussed in connection with GH and similar conditions (page 180). Following removal of a cup or of a Thompson or Judet prosthesis, a bone cavity always results but this cavity is significantly smaller than that following removal of a TP. Usually the greater trochanter can be smoothed off and inserted into the acetabulum.

Countless operations have been recommended in the last 10 years for these difficult cases such as: abduction arthrodesis (45°–90°) followed 6 weeks later by subtrochanteric correction osteotomy (Abbott, Fischer, Lucas); nail arthrodesis (Thompson, Lange) with additional pelvic graft; ischiofemoral arthrodesis (Bosworth), intra-articular and para-articular hip arthrodesis, corticocancellous graft from the iliac crest (Rinaldi), arthrodesis with homologous bone grafting and screw fixation of the greater trochanter (Guilleminet and Desdrosses; nail arthrodesis with additional ischiofemoral or iliofemoral grafting (Merle D'Aubigné and Postel). The great disadvantage of all these procedures is the prolonged immobilisation in a cast (average 3–5 months). If at all possible we prefer rigid internal fixation, even in these cases. Usually the medial displacement following PO suffices to

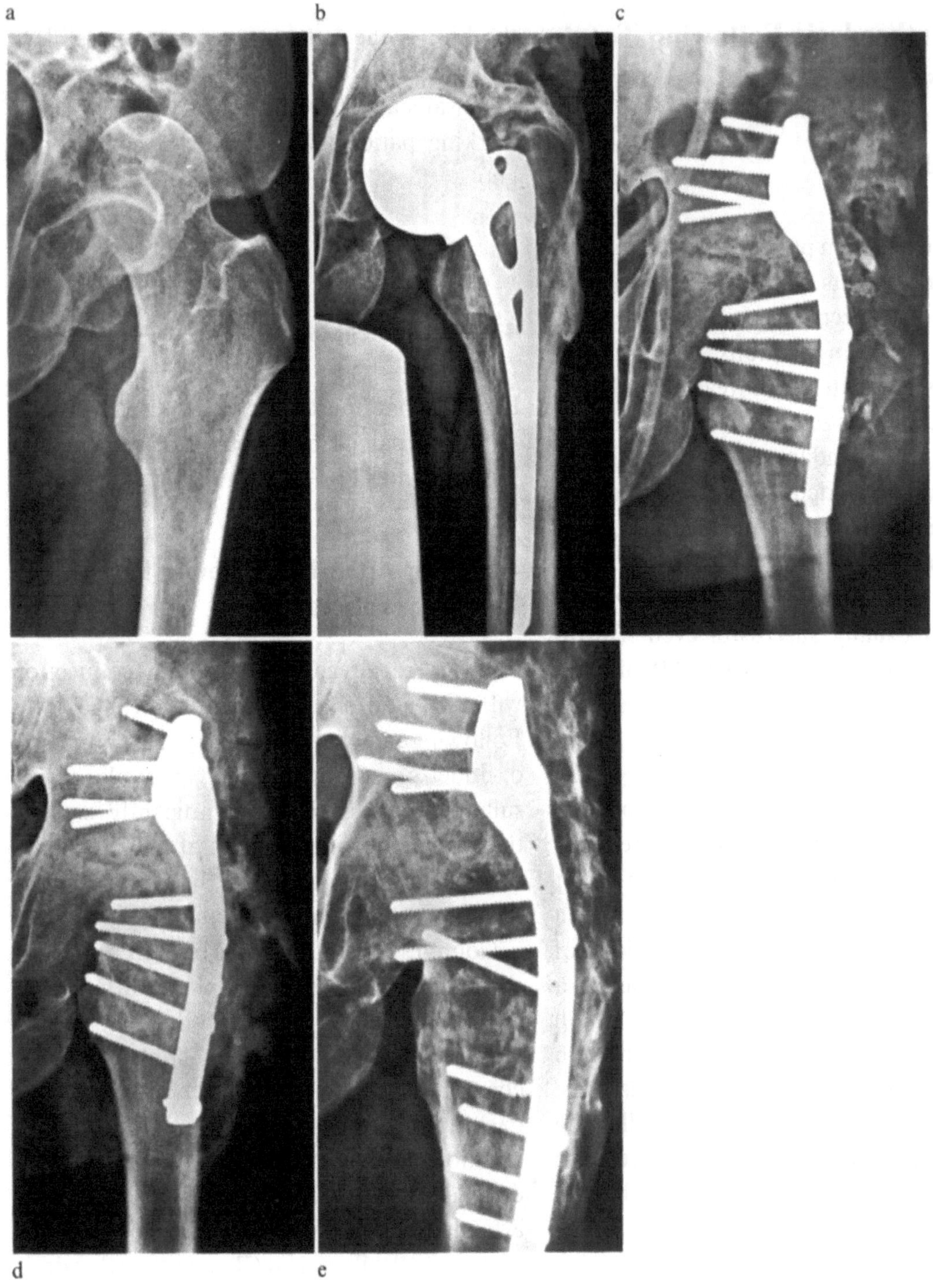
a
b
c
d
e

create a sufficiently large area of contact between the freshened trochanter and the pelvis. The way is then clear for HA using rigid internal fixation. (Figs. 218, 219). Sometimes following partial joint prosthesis implantation, partial ankylosis occurs without joint deformity; in such cases the implant material may be left in situ, and the ankylosis may be completed by rigid internal fixation (Fig. 220).

4.2.2 Hip Arthrodesis Following Total Prosthesis

Here the local factors present considerably greater problems. A considerable bone cavity results from removal of the implant and particularly from removal of the bone cement. There is hardly any cancellous bone left in the trochanter or in the proximal femur. The bone is biologically inferior, the blood supply is reduced and the danger of subclinical infection is always present.

The severe changes in bone structure which are usually present around the acetabulum make PO inadvisable. One can also expect considerable leg shortening. In the whole of the world literature we failed to find a publication on HA following (infected) TP and only one case occurred in our series (Fig. 221). If the operation is indicated we first attempt to fill the freshened acetabulum and the defect in the proximal femur with homologous and/or autologous corticocancellous grafts. One or more femoral heads excised during a TP operation would be particularly suitable. The second step comprises either an abduction arthrodesis followed later by subtrochanteric corrective osteotomy or HA with minimal internal fixation (bridging plate fixed to the pelvis and proximal femur).

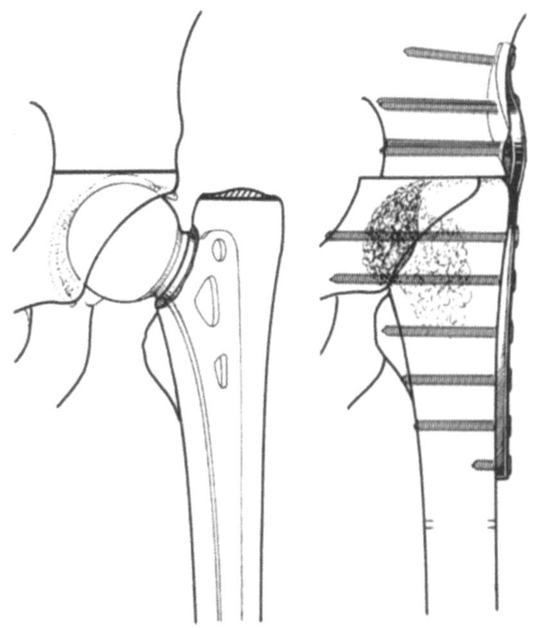

Fig. 219. *Principle of HA following partial hip replacement* (Diagrammatic representation of Figs. 218b and c.) The trochanter is freshened and the cavities in the acetabulum and proximal femur are filled with cancellous bone. PO is carried out with more or less marked medial displacement of the distal pelvic component in order to assure good contact between trochanter and pelvis. Rigid internal fixation with a cobra-head plate

Figs. 218–221. *HA following partial and total joint replacement*

Fig. 218. *Replacement of a Moore prosthesis by cobra-head plate arthrodesis.* J. D., ♀, aged 45 years, No. 102162.

a) Traumatic dislocation of the hip joint.

b) One year following implantation of a Moore prosthesis. 4.5 cm leg shortening. Severe limitation of hip mobility. 45° fixed external rotation deformity.

c) Cobra-head plate arthrodesis with PO. Inadequate correction of external rotation deformity.

d) Sixteen months later. Significant bone resorption around the proximal end of the plate. Severe calcification around the distal end of the plate. HA not united with certainty. Clinical evidence of PA (pain, standing on one leg impossible, lack of rigidity).

e) Six years after rearthrodesis with a longer cobra-head plate, cancellous bone plasty and corrective subtrochanteric osteotomy performed because of stiff PA and rotation deformity. The HA is united with good leg position. Correction of 5 cm leg shortening with orthopaedic shoe

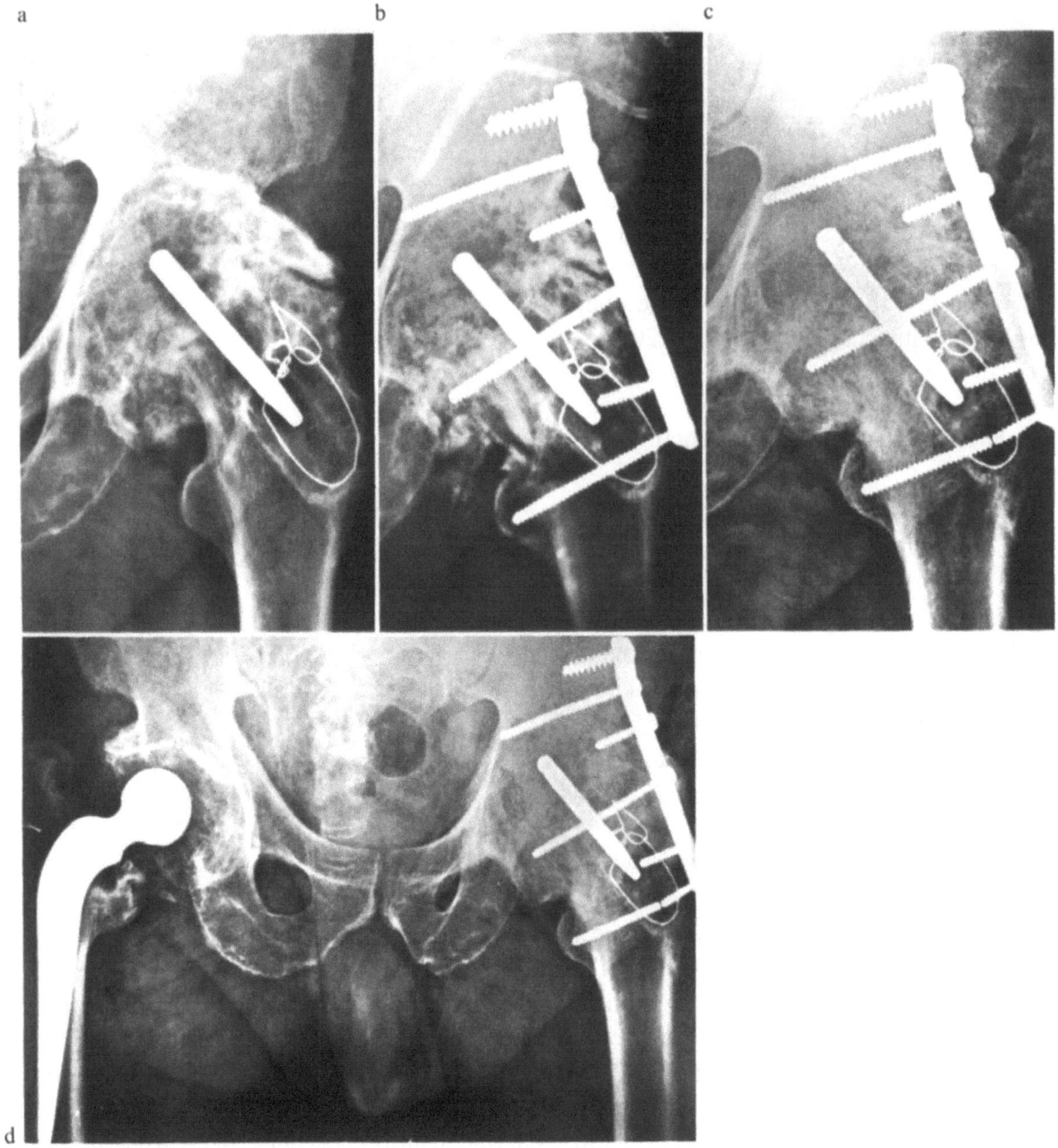

Fig. 220. *HA following Judet prosthesis*. B. F., ♂, aged 69 years, No. 103134.

a) Ten years after implantation of Judet prosthesis. Painful partial ankylosis.

b) HA. The prosthesis is left in place. A corticocancellous bone graft is taken from the iliac crest and inserted into a slot between the lateral pubic ramus and the femur along the femoral neck. Tension band plate.

c) Follow-up 6 years later. HA united with good leg position. Patient complaint-free.

d) Pelvic film from the same case. On the opposite side a 5 year old TP with perfect results. Abduction 50 cm. Flexion/extension 60 – 0 – 0°. Patient farms full time

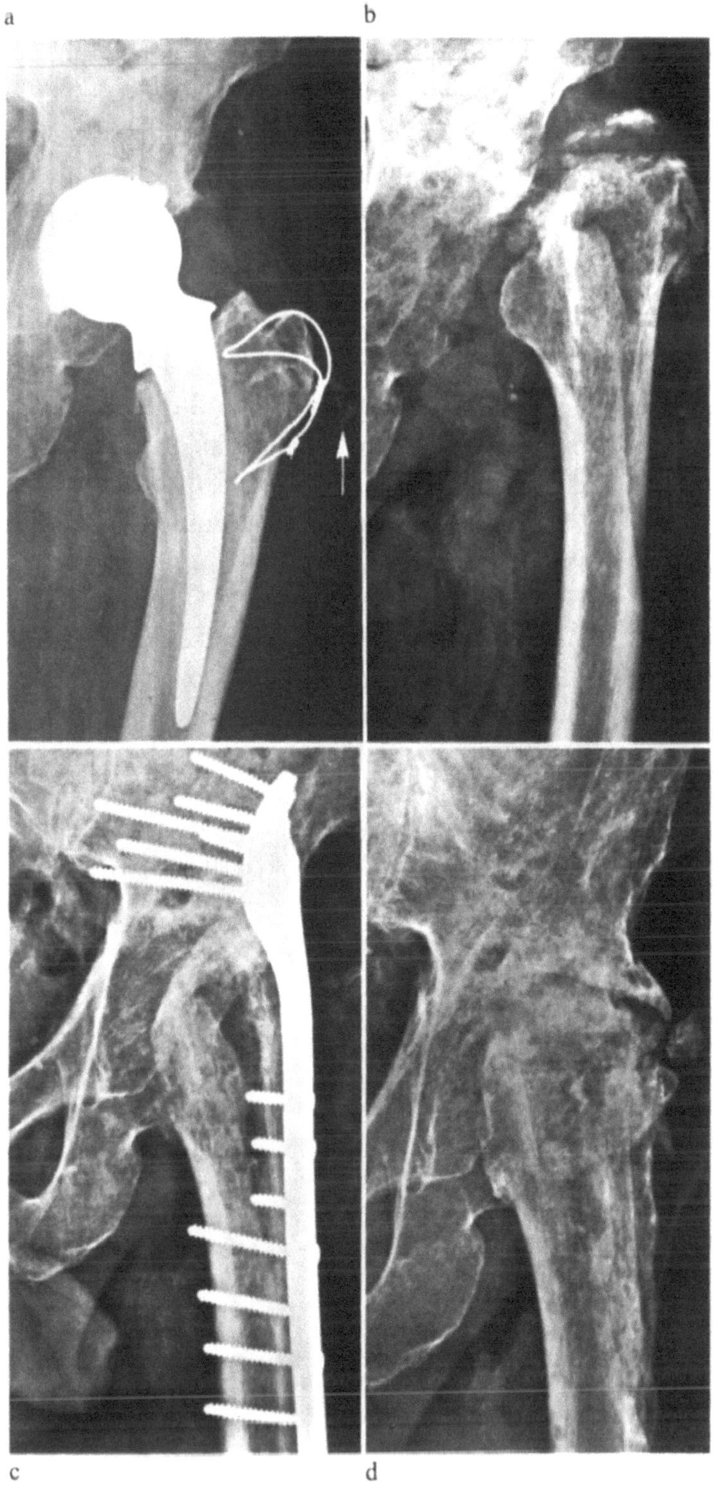

Fig. 221. *Cobra-head plate arthrodesis of a Girdlestone hip following removal of an infected prosthesis.* W. G., ♂, aged 69 years, No. 109080.

a) Four months after TP implantation. Wound fistula (see arrow).

b) Five months later. The infected TP has been removed. Girdlestone hip.

c) One month following HA with the leg in slight abduction.

d) One year following removal of the cobra-head plate and cancellous bone plasty because of painful fibrous ankylosis. The PA gap is still visible but bone union is commencing, particularly medially. Significant subjective improvement. Standing on one leg has been possible for several weeks

5 Summary

The combination of HA and TP is particularly to be recommended in young patients with severe bilateral hip disease. Usually the HA is the first operation and is performed on the more severely affected side. Despite the increased stress placed on the TP by the HA, the follow-up of our patients failed to show any effects detrimental to the TP.

Because of the considerable technical difficulties and increased risk to the patient associated with replacement of an arthrodesis by a total prosthesis, the operation is only indicated if severe problems have arisen, particularly in the LS, the knee joint or the contralateral hip. Despite arthrodesis lasting many years and the resulting disuse atrophy of the muscles, the abductors will resume their pelvic stabilising function following replacement of an HA by a TP as long as the abductor insertion is retained and there is no extensive muscle scarring. The results of the operation are very satisfying but the procedure is rendered more difficult by previous operations, differences in leg length, deformity and changes in the bone structure.

HA subsequent to TP is one of the problem operations in orthopaedic surgery. Following partial prosthetic replacement sufficient contact area between the pelvis and the proximal femur is assured by PO and medial displacement. This in turn allows the arthrodesis to be carried out by rigid internal fixation. In addition, bone cavities are, as far as possible, filled with cancellous bone.

We have only seen one case of HA following infected TP (Fig. 221). The extensive bone cavities, the biologically inferior bone and latent infection combine to present the surgeon with a difficult problem. From a biomechanical point of view, HA with primary rigid internal fixation is hardly possible.

IV. Complications

"1. If anything can go wrong, it will
2. When left to themselves, things go from bad to worse.
3. If two things can go wrong, the worst one will happen.
4. If something happens, it will be at the most inconvenient time.
5. Nature always sides with the hidden flaw in the system."

Anonymous

1 Introduction

The frequency of complications is an illustration of the challenge presented both to the doctor and to the patient by HA. In our series the most frequent complications are PA and malposition. This is a consequence of the considerable biomechanical load placed on the arthrodesed hip and the technical difficulties encountered in adjusting the leg position correctly at operation.

The next complication, in order of frequency, is infection which presents special problems in any orthopedic procedure. Luckily, these problems are easier to solve following HA than following partial prosthetic replacement.

With the development of CHARNLEY's arthrodesis technique and HA using rigid internal fixation, fatigue fractures have been added to the list of complications. Studies of our failed HA from 1961 to 1971 have allowed us to reach important conclusions concerning indications and techniques.

2 Pseudoarthrosis

This is the most important complication following HA (14.5%). In our series a significant reduction in PA frequency has occurred in recent years which may be associated with the type of fixation. The use of rigid internal fixation has improved the prognosis in respect of PA noticeably. A reduction in PA frequency already occurred on introduction of the double-plate technique. PA became even less common following the use of the cobra-head plate; only 16 PA occurred following 258 Type IV HA (6.2%) compared to 22% – 25% following Type I and Type II arthrodeses (Table 34).

Table 34. Pseudarthroses, radiologically nonunited HA and infections (1961 – 1971)

Arthrodesis type	Pseudarthroses	%	Radiol. nonunited	%	Infection	%
Freshening	10	31.2	3	9.4	3	0.9
Nailing	1	50.0	–	–	–	–
CHARNLEY	1	50.0		–	–	–
Type I	35	22.4	2	1.3	5	3.2
Type II	5	25.0	–	–	–	–
Type III	15	14.0	3	2.8	6	5.6
Type IV	16	6.2	6	2.3	9	4.2
Atypical	1	20.0	–	–	1	20.0
Total	84	14.5	14	2.4	24	4.1

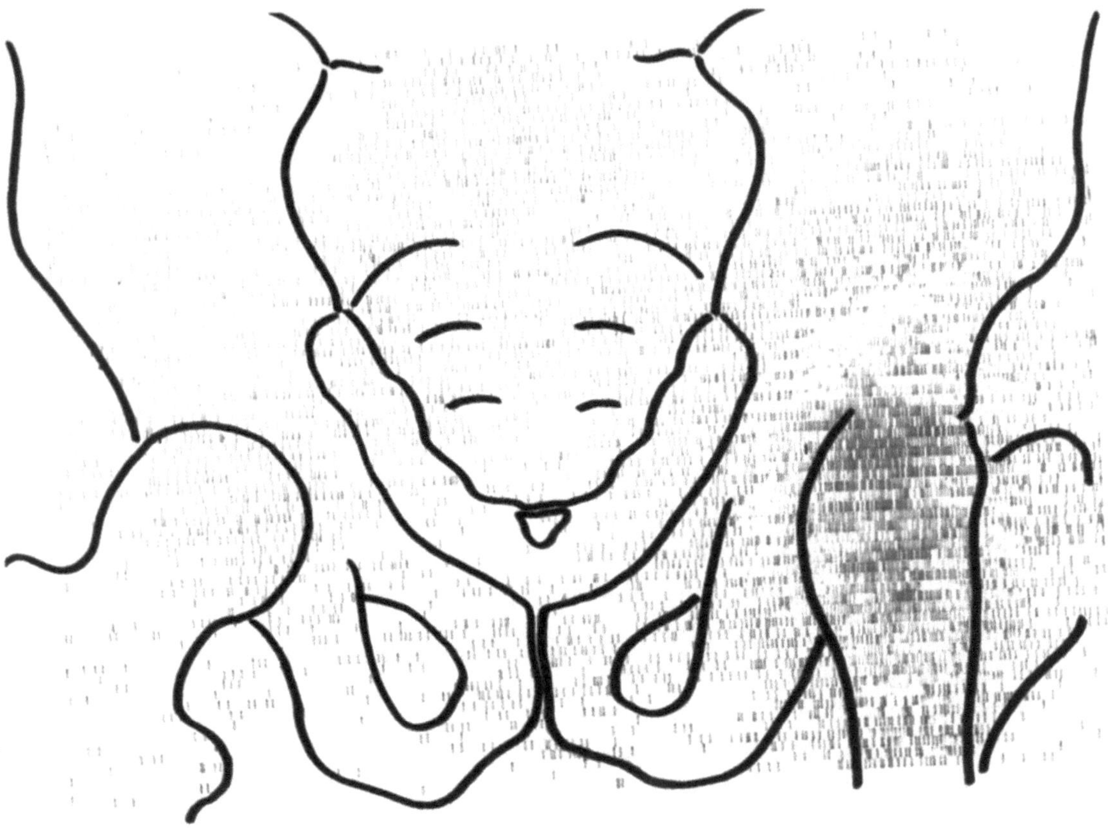

Fig. 222. *Scintigram of a pseudarthrotic HA*. W. G., ♂, aged 71 years, No. 109080. Markedly increased activity in the PA when compared with the opposite side

This proves that HA is only followed by PA if there is inadequate rigidity.

Pseudoarthrosis in a HA or in an IO which accompanies HA behaves in a biologically similar manner to fracture PA. It results either from inadequate rigidity or from infection. Pseudoarthroses are usually *reactive or proliferative with a pronounced tendency to healing* so that rigid internal fixation suffices to bring about union. The osteoporotic and regenerative features of PA can be demonstrated scintigraphically and scintimetrically (SEGMÜLLER) (Fig. 222).

Infected PA subsequent to an orthopedic operation requires the same treatment as infected PA following a fracture, i.e., debridement, sequesterotomy, stabilisation, cancellous bone plasty and drainage (WEBER, CECH).

2.1 Noninfected Pseudoarthrosis

2.1.1 Stabilisation of the Pseudoarthrosis

Basically, compression internal fixation suffices in the treatment of noninfected PA.

a) Compression Internal Fixation

In the treatment of PA, fixation is best brought about using the *cobra-head plate*. This technique is therefore used in the majority of cases (PA subsequent to Type I, Type II and Type III).

If possible, a cobra-head plate arthrodesis is also performed for PA following Type IV arthrodesis.

However, if there is inadequate pelvic anchorage for the cobra-head plate, *HA with two plates* is carried out.

If PA occurs at the level of the subtrochanteric osteotomy only one plate is used. In selected cases the stiff PA can be treated using only one plate which functions as a tension band.

Case Material

I. PA at the level of the HA:
   1. Cobra-head fixation (Figs. 223 – 229)
   2. Fixation with two plates (Figs. 230 – 235)
   3. Fixation with one plate (Figs. 236 – 238)

II. PA of the subtrochanteric or intertrochanteric osteotomy
   1. Cobra-head plate fixation (Figs. 239 – 242)
   2. Fixation with two plates (Figs. 243 – 245)
   3. Fixation with one plate (Fig. 246)

b) Bone Grafting

Bone union may be accelerated by simultaneous cancellous bone plasty. This may be performed in two ways:

1. Insertion into a slot of a corticocancellous graft taken from the iliac crest. This should cross the ventral aspect of the pseudoarthrotic gap (Fig. 247a).
2. Filling of a ventrally prepared decorticated pocket with cancellous bone chips (Fig. 247b).

a b c

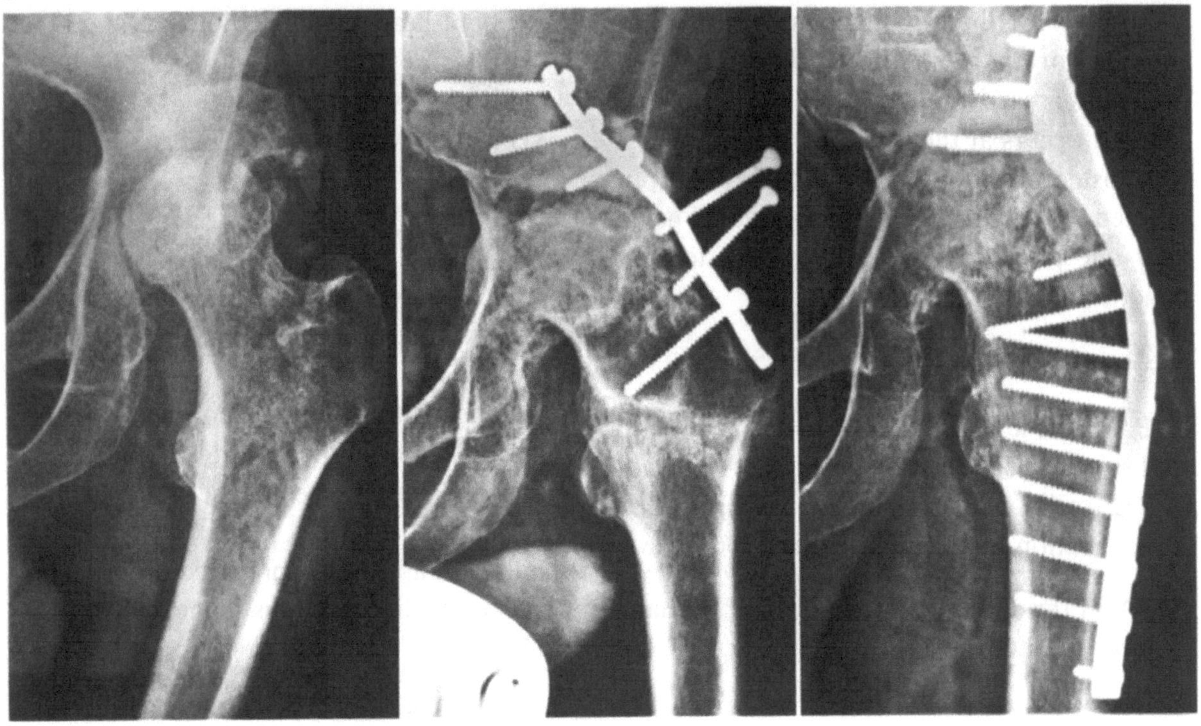

Fig. 223. *PA at the level of the HA*. Sch. A., ♂, aged 37 years, No. 111171.

a) Three months following fracture dislocation of the hip treated by traction.

b) Thirteen months following Type II arthrodesis. Intertrochanteric osteotomy united; HA pseudarthrotic.

c) One year following rearthrodesis with a cobra-head plate. PA united. Ideal leg position

a b c

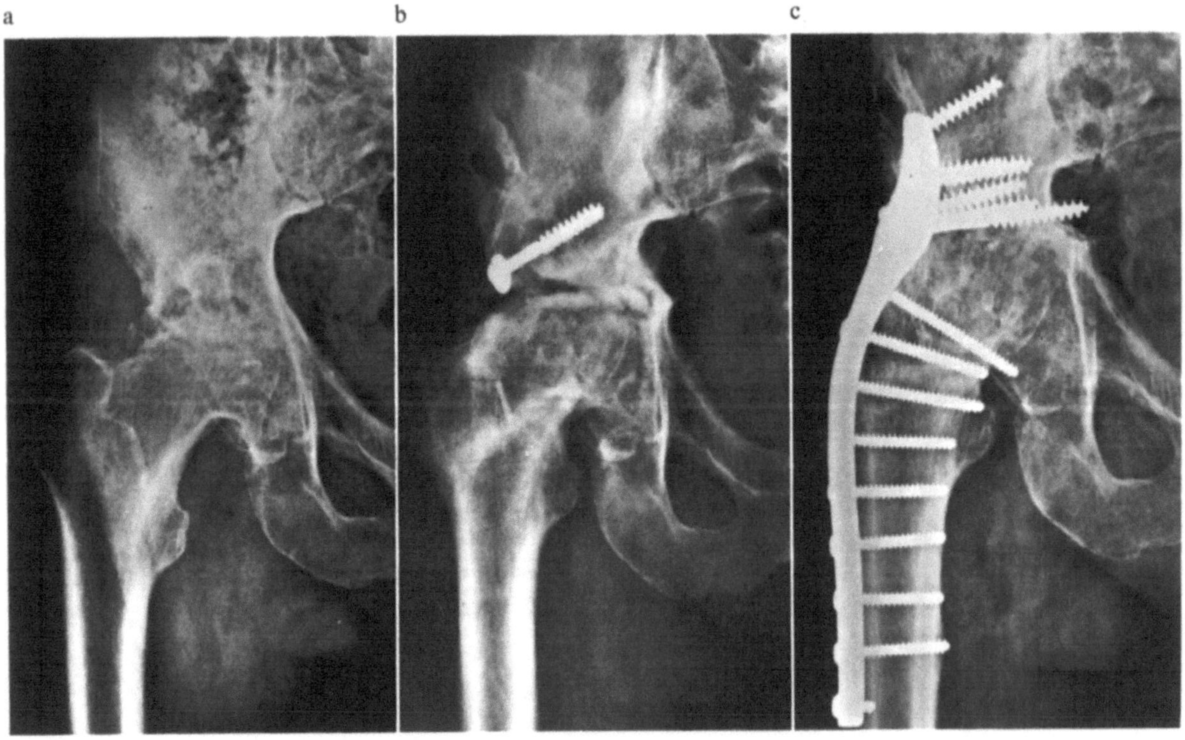

a b

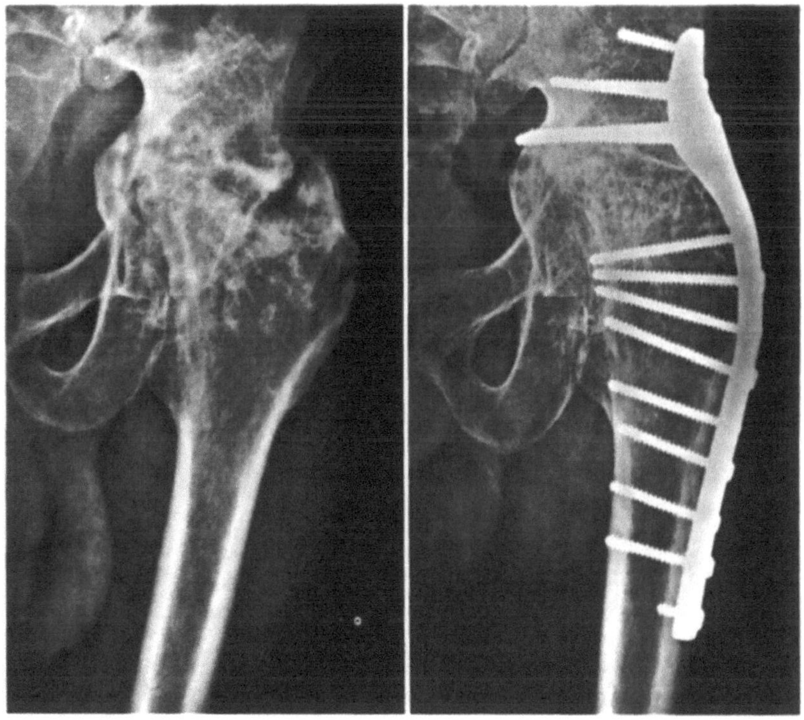

Fig. 225. *PA following decortication arthrodesis.* K. P., ♂, aged 44 years, No. 112227.

a) PA 8 years following decortication arthrodesis for NHF secondary to trauma.

b) Thirty-eight months following rearthrodesis with a cobra-head plate. PA united. Ideal leg position. 1 cm leg shortening

←

Fig. 224. *PA following Type I HA.* K. M., ♂, aged 57 years, No. 91008.

a) Advanced arthrosis of the hip with the joint fixed in 30° flexion, 5° abduction and 20° external rotation.

b) Sixteen months following Type I HA. Intertrochanteric osteotomy united with PA at the level of the PO.

c) Thirteen months following rearthrodesis with a cobra-head plate. PA united. Patient working full time as a farmer

a b c

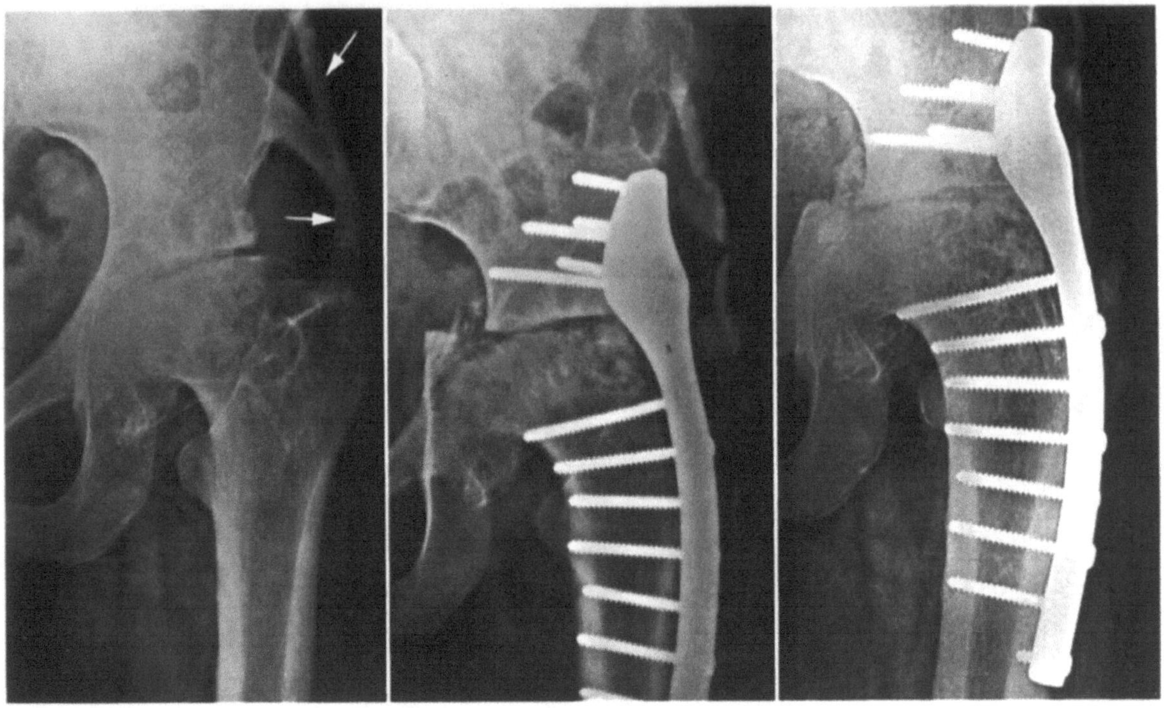

Fig. 226. *PA following extra-articular bridge-graft arthrodesis.* R. M., aged 57 years, No. 109646.

a) Eighteen years following attempted HA. PA of the distal part of the iliofemoral graft. Joint space still present. The patient can flex the leg to 20°.

b) Three weeks following cobra-head arthrodesis with PO.

c) Eight months later. Ideal union

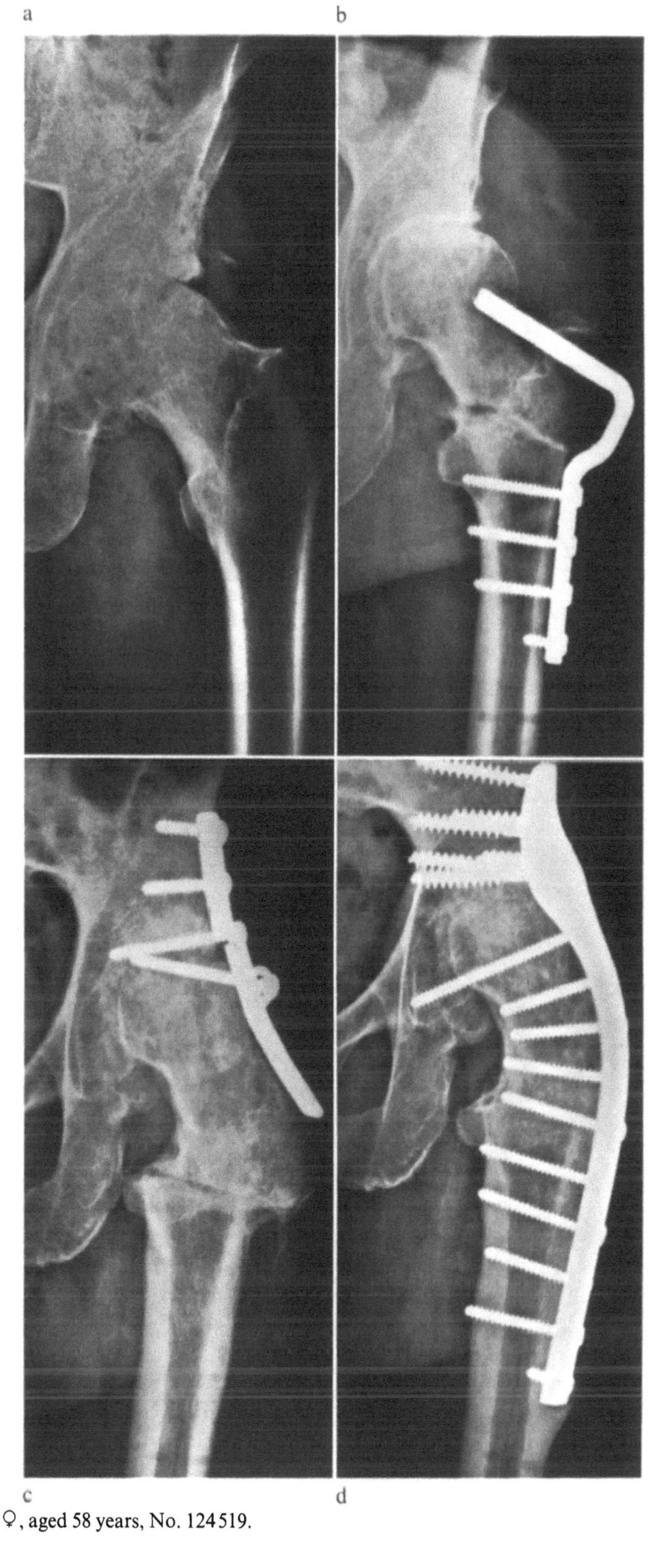

Fig. 227. *PA following buttress-plate arthrodesis.* R. L., ♀, aged 58 years, No. 124519.

a) Advanced arthrosis of the hip.

b) Intertrochanteric valgus osteotomy. The plate has been inserted too high up.

c) Five months following attempted arthrodesis for joint infection following intertrochanteric osteotomy. Intertrochanteric osteotomy united. Plate fracture at the level of the PA.

d) Nine months following rearthrodesis with a cobra-head plate. PA clinically and radiologically reunited

a b

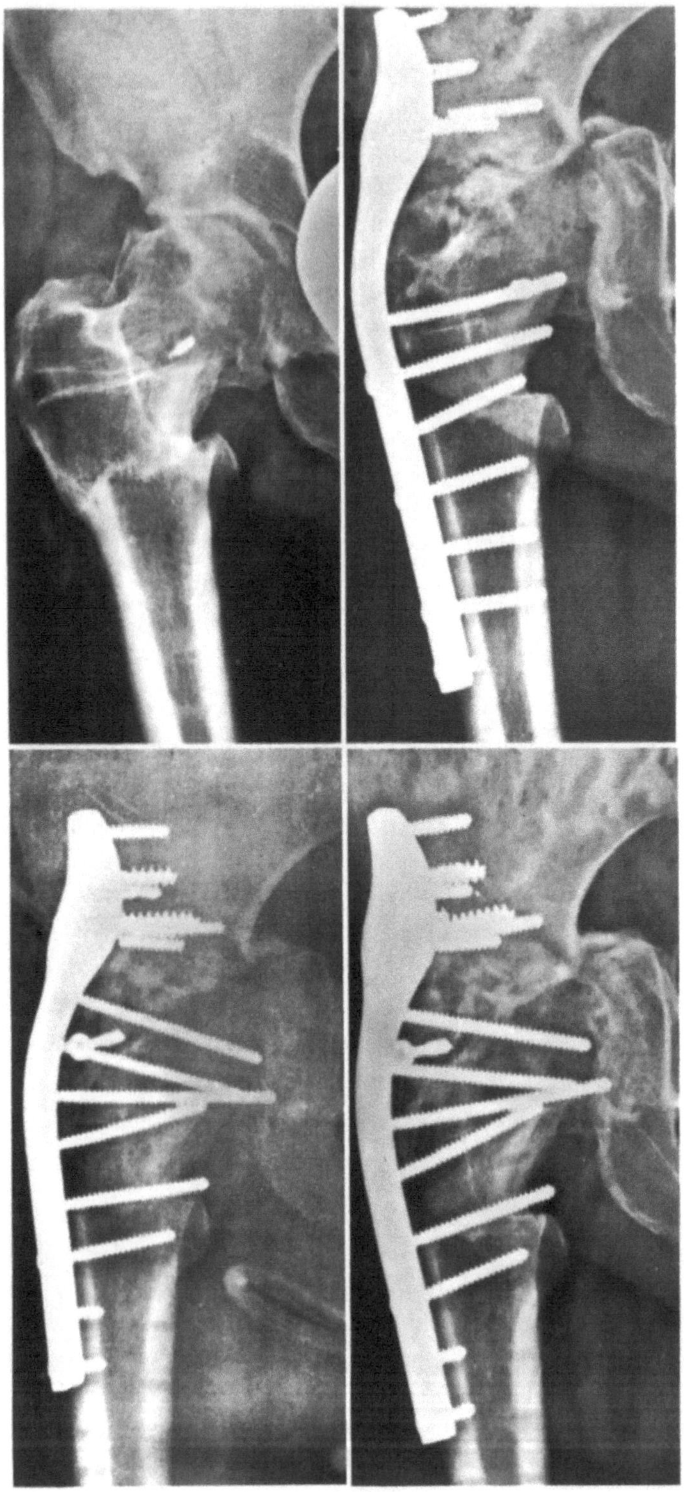

c d

Fig. 228. *PA following attempted arthrodesis with a cobra-head plate*. L. T., ♀, aged 37 years, No. 120237.

a) One year following intertrochanteric osteotomy for arthrosis of the hip. Extensive osteophyte formation. Total loss of joint congruence.

b) Four months following Type IV HA with PO. Screw fracture, increase radiolucency in the region of the osteotomy and unequivocal clinical evidence of PA.

c) Radiograph immediately following rearthrodesis. A large graft which was taken from the anterior iliac crest was applied anteriorly and fixed with a screw so as to bridge the osteotomy gap.

d) Three months later. Good bone union. Full weight bearing possible with no subjective complaints

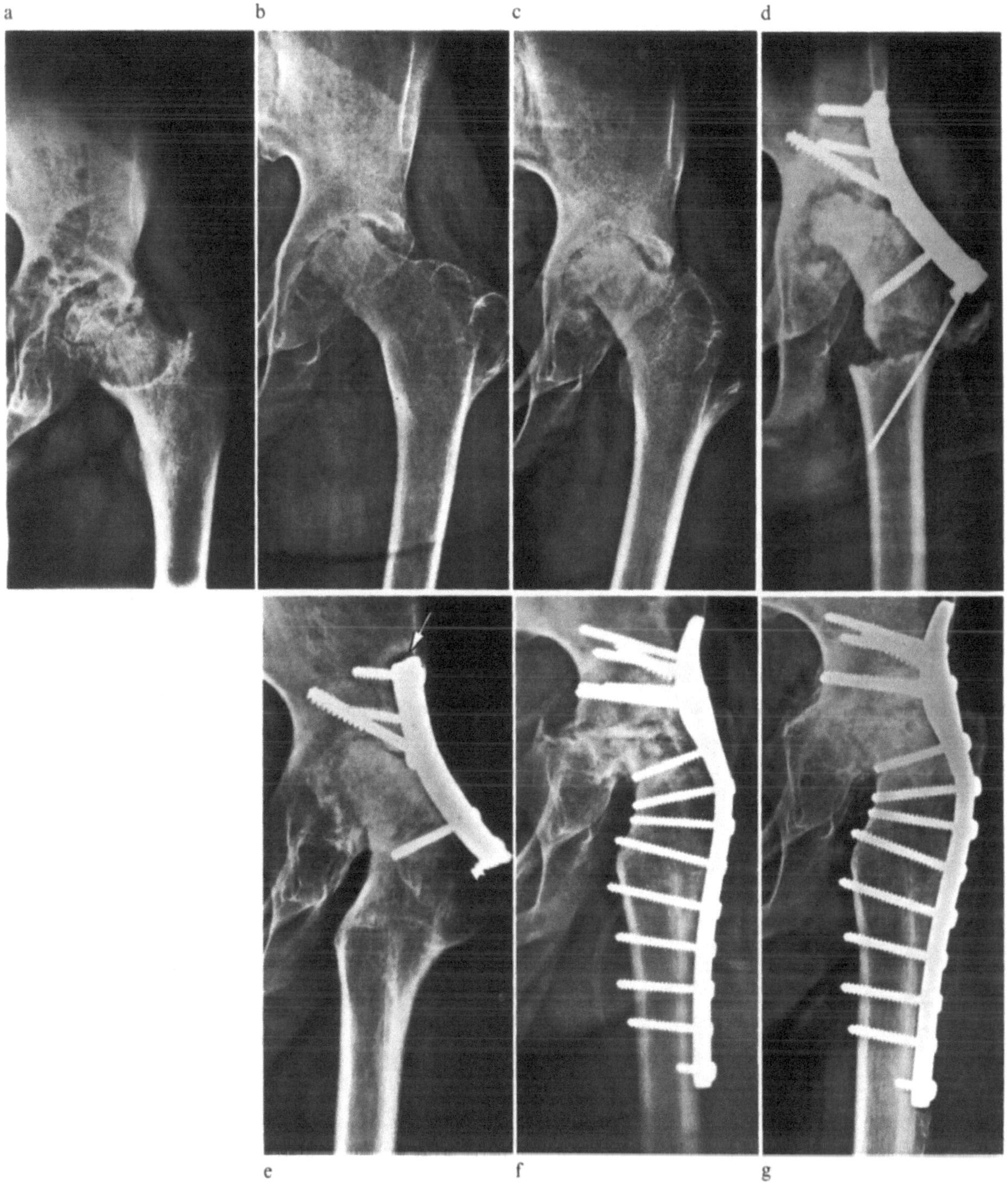

Fig. 229. *PA following Type II HA*. F. R., ♀, aged 18 years, No. 70856.

a) Two years following traumatic dislocation of the hip. Femoral head necrosis

b) Seven months following implantation of a Silastic membrane. 3.5 cm leg shortening.

c) Fourteen months later. Painful and almost total ankylosis. 5 cm leg shortening.

d) Type II HA.

e) Six years later. Painful PA. Increased radiolucency around the plate and screw indicates loosening.

f) Immediately following rearthrodesis with a cobra-had plate and PO.

g) Six months later. Subjective and objective union of the PA

a b c

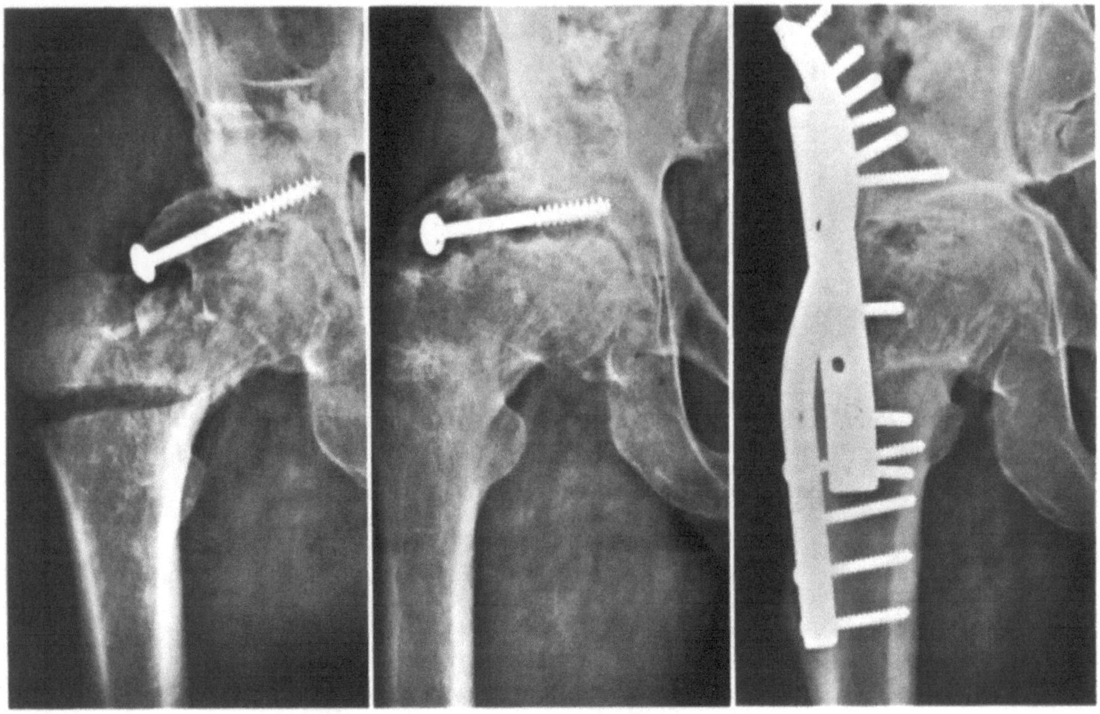

Fig. 230. *PA following Type I HA*. M. J., ♂, aged 51 years, No. 84908.

a) Type I HA performed for hip arthrosis with almost complete ankylosis.

b) Ten months later. Intertrochanteric osteotomy united. Loosening of the screw. Painful PA.

c) Sixteen months following rearthrodesis with two plates. PA united. Patient complaint free and working full time as a farmer

a b c

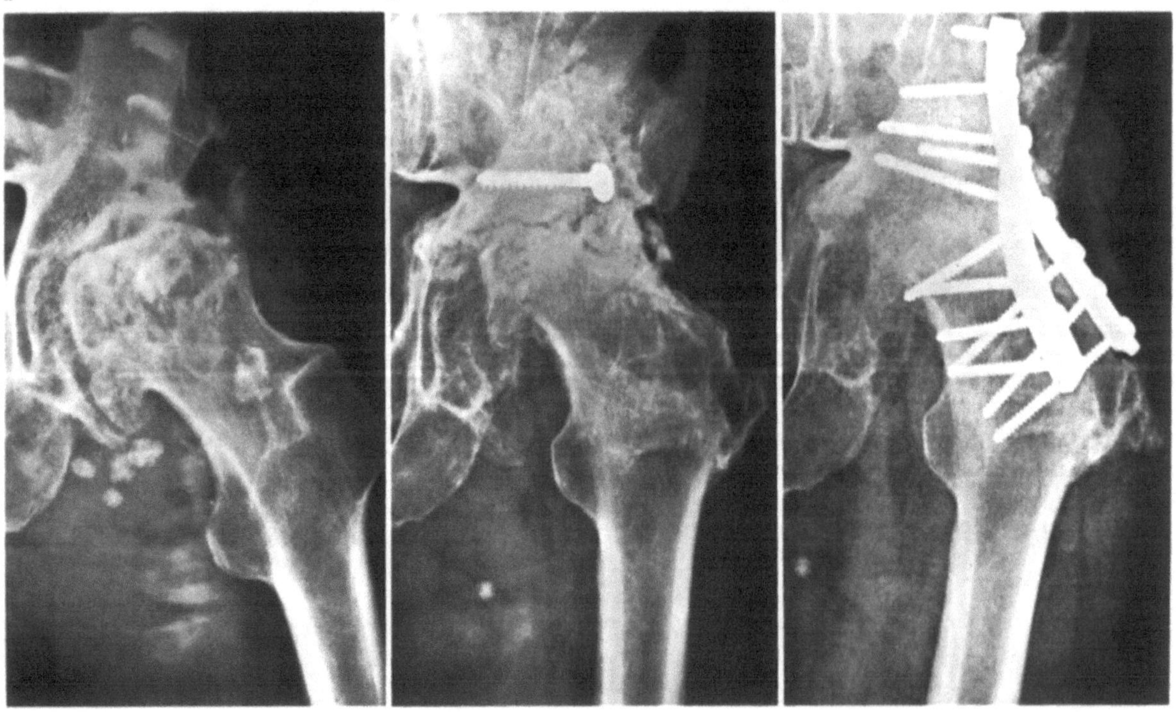

a b c

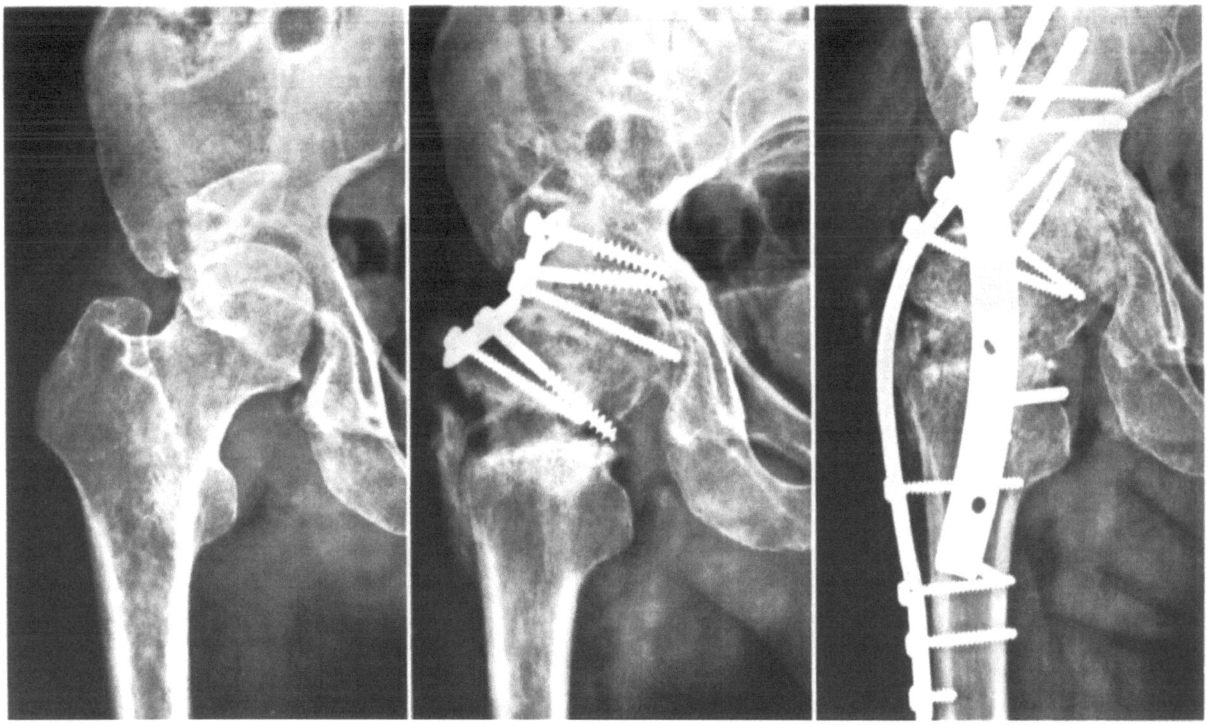

Fig. 232. *PA following Type II HA*. C. T., ♀, aged 59 years, No. 99118.

a) Seven months old traumatic dislocation of the hip on the right side with fracture of the acetabular roof.

b) Eight months following Type II HA. Intertrochanteric osteotomy united. Painful PA of the HA.

c) Three months following rearthrodesis with a cobra-head plate. The straight plate has been made concave so as to hold cancellous bone graft in place. PA united. Patient complaint-free

Fig. 231. *PA following Type I HA*. G. R., ♂, aged 46 years, No. 91783.

a) Preoperative radiograph. Severe arthrosis of the hip.

b) Six months following Type I HA with PO. Pseudarthrosis.

c) Five months following double-plate arthrodesis. PA united. Patient working full time as construction labourer

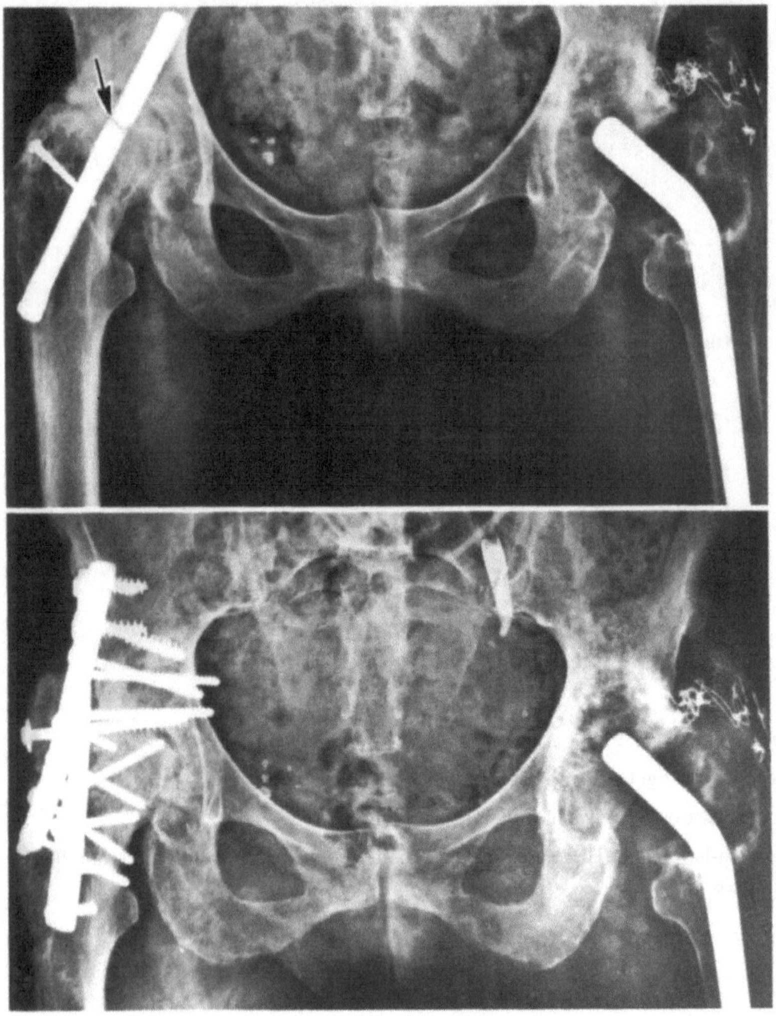

a b

Fig. 233. *PA following attempted arthrodesis by transarticular nailing*. E. M., ♀, aged 67 years, No. 75908.

a) Three years following Merle d'Aubigné plasty of the left hip and 6 years following arthrodesis of the right hip. The nail has fractured and there is a painful PA.

b) Six months following double-plate arthrodesis. Subjective and objective union of the PA

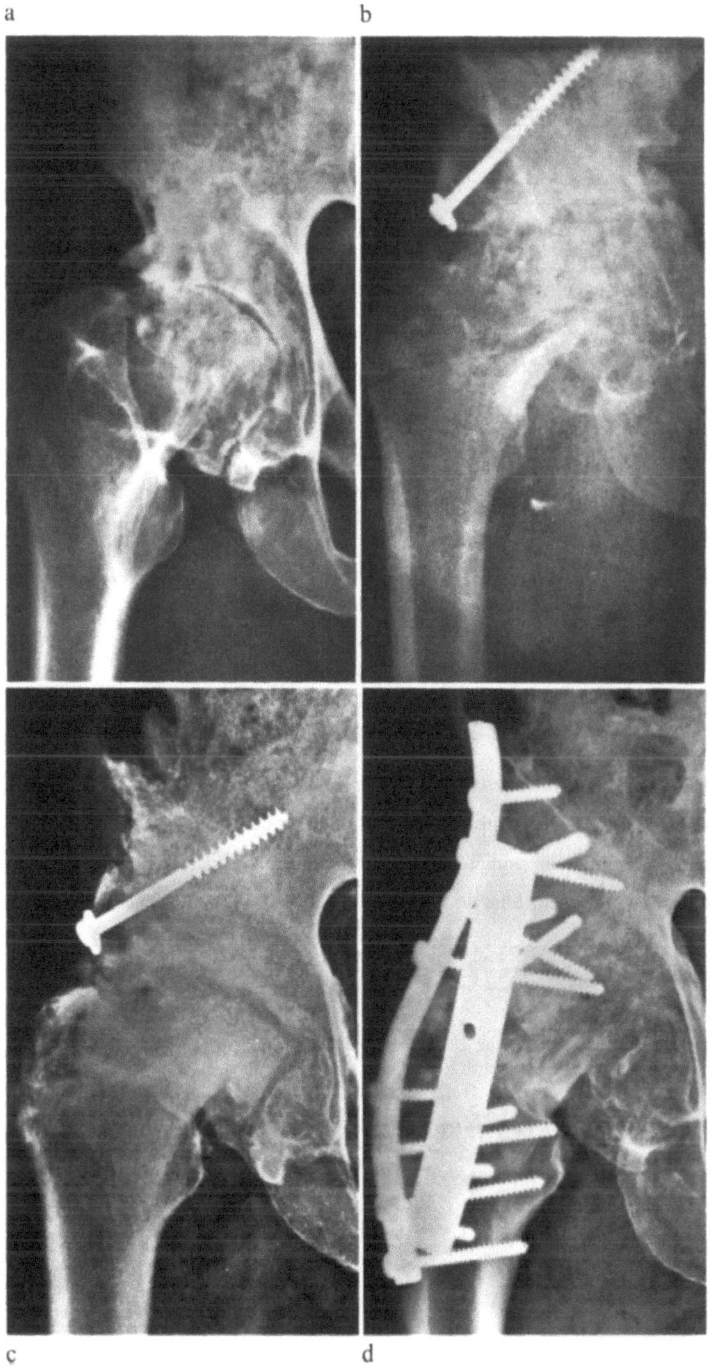

Fig. 234. *PA following Type I HA*. K. H., ♂, aged 57 years, No. 78471.

a) Severe hip arthrosis.

b) Type I HA with excessively high intertrochanteric osteotomy.

c) Twelve months later a very painful PA has developed.

d) Twenty months following rearthrodesis with two plates. The PA has united. The patient is complaint-free and working full-time in an automobile paint shop

a b c

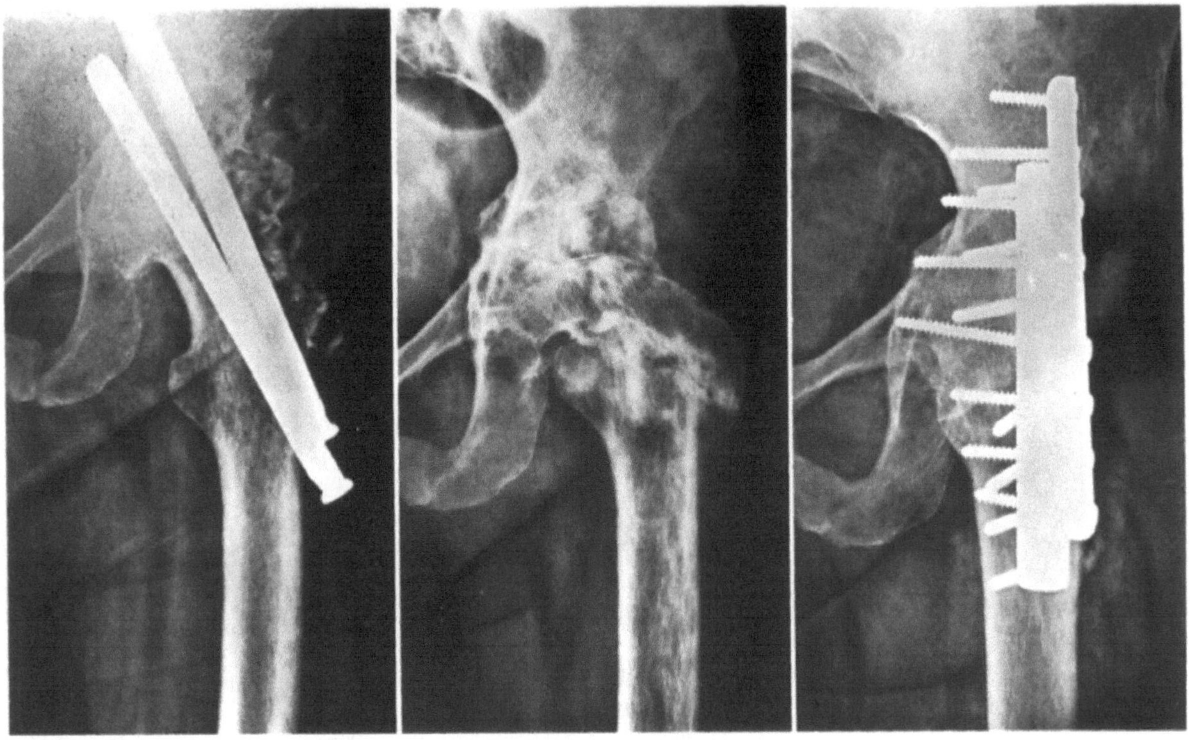

Fig. 235. *Double-plate arthrodesis following two attempts at HA*. R. B., ♀, aged 43 years, No. 5350.

a) Nail arthrodesis performed for NHF following central dislocation of the hip. PA had occurred.

b) PA 5 months following renewed decortication arthrodesis with intertrochanteric osteotomy.

c) Follow-up 9 years after double-plate arthrodesis. PA united with good leg position

a b c

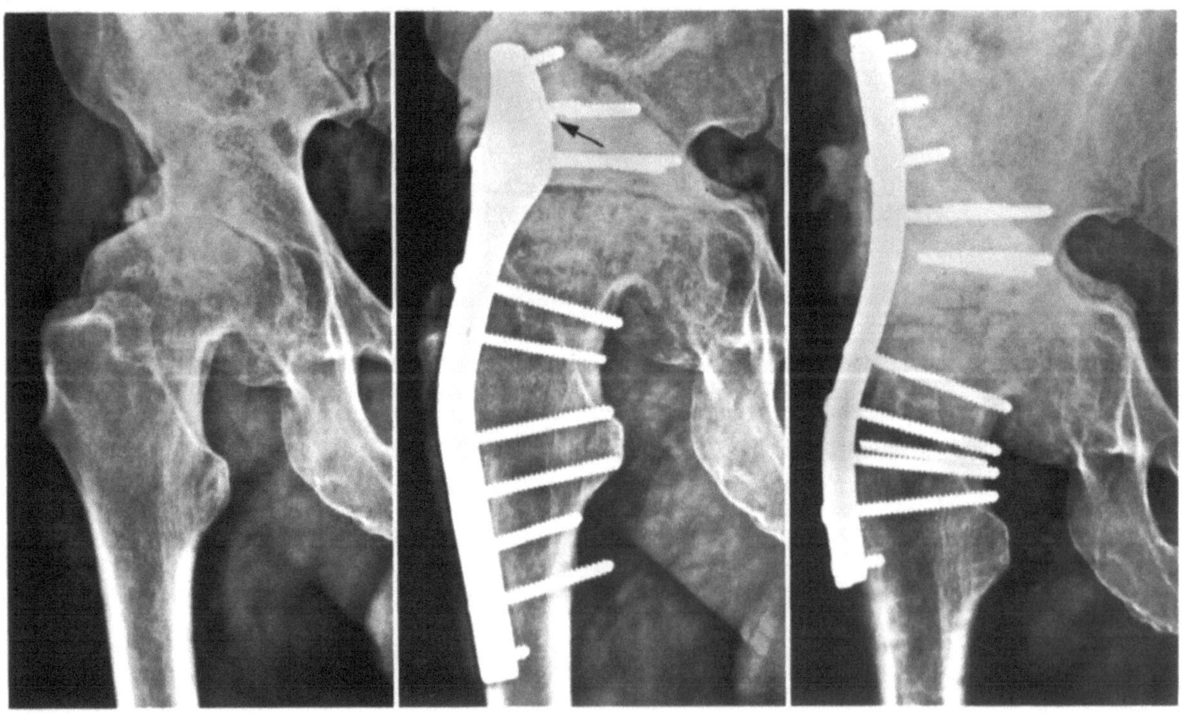

a b c

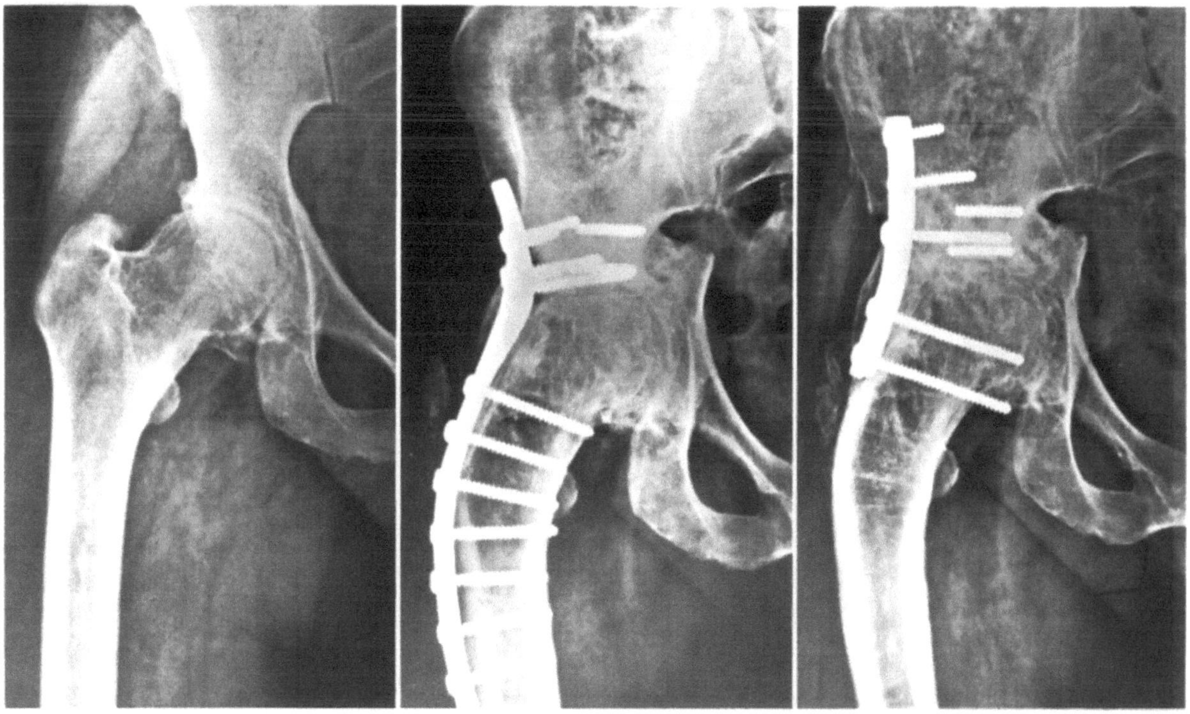

Fig. 237. *PA following Type IV HA.* G. M., ♀, aged 53 years, No. 98582.

a) Preoperative film.

b) Twenty months following attempted arthrodesis with a cobra-head plate and PO. Unequivocal clinical and radiological evidence of PA. Screw fracture.

c) Fifteen months following rearthrodesis. A graft was taken from the iliac crest and inserted into a slot across the arthrodesis; a compression plate was then applied. The PA has united

Fig. 236. *PA following Type IV HA.* C. L., ♂, aged 45 years, No. 143441.

a) Arthrosis of the hip secondary to CDH.

b) One year following femoral head plate arthrodesis of the hip. Unequivocal evidence of PA with screw fracture.

c) Three months following Type II rearthrodesis. Bone union is radiologically incomplete. Clinically the arthrodesis is united with good leg position

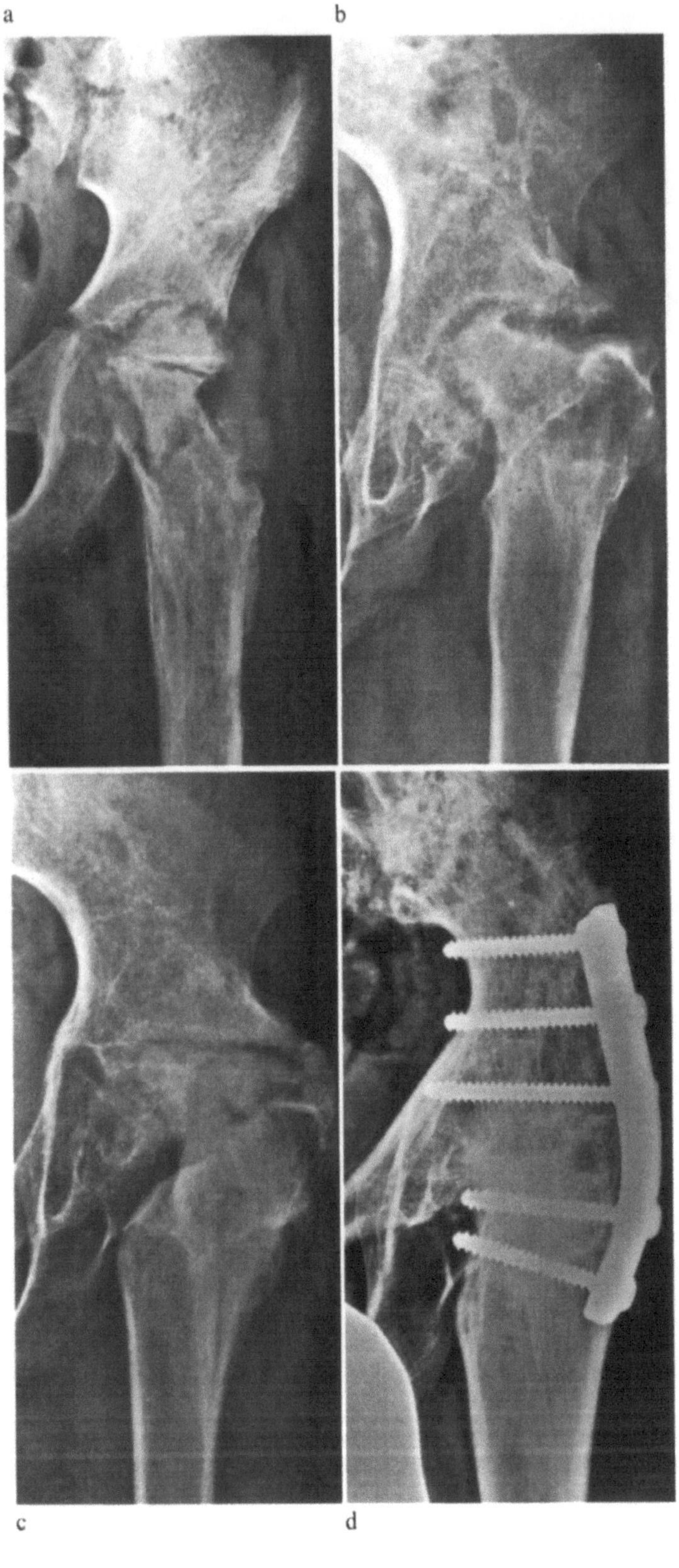

Fig. 238. *PA following two attempts at freshening arthrodesis*. S. V., ♂, aged 16 years, No. 52851.

a) Severe destruction of the hip joint (Purulent arthritis).

b) Four months following evacuation of the abcess and freshening arthrodesis. Pseudarthrosis.

c) Four months following rearthrodesis with PO and transverse intertrochanteric osteotomy. Union of the PO has failed to occur.

d) Six months following Type II rearthrodesis and clamping of an iliac crest graft in an anterior slot. Subjective and objective union of the PA.

a b c

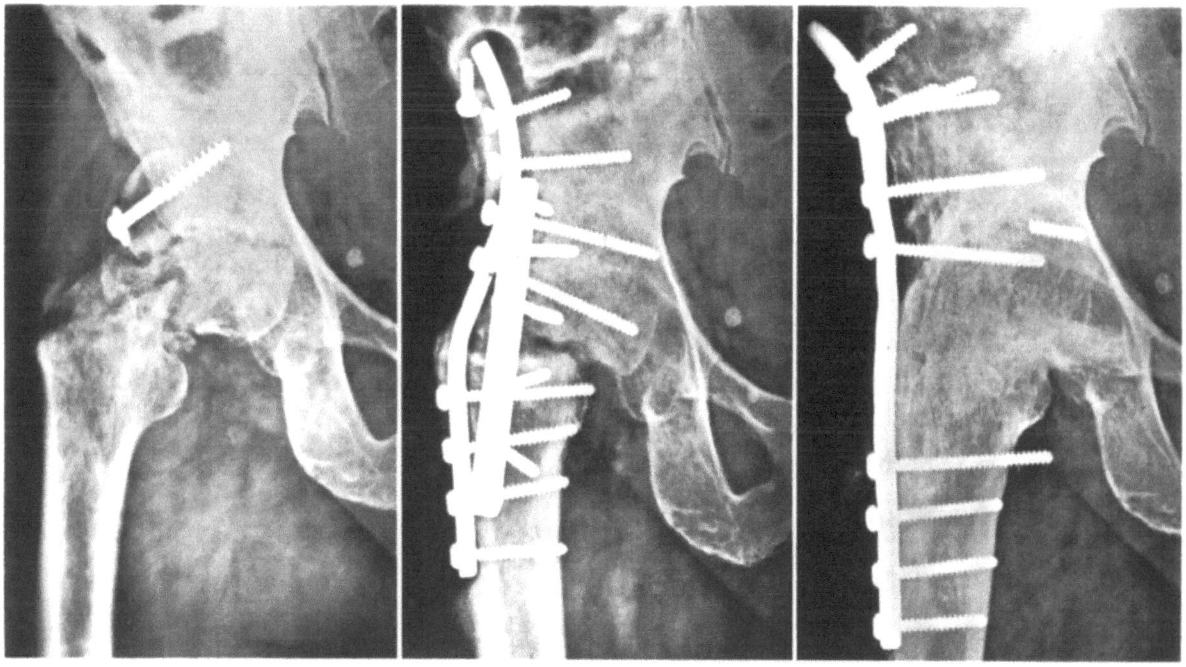

Fig. 239. *PA of the intertrochanteric osteotomy following HA.* W. A., ♀, aged 48 years, No. 97064.

a) Three months following Type I HA performed for hip arthrosis. PA of the HA and of the intertrochanteric osteotomy.

b) Eight months following rearthrodesis with two plates. The HA has united but there is PA of the intertrochanteric osteotomy with implant loosening and fracture of a screw.

c) Five years following further arthrodesis with a cobra-head plate and bone graft. PA united with good leg position

a b c

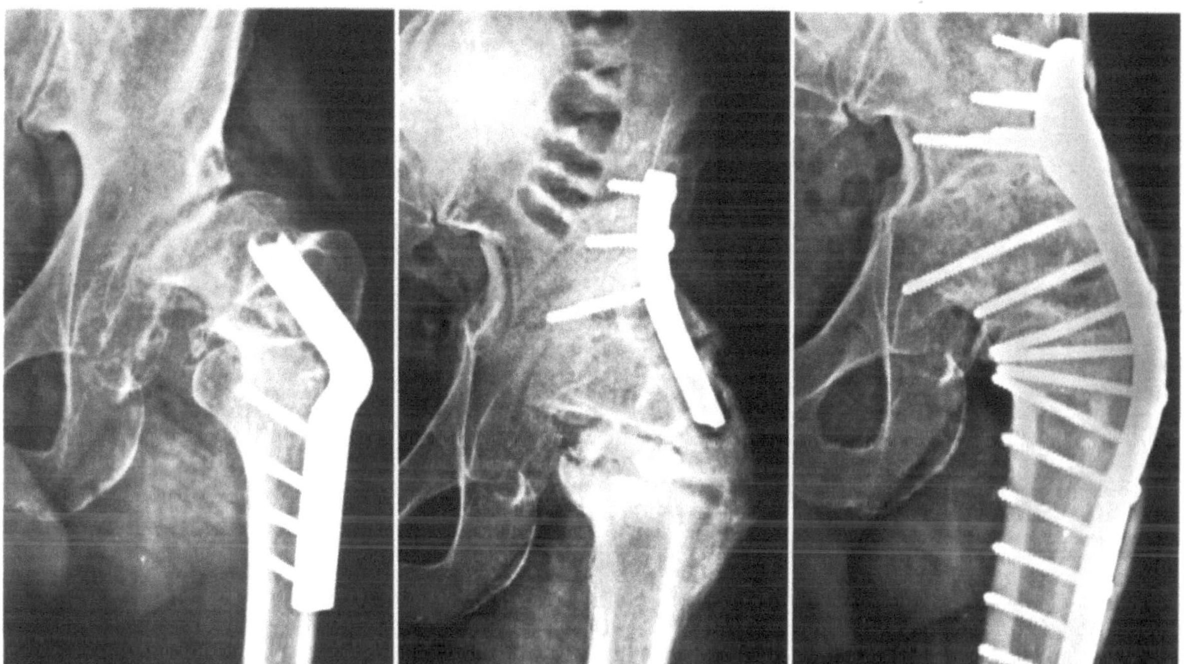

Fig. 240. *Pseudarthrotic intertrochanteric osteotomy following atypical HA.* W. W., ♂, aged 52 years, No. 110275.

a) Septic arthritis following intertrochanteric osteotomy performed for hip arthrosis secondary to Perthes disease.

b) Seven months following attempted HA; the HA is almost completely united. PA of the intertrochanteric osteotomy.

c) Follow-up 4 years following internal compression fixation with a cobra-head plate. The PA is united and there is 3.5 cm leg shortening. The patient is complaint-free and working full time as a construction foreman

a b

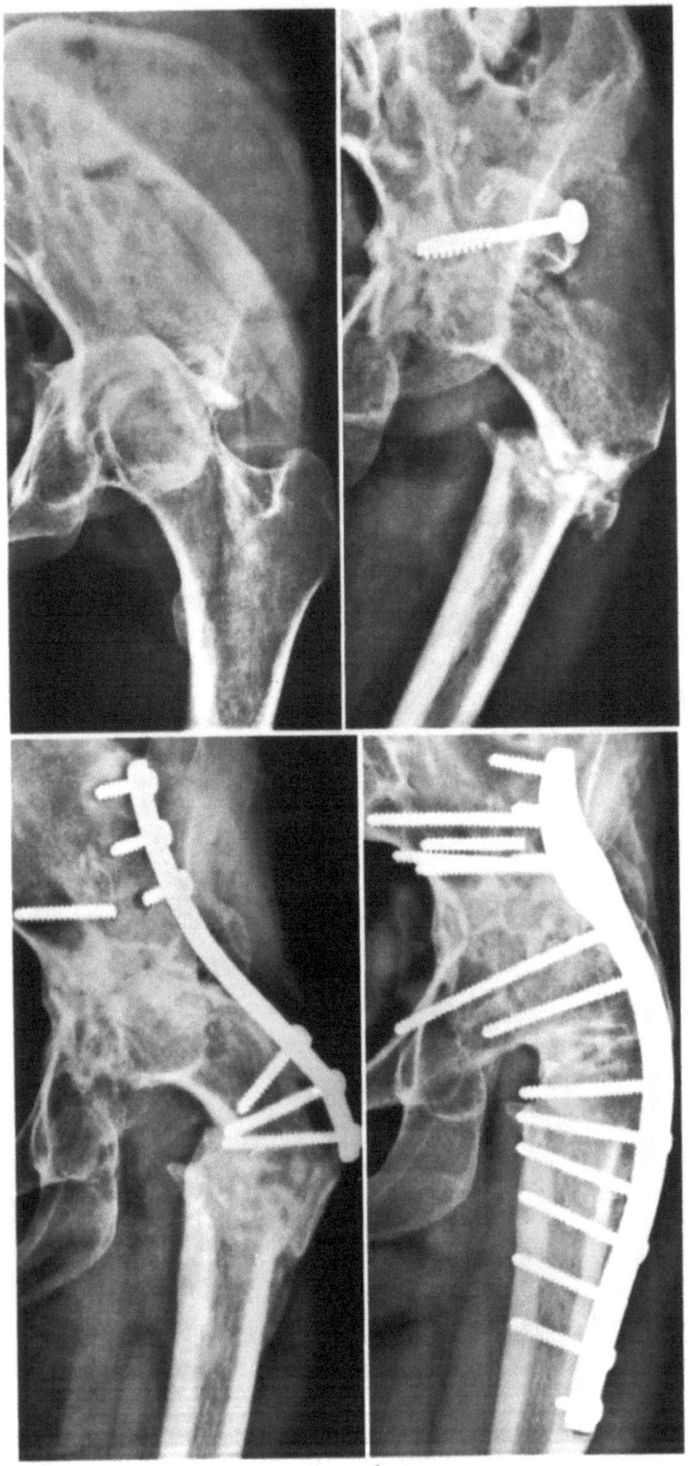

c d

Fig. 241. *PA of the HA as well as the intertrochanteric osteotomy*. D. M., ♀, aged 23 years, No. 115634.

a) Post-traumatic hip arthrosis 3 years after acetabular fracture.

b) Three months following Type I HA. Both the HA and the subtrochanteric osteotomy are pseudarthrotic. Adduction deformity with varus deformity of the proximal femur.

c) Ten months following Type II rearthrodesis with extensive freshening of the bone and insertion of a cancellous bone graft at the level of the subtrochanteric osteotomy. The latter is united but PA of the HA persists with loosening of the metal and screw fracture.

d) Thirteen months following treatment of PA and adduction deformity by rearthrodesis with a cobra-head plate. The PA has united and the angle of arthrodesis is satisfactory. The patient is complaint-free and working full time

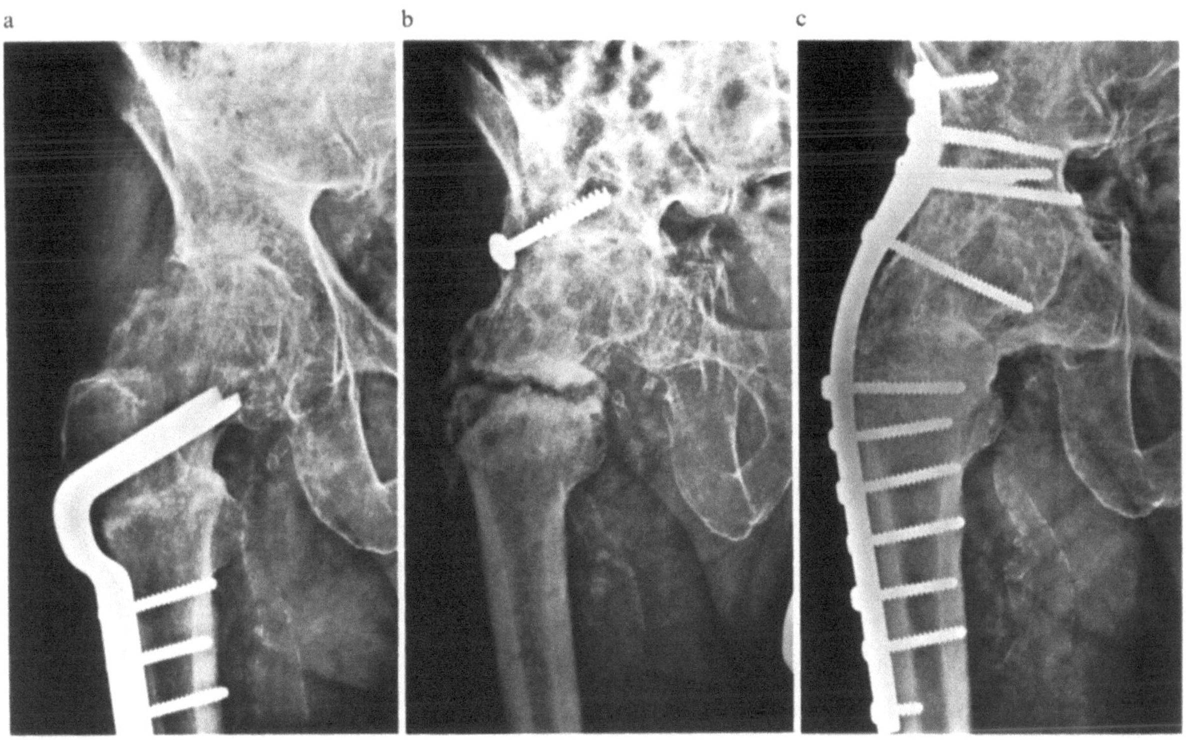

Fig. 242. *PA of the intertrochanteric osteotomy following Type I HA*. E. A., ♂, aged 65 years, No. 76176.

a) Nine months following intertrochanteric osteotomy performed for arthrosis of the hip. The hip is painful and almost ankylosed.

b) Nine months following Type I HA. PA of the intertrochanteric osteotomy.

c) Follow-up 7 years following internal compression fixation with a cobra-head plate. The PA is united and the patient is working full time as a baker

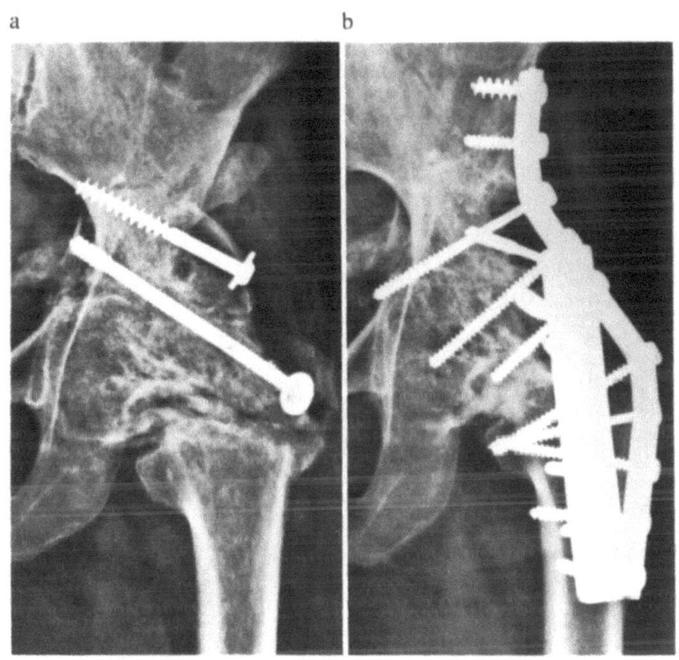

Fig. 243. *PA of the intertrochanteric osteotomy following Type I HA*. B. V., ♀, aged 39 years, No. 70824.

a) Nine months following HA performed for severe hip arthrosis secondary to septic arthritis and osteomyelitis. The PO is united and the intertrochanteric osteotomy is pseudarthrotic.

b) Twelve months following internal compression fixation with two plates. The PA is united

a b c

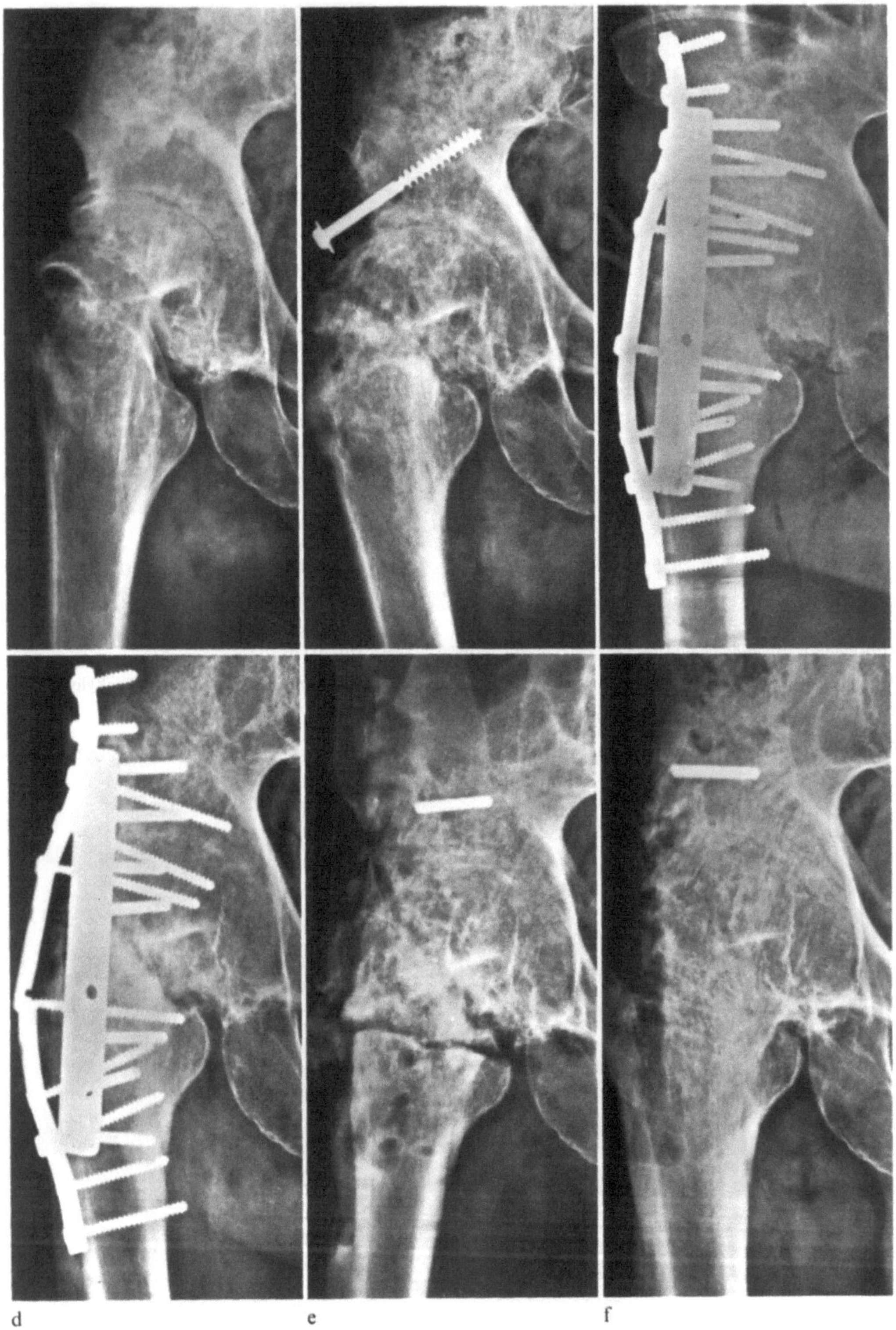

d e f

Fig. 244. *PA of the intertrochanteric osteotomy following Type I HA*. K. S., ♂, age 59 years, No. 71 859.

a) Severe hip arthrosis with almost complete ankylosis in external rotation.

b) Ten months following Type I HA. PA of the intertrochanteric osteotomy and adduction deformity.

c) Internal compression fixation with two plates.

d) Thirteen months later a painful PA is still present with fracture of the plate.

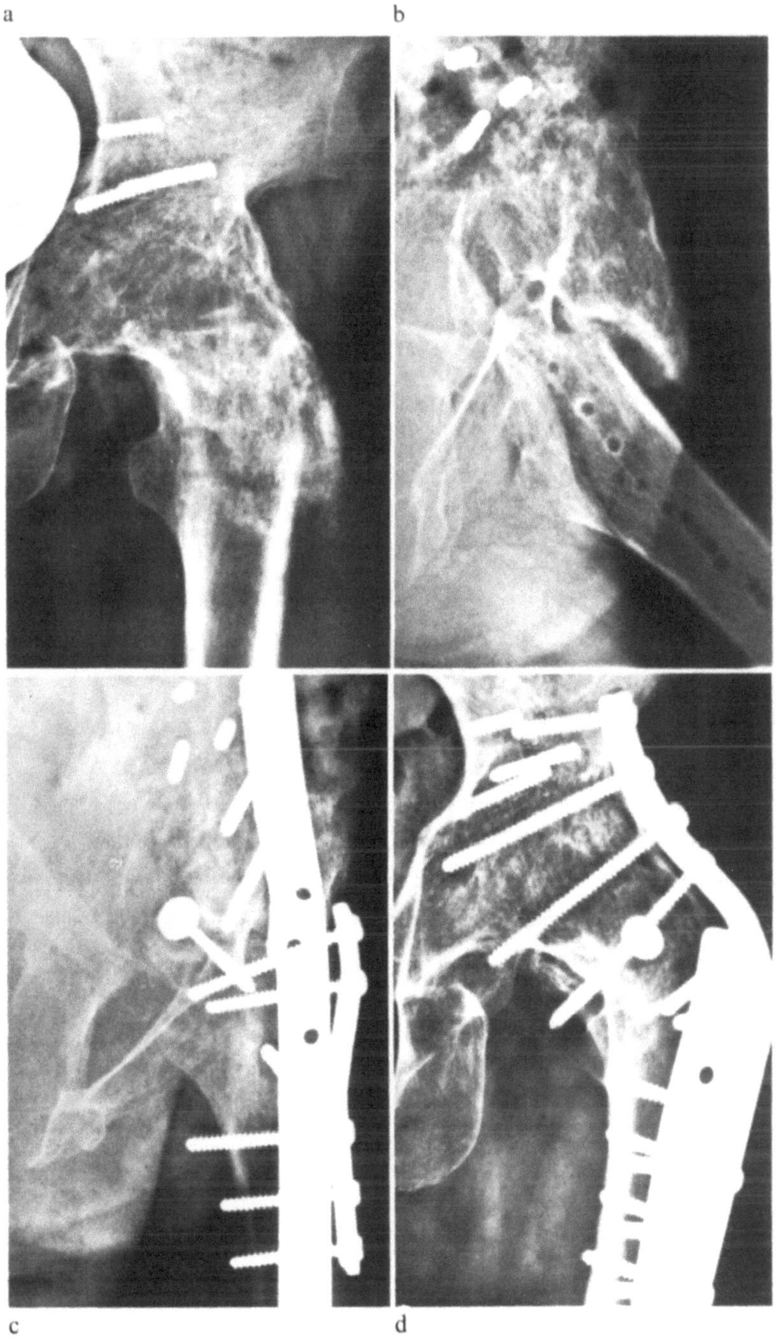

Fig. 245. *PA of the intertrochanteric osteotomy following Type IV HA*. D. H., ♀, aged 45 years, No. 141850.

a and b) Five months following removal of the cobra-head plate. PA of the intertrochanteric osteotomy.

c) One month later. Internal compression fixation with two plates.

d) One year later. PA united. Full painless weight bearing possible

---

e) Implant removal, freshening of the bone, cancellous bone plasty. Hip spica for 3 months. Walking with partial weight bearing using cane for 18 months.

f) Follow-up 6 years later. The PA is united and the HA is united at the correct angle. Correction of 4 cm leg shortening by orthopaedic shoe. The patient, a farmer, has returned to full-time work

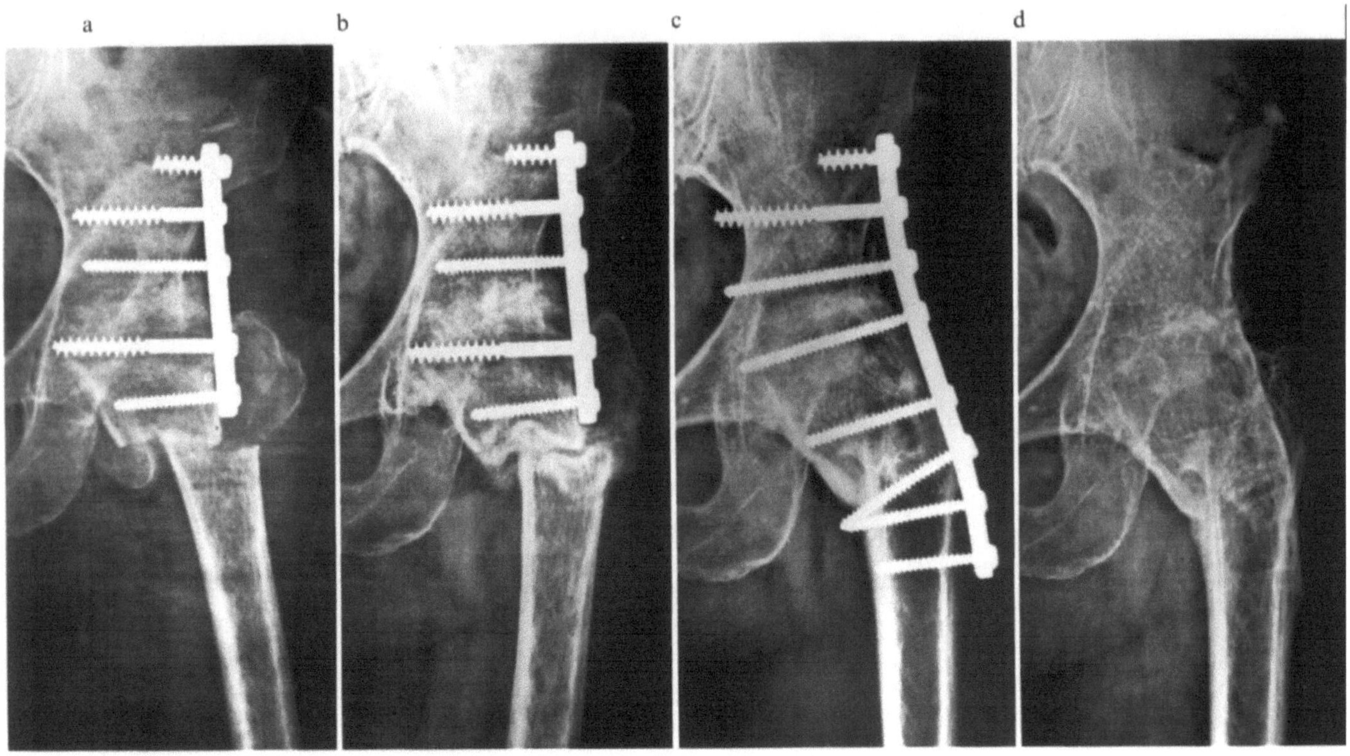

Fig. 246. *PA of the subtrochanteric osteotomy following Type II HA*. M. H., ♀, aged 52 years, No. 90409.

a) Ten days following Type II HA without PO; the operation was performed for NHF secondary to nailing of the femoral neck.

b) Four months later. The HA is united. There is PA of the subtrochanteric osteotomy.

c) Thirteen months following internal compression plate fixation. The PA has united.

d) Following implant removal

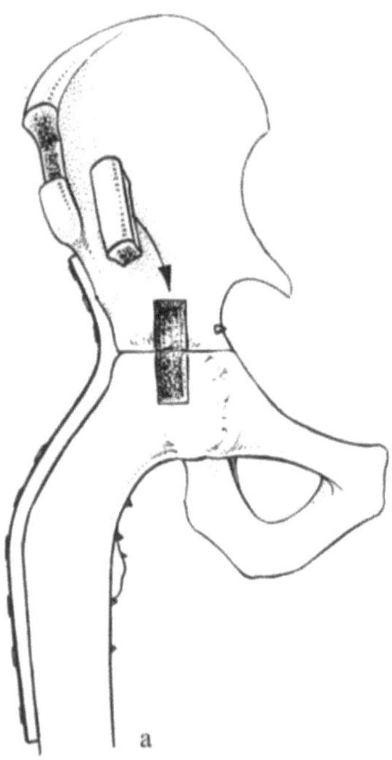

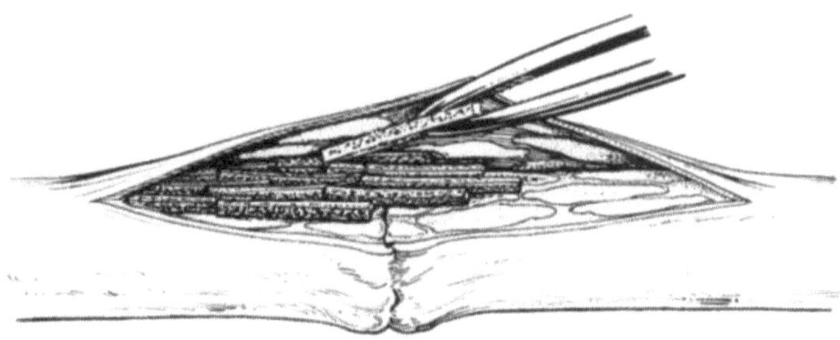

Fig. 247. *Use of bone grafts to accelerate healing of a PA*.

a) The PA is stabilized with a „bridging plate.“ One or two firm corticocancellous blocks are taken from the anterior aspect of the iliac crest and are wedged into a groove which crosses the PA.

b) By extensive freshening of the bone a pocket is formed in the bone which is then filled with autologous cancellous grafts

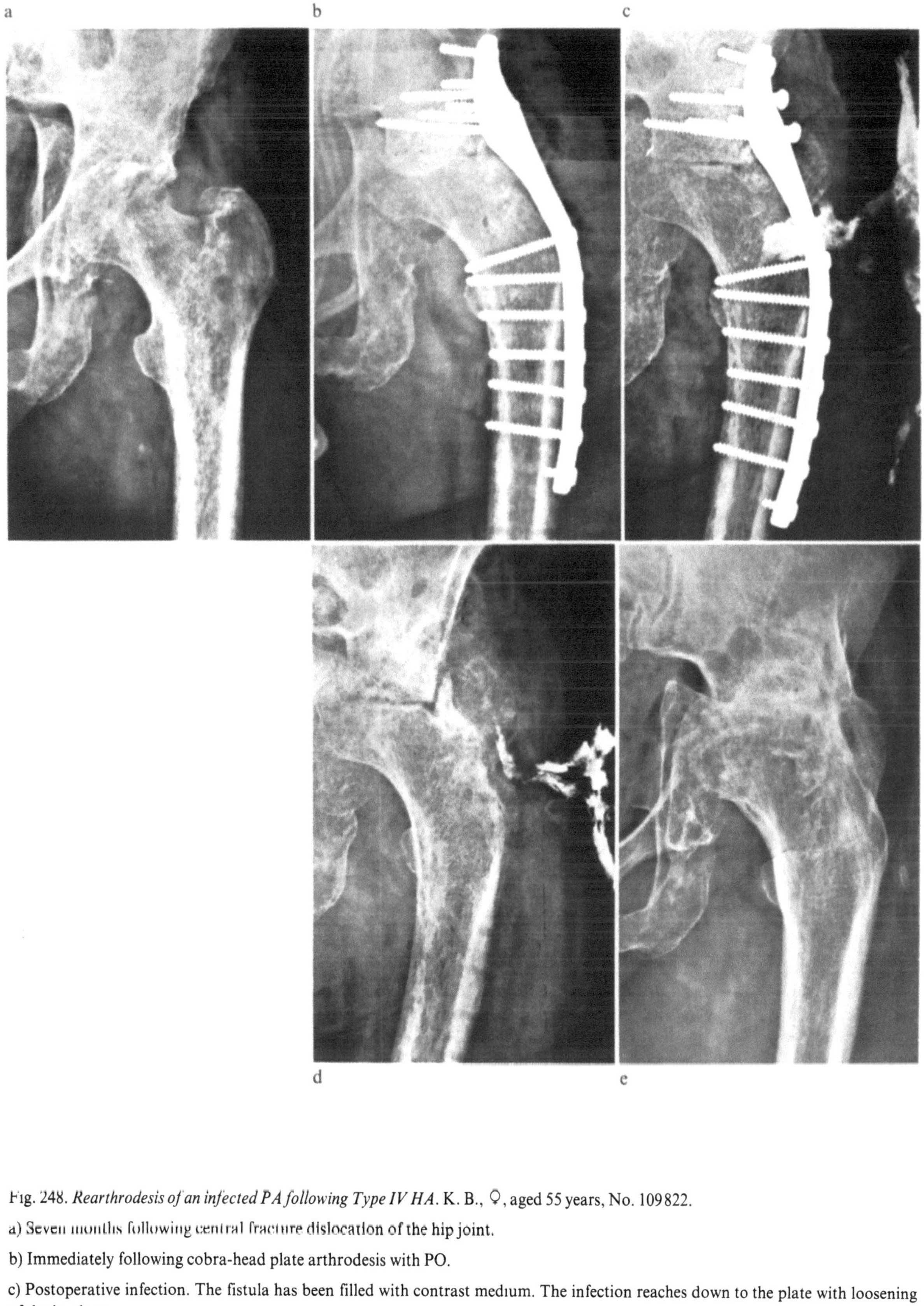

Fig. 248. *Rearthrodesis of an infected PA following Type IV HA.* K. B., ♀, aged 55 years, No. 109822.

a) Seven months following central fracture dislocation of the hip joint.

b) Immediately following cobra-head plate arthrodesis with PO.

c) Postoperative infection. The fistula has been filled with contrast medium. The infection reaches down to the plate with loosening of the implant.

d) Repeat contrast filling of the fistula 3 months following implant removal, debridement and drainage. The fistula still extends to the area of the greater trochanter. Incipient bone union of the medial part of the osteotomy.

e) Result 2 years later. The PA is united at the ideal angle. The patient is complaint-free and working full time

2.2 Infected Pseudoarthrosis

In our series we have a total of 24 infections following HA with only one infected PA.

The infected PA following HA is treated by removal of the metal, thorough debridement, autologous cancellous bone plasty and drainage with appropriate antibiotic therapy. A hip spica is applied to immobilise the joint. As in the infected hip, rearthrodesis with minimal internal fixation may be carried out immediately in the presence of quiescent infection.

Otherwise, following failure of bone union and healing of the infection, rearthrodesis with minimal internal fixation is performed at a later stage and is usually combined with intertrochanteric osteotomy and, if necessary, further cancellous bone plasty (Fig. 248).

3 Malposition

In our series, malposition occurred in 13.8% of cases (Table 35).

It can be seen from the Table that adduction is the most frequent of the deformities (7.7%) followed by external rotation (3.4%), internal rotation (1.5%) and abduction (1.0%). The two latter malpositions are rare but have serious consequences.

The greatest frequency of malposition was associated with Type IV cobra-head plate arthrodeses (17.0%); the majority were adduction or external rotation deformities.

This high percentage shows that too little attention was paid to correct positioning of the leg during the operation.

In 21 of our 80 cases in which HA resulted in malposition, corrective osteotomy had to be carried out. In another 59 cases, the malposition did not present a significant problem and the patients were satisfied with the results of arthrodesis (Figs. 249, 250).

Table 35. Arthrodeses and hip deformity

Arthrodesis type (number of cases)		Adduction	Abduction	External rotation	Internal rotation	Total	%
Freshening	(32)	–	4	–	1	5	15.6
Nailing	(2)	–	–	–	–	–	–
CHARNLEY	(2)	–	–	–	–	–	–
Type I	(156)	10	–	5	1	16	10.2
Type II	(20)	3	–	–	–	3	15.0
Type III	(108)	8	–	–	3	11	10.2
Type IV	(258)	23	2	15	4	44	17.0
Atypical	(5)	1	–	–	–	1	20.0
Total	(583)	45	6	20	9	80	
Percent	(100)	7.7	1.0	3.4	1.5	13.8	

Fig. 249. *Osteotomy for correction of flexion deformity following HA*. B. D., ♂, aged 15 years, No. 94606.

a) Six months following valgus osteotomy of a rheumatoid hip (bilateral congenital hip dislocation was also present). Painful partial ankylosis of the joint.

b) Immediately following HA.

c) Two years later. The HA is united with 35° of flexion deformity and is otherwise perfect.

d) Fourteen months following extension osteotomy (flexion reduced by 20°). The angle of the HA is now perfect, with 1 cm leg shortening. The patient, a telephone operator, is complaint-free and working full time

a b

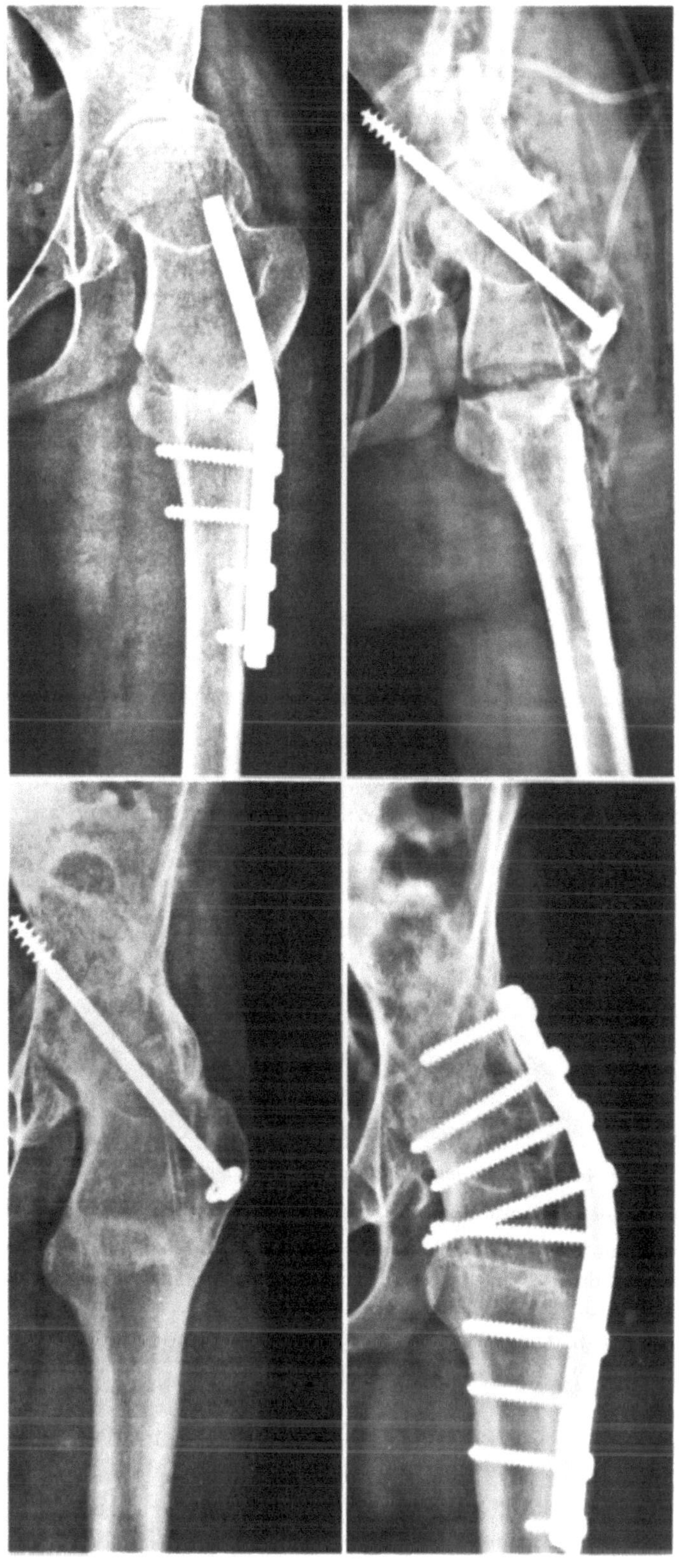

c d

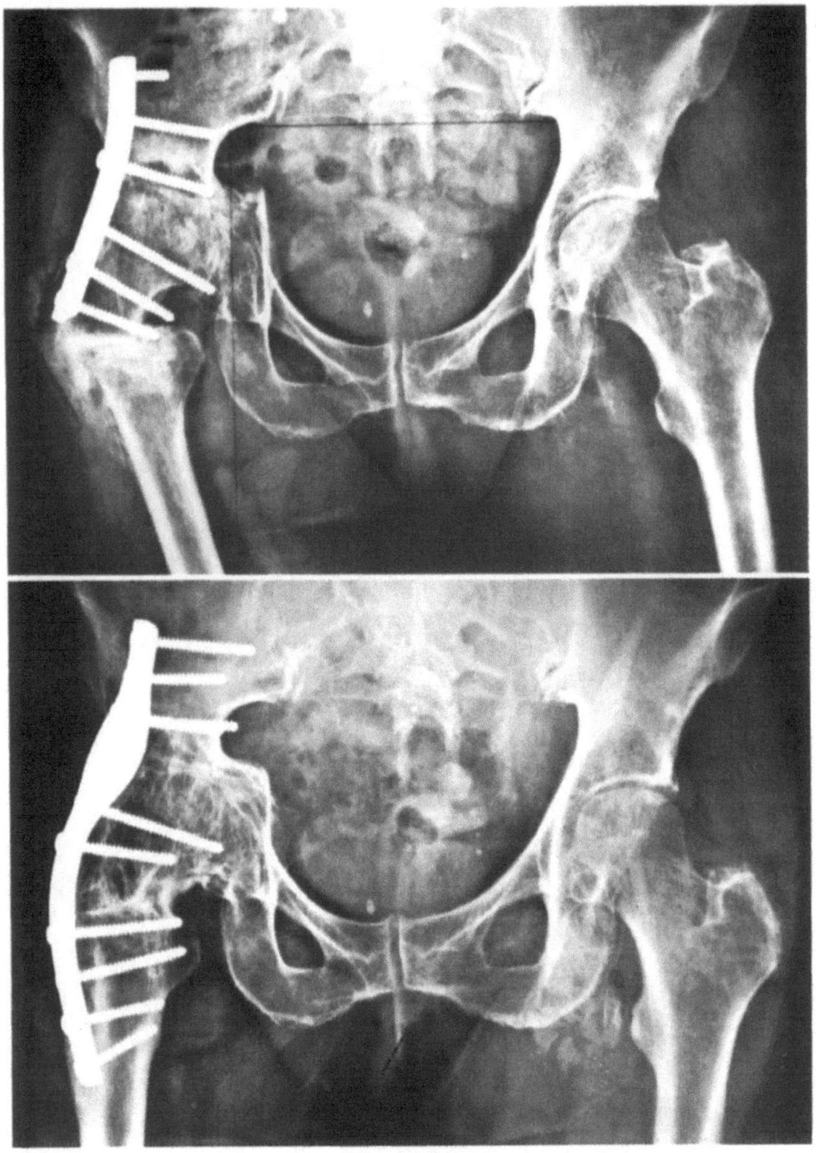

a

b

Fig. 250. *Adduction deformity following HA*. E. A., ♀, aged 56 years, No. 93970.

a) Six months following Type II HA with PO. Severe adduction deformity (18°) with 8 cm leg shortening.

b) Result 5 years following correction of the angle by intertrochanteric osteotomy and cobra-head plate fixation. The HA is united with perfect angulation and 1 cm leg shortening. Patient is working full time as a nurse

4 Infections

Postoperative infection followed 24 of our HA (4.1%).

4.1 Hematoma Considered as Potential Infection

The direct correlation between infection and hematoma is noticeable (Table 17).

Eleven out of 29 hematomas resulted in infection. Only six had been immediately evacuated. We have drawn the following conclusions:

- Careful attention must be paid to hemostasis during the operation.
- All layers of the surgical wound must be adequately drained with suction drains.
- Occurrence of a hematoma is an indication for immediate revision of the whole wound with evacuation of the hematoma.

4.2 Fresh Postoperative Infections

Fresh postoperative infections are also indications for immediate revision with thorough débridement. The internal fixation material is left in place and suction and perfusion drains (Fig. 251) are left in place.

Appropriate antibiotic therapy is started, both parenterally and via the perfusion fluid.

We use Ringer solution for perfusion. We have obtained good results with the following perfusion fluid formula:

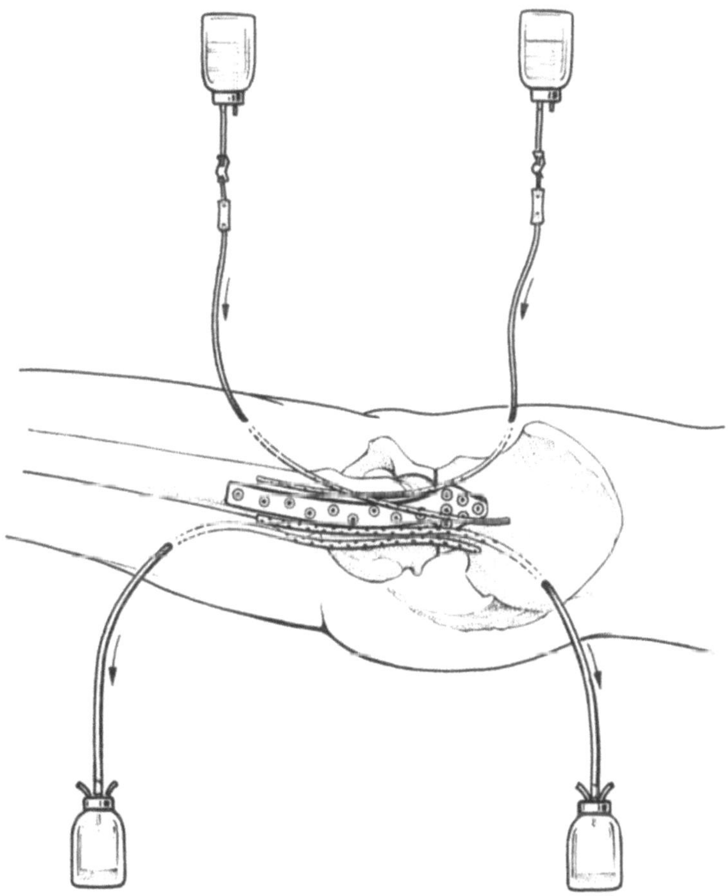

Fig. 251. *Perfusion-drainage of an infected cobra-head plate arthrodesis.* The perfusion fluid is delivered to the desired site of action (particularly along the implant) by thin perforated drains. At least two large-calibre suction drains are used to evacuate the perfusion fluid

Ringer solution 1600 ml/day
Alevaire (Winthrop Laboratories): 400 ml/day
aqueous solution containing
- Superinone 0.125% (a nontoxic detergent)
- sodium bicarbonate 2%
- glycerine 5%

or

Ringer solution without Alevaire 2000 ml/day

Depending on the results of bacteriological sensitivity tests, antibiotics are added to the perfusion fluid as follows (quantities per liter fluid):

- Cephalothin, 2 g
  or
- Lincomycin, 600 mg
  or
- Penicillin G, 5 megaunits, combined with Alevaire to inhibit penicillinase
  or
- Polybactrin Soluble UG, 1–2 ampoules (1 ampoule contains:
  Polymixin B sulphate 15,000 IU
  Bacitracin 2,500 IU
  Neomycin sulphate 4,000 IU)

The wound is always approximated with deep mattress sutures and the skin is closed with eversion sutures.

By this means infection is usually either completely eradicated or the fresh infection becomes quiescent, in some cases with a residual fistula (Fig. 252).

4.3 Quiescent Infection

In these cases one waits for bony union of the HA to occur. When this is completed, the metal is removed, débridement of the wound with excision of the fistula is carried out and suction drains are left in place.

The procedure is the same as for infected PA if the infection does not heal and signs of metal loosening appear (Figs. 253–255).

Fig. 252. *Postoperative infection following cobra-head plate arthrodesis*. F. W. ♂, aged 34 years, No. 135798.

a) Six months following treatment of an extremely painful hip arthrosis secondary to Perthes disease by intertrochanteric osteotomy. Subjective complaints remain unchanged.

b) Immediately following cobra-head plate arthrodesis with PO and a marked degree of medial displacement.

c) Five months later. Increasing pain in the left thigh with marked swelling and reddening around the site of the incision. The radiographs show bone resorption with loosening of the plate and screws secondary to late infection.

d) One day later, following implant removal, clearing out of the abcess (Staphylococcus aureus) and perfusion-drainage for 17 days. Primary wound healing.

e) Follow-up 1 year later. The HA is united at the correct angle. The appearance of the scar is normal. No pain

a b c

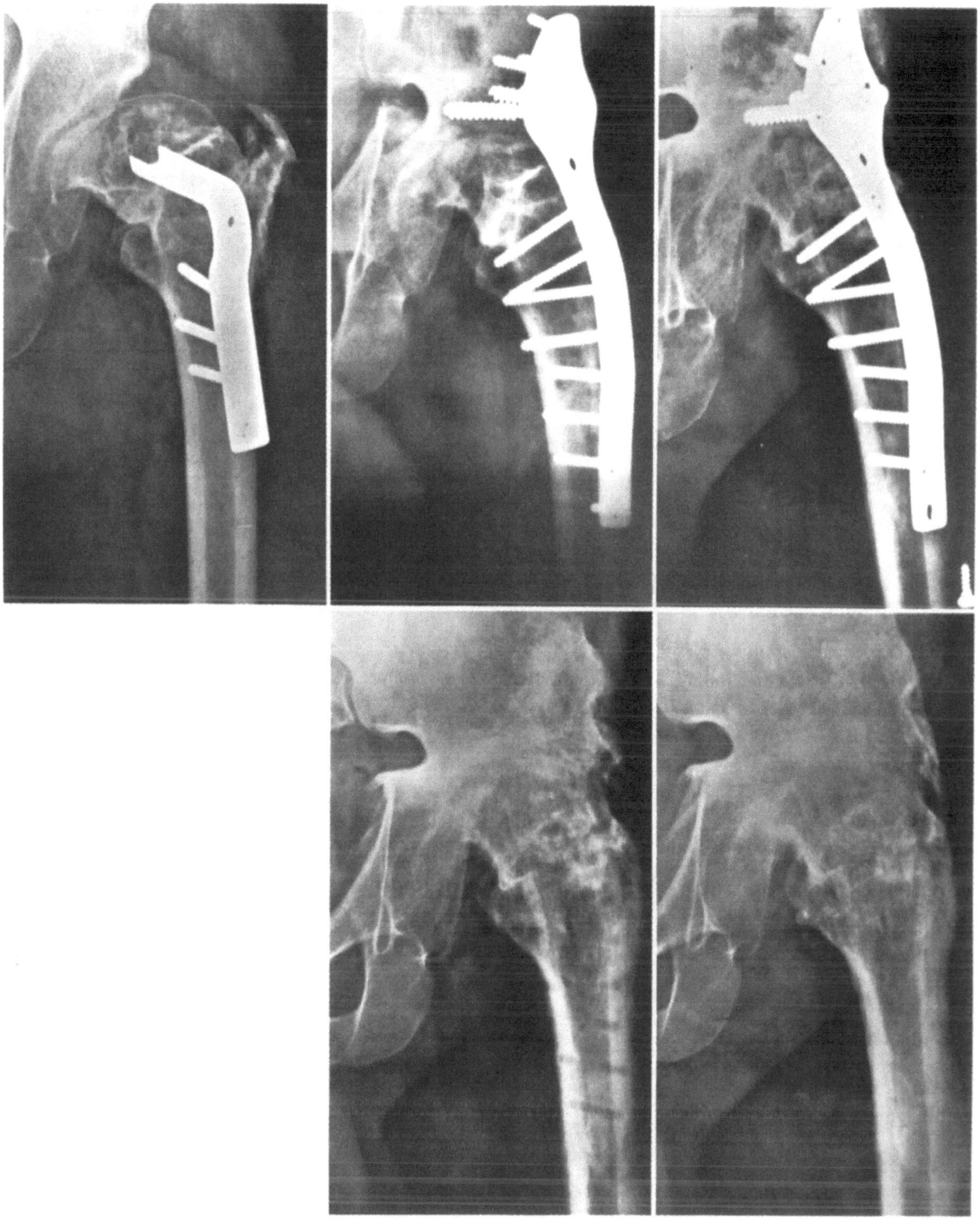

d e

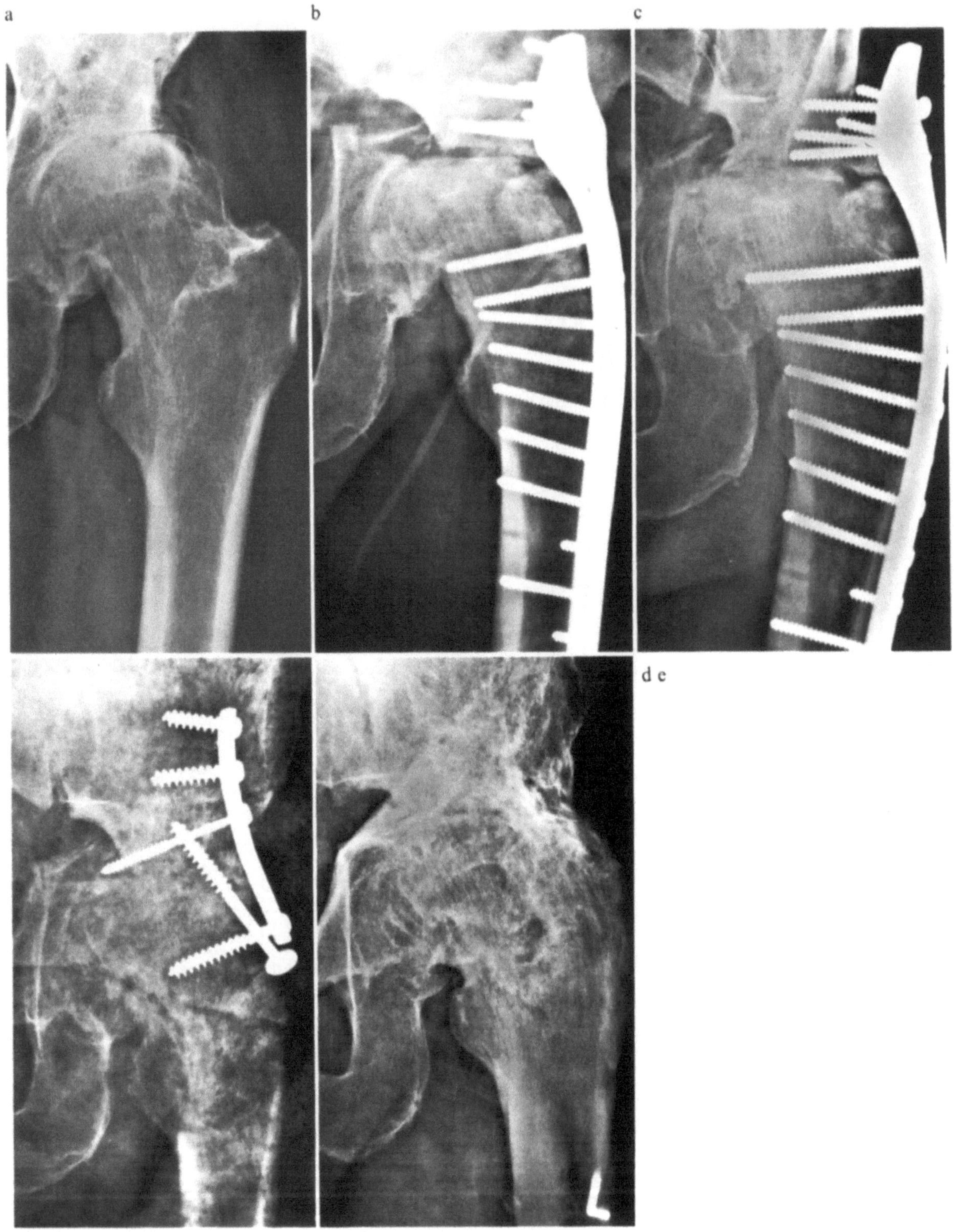

Fig. 253. *Infection following Type IV HA*. F. H., ♂, aged 57 years, No. 137904.

a) Before operation.

b) Immediately following cobra-head plate arthrodesis with PO.

c) Three weeks later. The arthrodesis has collapsed.

d) One month following Type II rearthrodesis. The wound swab taken at operation grew Pseudomonas pyocyaneus. Ten days postoperatively a fistula formed at the upper end of the wound. Following union of the intertrochanteric osteotomy and of the HA the fistula was excised, the abcess was cleared out and the implant was removed.

e) Follow-up 3 years postoperatively. The scar is of normal appearance and infection is no longer present. Perfect HA

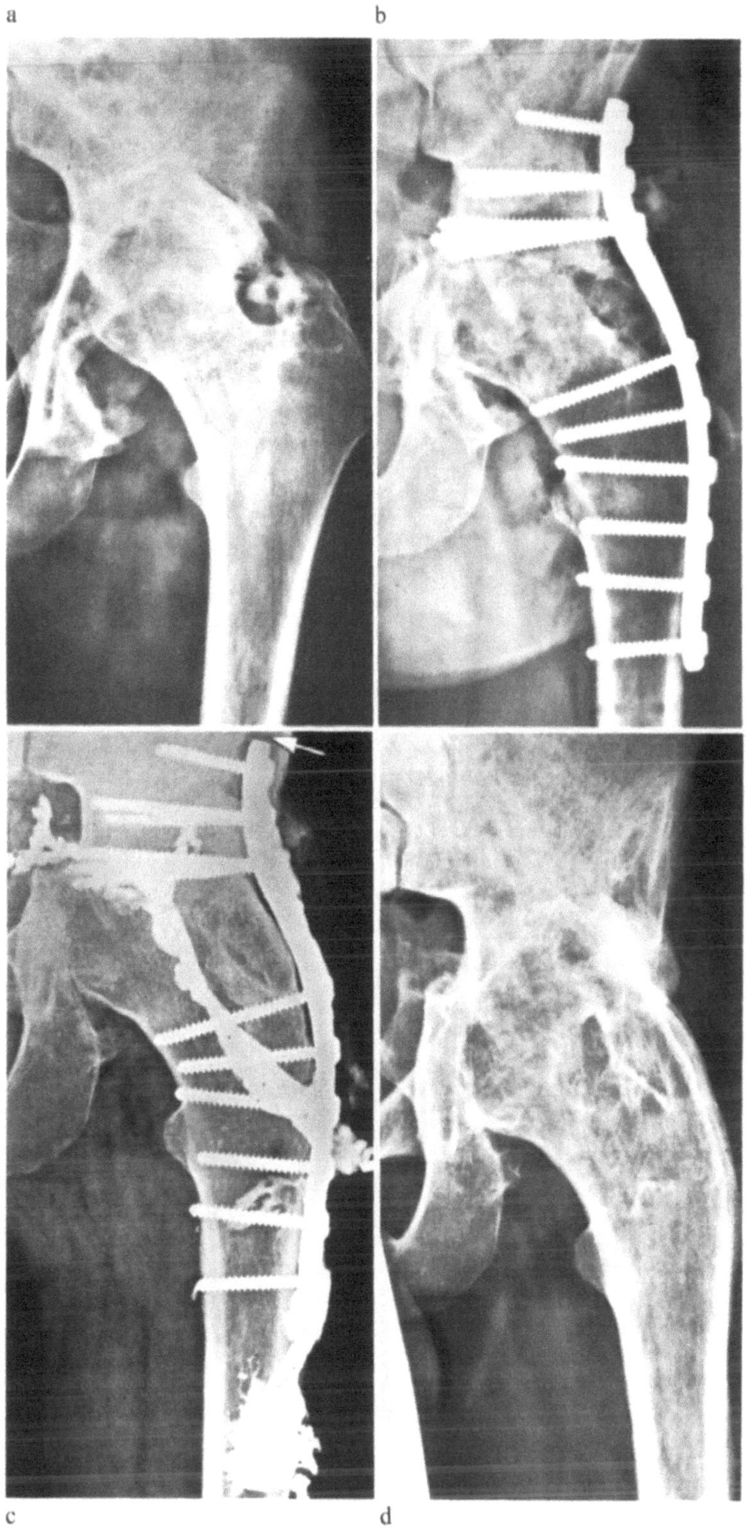

Fig. 254. *Bone infection following Type IV HA*. A. T., ♀, aged 21 years, No. 93295.

a) Post-traumatic arthrosis of the hip 2 years following high posterior dislocation of the hip with comminuted fracture of the acetabulum.

b) Type IV HA with PO.

c) Contrast radiograph showing the fistula 7 months later. The contrast medium extends as far as the osteotomy and the plate. There is loosening of the implant.

d) Result 1 year following excision of the fistula, cancellous bone plasty and perfusion-drainage. The HA is united at the correct angle. The infection is no longer present. The patient is working full time

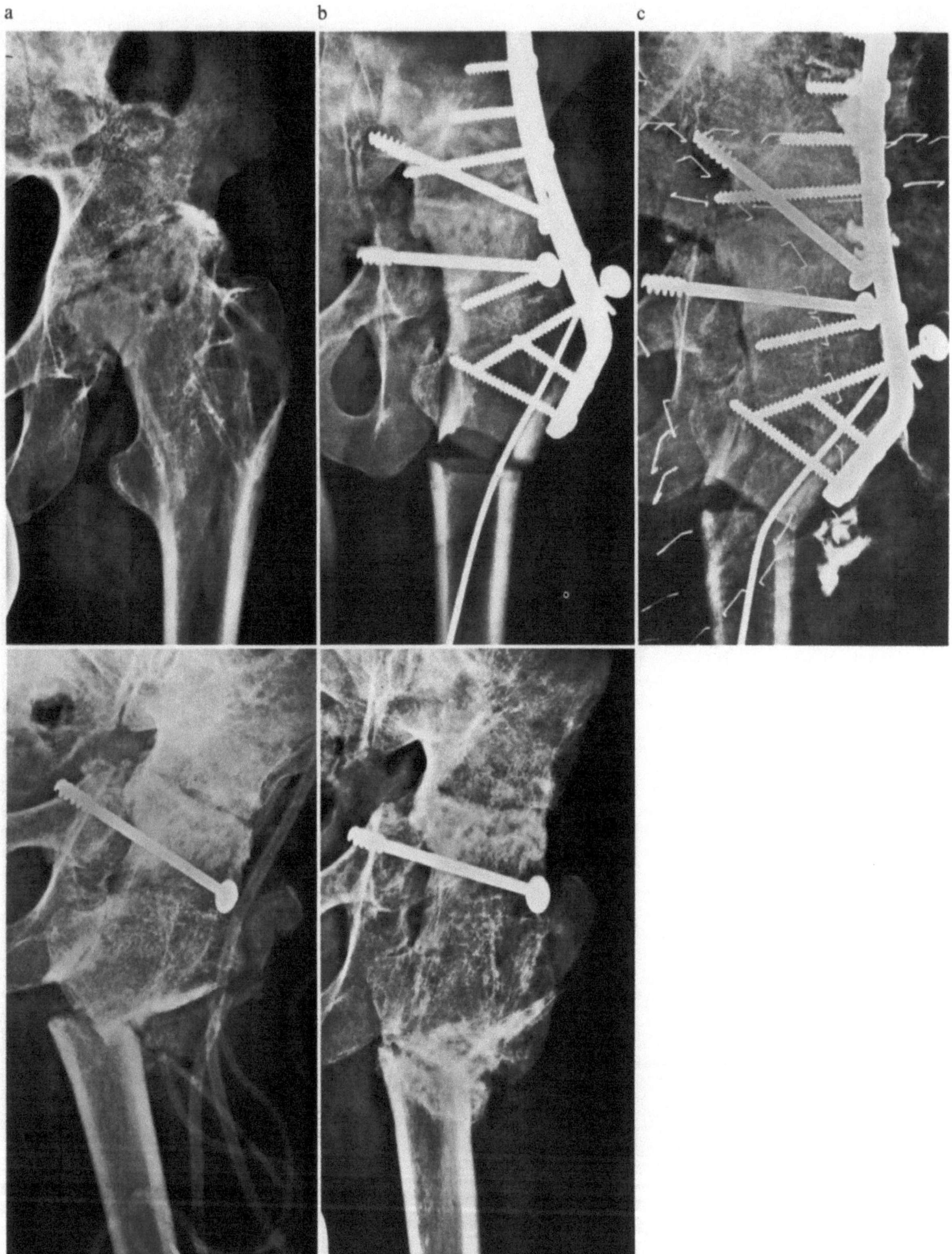

a
b
c
d
e

5 Fatigue Fractures

There were six genuine fatigue fractures following HA in our series, one of which occurred following HA in another hospital (1%).

Three further fractures occurred following trauma (one in our clinic, two in other hospitals).

The localisation was as follows:

- Femoral diaphysis (distal end of the plate): five cases
- Femoral neck: one case

Only one fracture could have been said to be caused by genuine trauma.

5.1 Femoral Diaphyseal Fractures

5.1.1 Mechanism of Fatigue Fracture

Following internal plate fixation, elasticity of the bone around the plate is always partially reduced.

The bone thus becomes divided into two segments with differing elasticities. Stress peaks occur at the border between the segments. Bone remodelling occurs which is seen radiologically in this area as thickening of the cortex (Figs. 256, 257).

In this way, the bone compensates for the increased load. If the stress is too great, bone resorption occurs (atrophy, fibrosis) and fatigue fracture results. The tendency to bone union following fatigue fracture is good and in these cases internal compression-plate fixation is the treatment of choice.

5.1.2 Visualisation of Tension Lines Using Polarised Light

The factors determining the course of the fracture line were mentioned in the chapter on elastometry and are briefly summarised:

a) If the distal screw is short, the tension peaks occur laterally around that screw and medially around the tip of the screw proximal to it. The fracture line almost always joins the tension peaks (Figs. 258, 259).

b) If the distal screw is long, the tension peaks occur medially and laterally at the points of contact between the screw and the bone. Here, the fracture line joins these points of contact with a triangular wedge which is directed downwards (Fig. 260).

5.2 Femoral Neck Fracture

This fracture rarely occurs following arthrodeses using our techniques. We have only one case in our series. Conversely, it is a known complication of the CHARNLEY-type HA with central dislocation (See Biomechanics, Elastometry, p. 12 ff.) (Fig. 261).

5.3 Fractures Following Trauma

In all three cases, the fractures resulted from considerable trauma. However, the histories of the two cases in which the fracture line occurred at the level of the arthrodesis are

Fig. 255. *Postoperative infection in an HA in a case of sepsis and NHF secondary to nailing of a fracture of the femoral neck.* F. F. ♂, aged 31 years, No. 164465.

a) Painful fibrous ankylosis.

b) HA; the proximal femoral component has been brought into a vertical position.

c) Contrast radiograph taken 1 month later. The fistula has been filled with contrast medium which reaches down to the metal. For this reason almost all the implant material was removed leaving one cancellous screw.

d) Two weeks later. Evacuation of the abcess with perfusion-drainage, cancellous bone plasty and application of a cast.

e) Three months later following removal of the cast. The intertrochanteric osteotomy and HA have united. With 8° abduction deformity; the resulting increase in knee valgus has caused painful knee problems. With 4 cm leg shortening interesting. In both cases the metal was removed shortly before the accident (2 months and 3 months, respectively). Bone remodelling was still taking place and the bone was not yet capable of full weight bearing. For this reason, following removal of implant material weight bearing should be gradually and carefully incremented.

The third case is, in point of fact, not a fatigue fracture but is shown as a curiosity. There is a longitudinal fracture of the ala (Figs. 262 – 264).

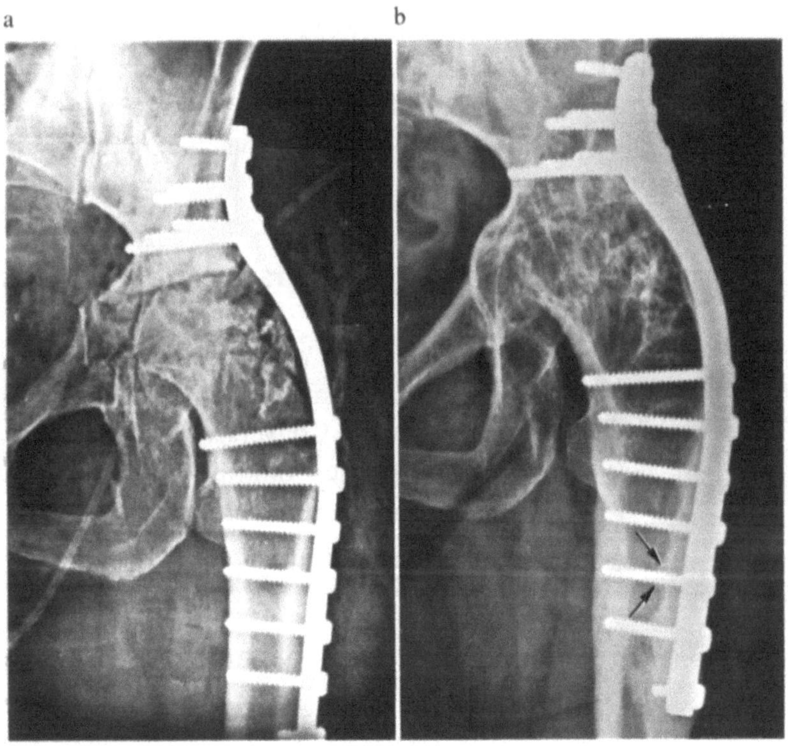

Fig. 256. *Increase in cortex thickness as a result of increased load on the bone.* B. B., ♀, aged 50 years, No. 104691.

a) Cobra-head plate arthrodesis with PO performed for hip arthrosis. Notice the normal cortex.

b) Follow-up 63 months later. The HA has united. There is marked thickening of the cortex at the distal end of the plate and round the screws

a b

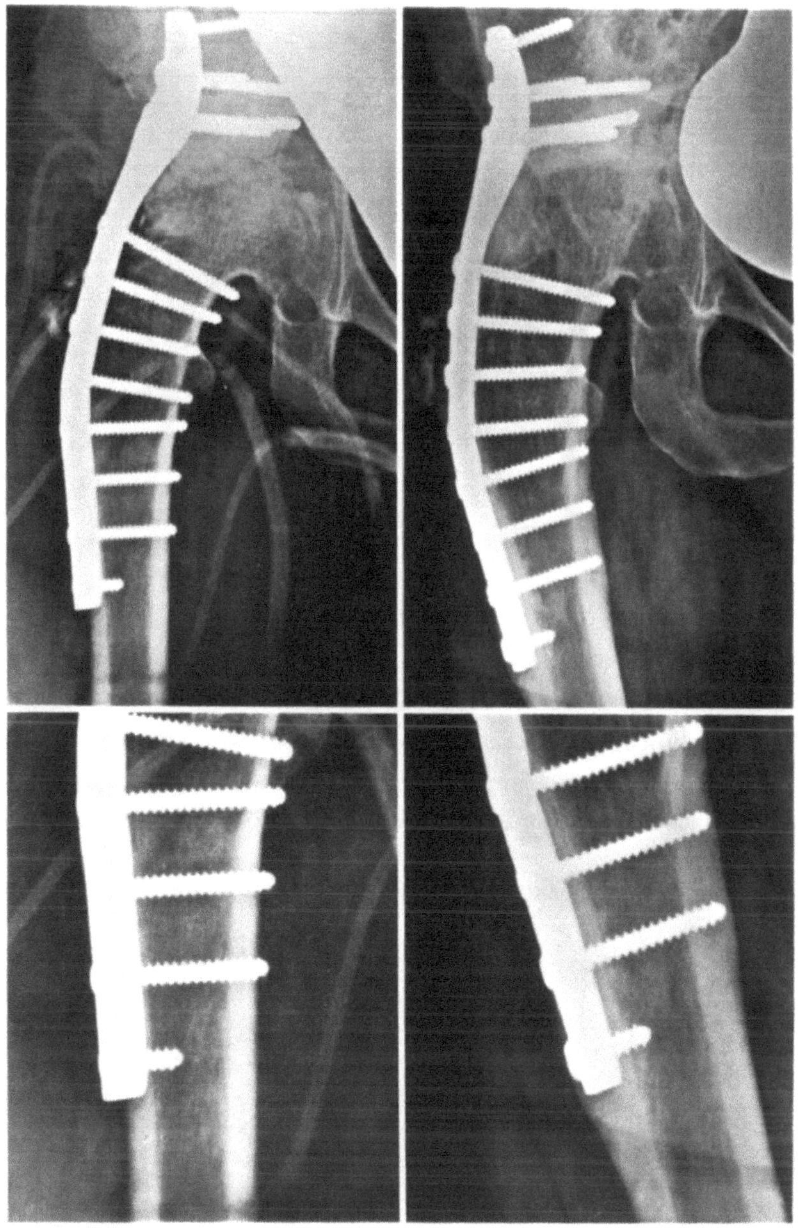

c d

Fig. 257. *Effect of increased load on the bone*. Fch. R., ♀, aged 36 years, No. 81 621.

a) Type IV HA. Cortex of normal appearance

b) Follow-up $4^1/_2$ years later. The arthrodesis has united. There is marked thickening of the cortex around the distal end of the plate. On the medial side the cortical thickening is decreased distal to the last of the screws which pass through both cortices.

c and d) Magnified view of the latter

a b c

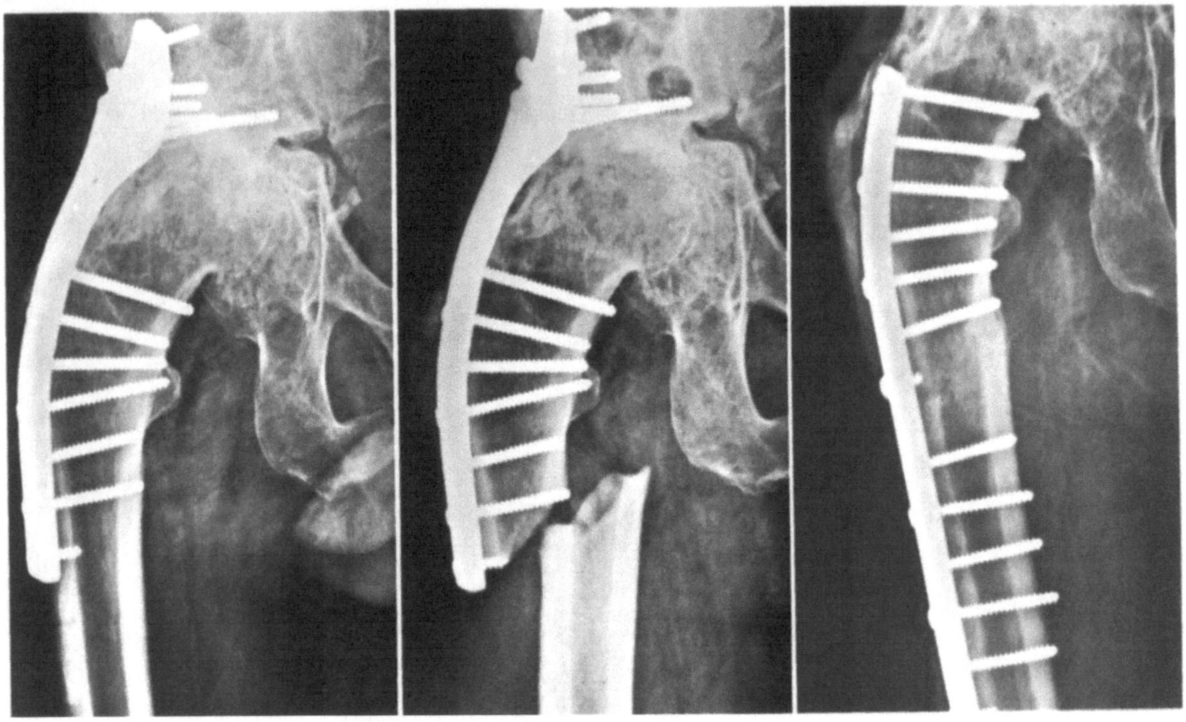

Fig. 258. *Fatigue fracture at the distal end of the cobra-head plate*. W. J., ♂, aged 57 years, No. 113844.

a) Fourteen months following Type IV HA. Arthrodesis united at the correct angle.

b) Two months later (following a fall at home). Fracture of the femoral diaphysis; the fracture line passes between the tips of the two distal screws.

c) One year following rigid internal fixation with a 14-hole AO plate. Complete fracture union

a b c

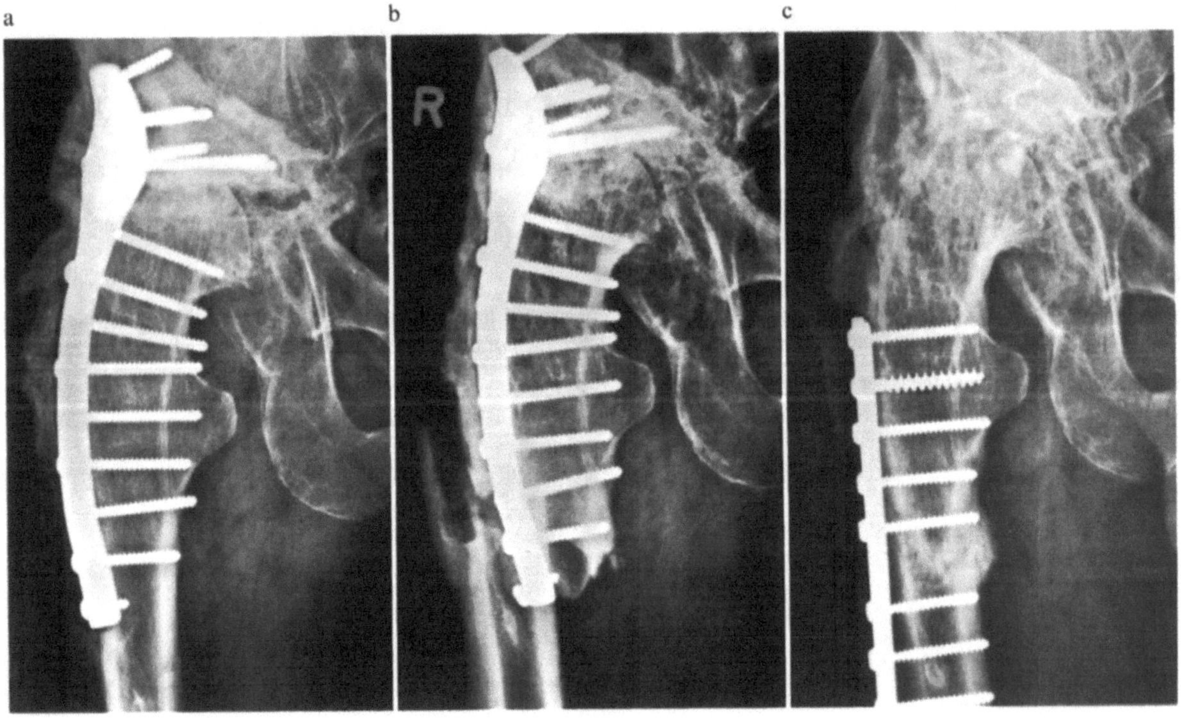

a b c

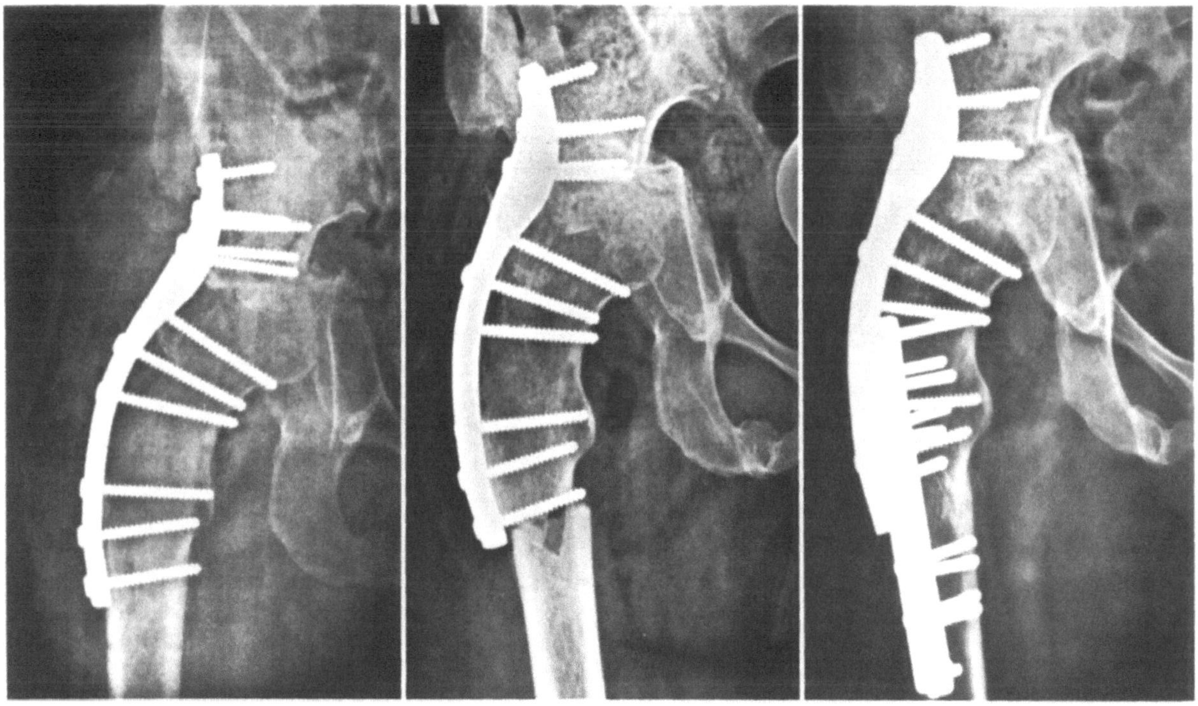

Fig. 260. *Fracture of the femoral diaphysis resulting from severe trauma following Type IV hip arthrodesis.* C. G., ♀, aged 29 years, No. 89861.

a) Type IV cobra-head plate arthrodesis with PO.

b) A severe fall on the right hip has resulted in fracture of the femoral diaphysis; the typical fracture line following use of long distal screws is seen.

c) Five months following rigid internal fixation. The fracture is united

←

Fig. 259. *Fracture of femoral diaphysis at the distal end of the cobra-head plate.* M. J., ♂, aged 57 years, No. 115300.

a) Seven months following Type IV HA.

b) Three years later following a severe fall on the hip. Fracture of the femoral diaphysis at the distal end of the plate.

c) Four months following rigid internal fixation with a straight 9-hole AO plate. The fracture is united

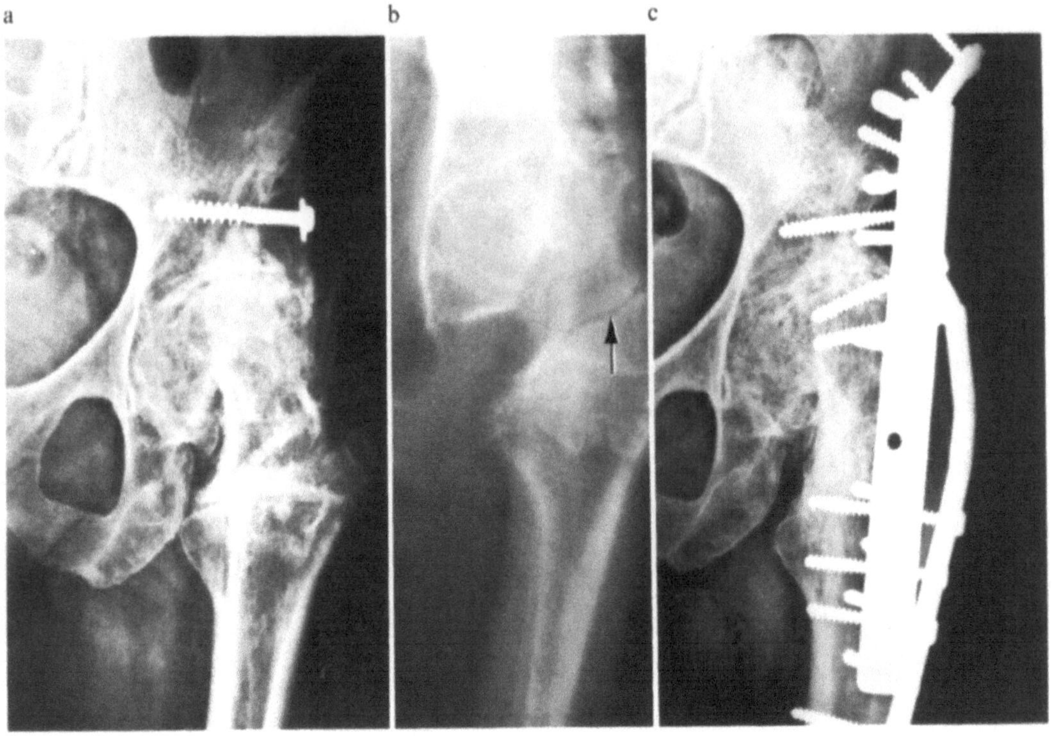

Fig. 261. *Femoral neck fracture following Type I HA*. K. N., ♀, aged 48 years, No. 82878.

a) Three months following Type I HA. There is adequate bone union at the osteotomy and the HA. The patient is complaint-free.

b) Three weeks later. Sudden onset of severe pain without history of trauma. The fracture line is clearly visible across the femoral neck.

c) Follow-up 13 months following rigid internal fixation with plate. The HA, the femoral neck fracture and the osteotomy are united

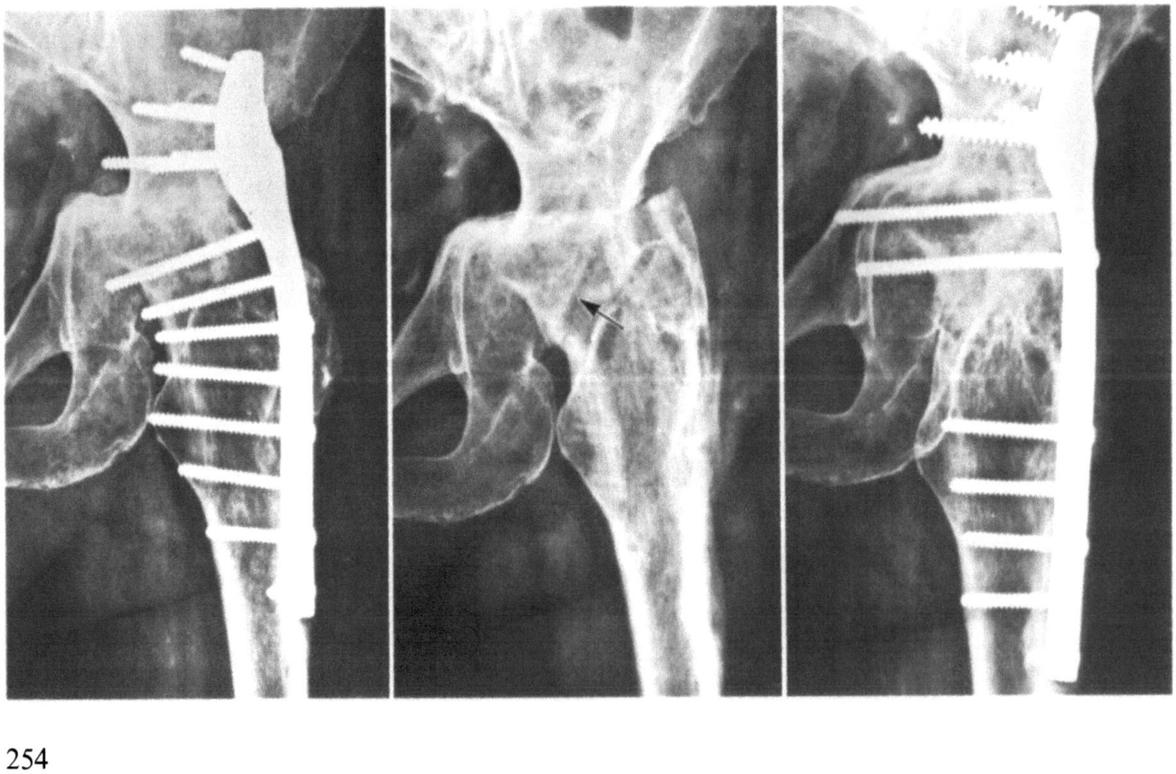

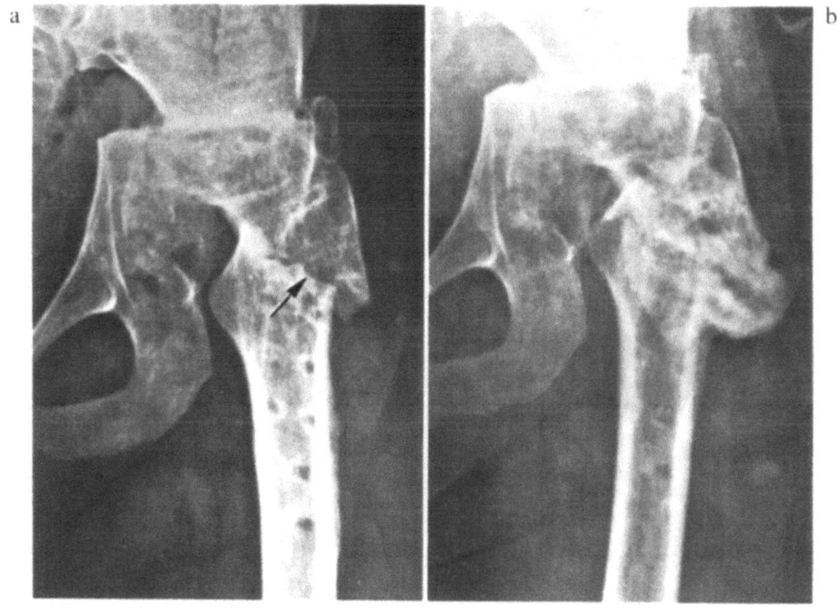

Fig. 263. *Pertrochanteric fracture resulting from severe trauma 2 months following implant removal.* K. O., ♀, aged 48 years, No. P-2630.

a) Fracture following fall 2 months after implant removal.

b) After 8 weeks in a cast there is massive callus formation and the fracture is united

Fig. 262. *Pertrochanteric fatigue fracture following implant removal (cobra-head plate arthrodesis).* I. L., ♀, aged 67 years, No. 124786.

a) One year following Type IV HA. Bone union is complete.

b) Fracture following severe fall 3 months after implant removal.

c) Four months following internal fixation with the cobra-head plate. The fracture has united

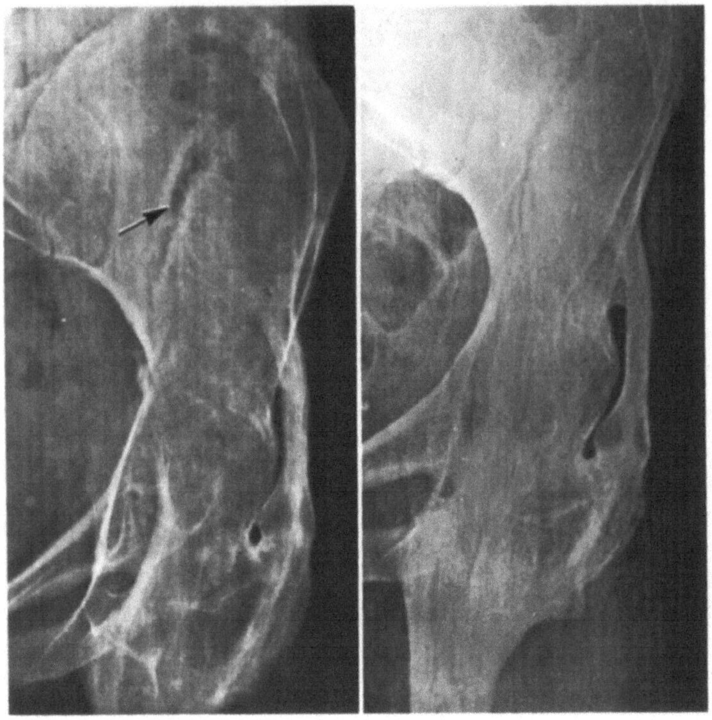

a b

Fig. 264. *Fatigue fracture of the iliac bone following iliofemoral graft arthrodesis.* T. E., ♀, aged 35 years, No. P-3519.

a) Longitudinal fracture of the iliac bone following fall on the breech.

b) Following 2 months bed rest the fracture is largely united

6 Dislocation of the Symphysis

This complication occurred in five of our cases in which HA was combined with PO. The subluxations of the symphysis in our series always occurred in patients between 50 – 60 years of age and followed considerable medial displacement following PO.

Our patients were always complaint-free despite the considerable arthrotic changes visible in one case. The finding was noticed on radiological follow-up of our patients (Figs. 265, 266).

7 Summary

A study of the complications following HA furnishes us with the following information:

- The increased popularity of HA with rigid internal fixation has resulted in a reduction in frequency of PA. PA only occurs if the HA is unstable. In the majority of cases bone union can be brought about by internal compression fixation, if necessary combined with autologous cancellous bone plasty.
- Deformity (particularly adduction and external rotation) occurred in 13.8% of cases. Correction was necessary in only one-quarter of the patients.
- Postoperative infections followed 4.1% of our HA. Prophylactic measures are: careful hemostasis; adequate drainage of the surgical wound; immediate evacuation of postoperative hematoma. If infection occurs: wound revision; débridement; suction and perfusion drainage; appropriate antibiotic therapy.
- Fatigue fractures are rare (1.0%). They tend to heal rapidly. All cases were successfully treated by compression-plate fixation.
- Dislocation of the symphysis is rare and occurred in our series in association with marked medial displacement of the PO and in older patients. Treatment is unnecessary as the patients are complaint-free.

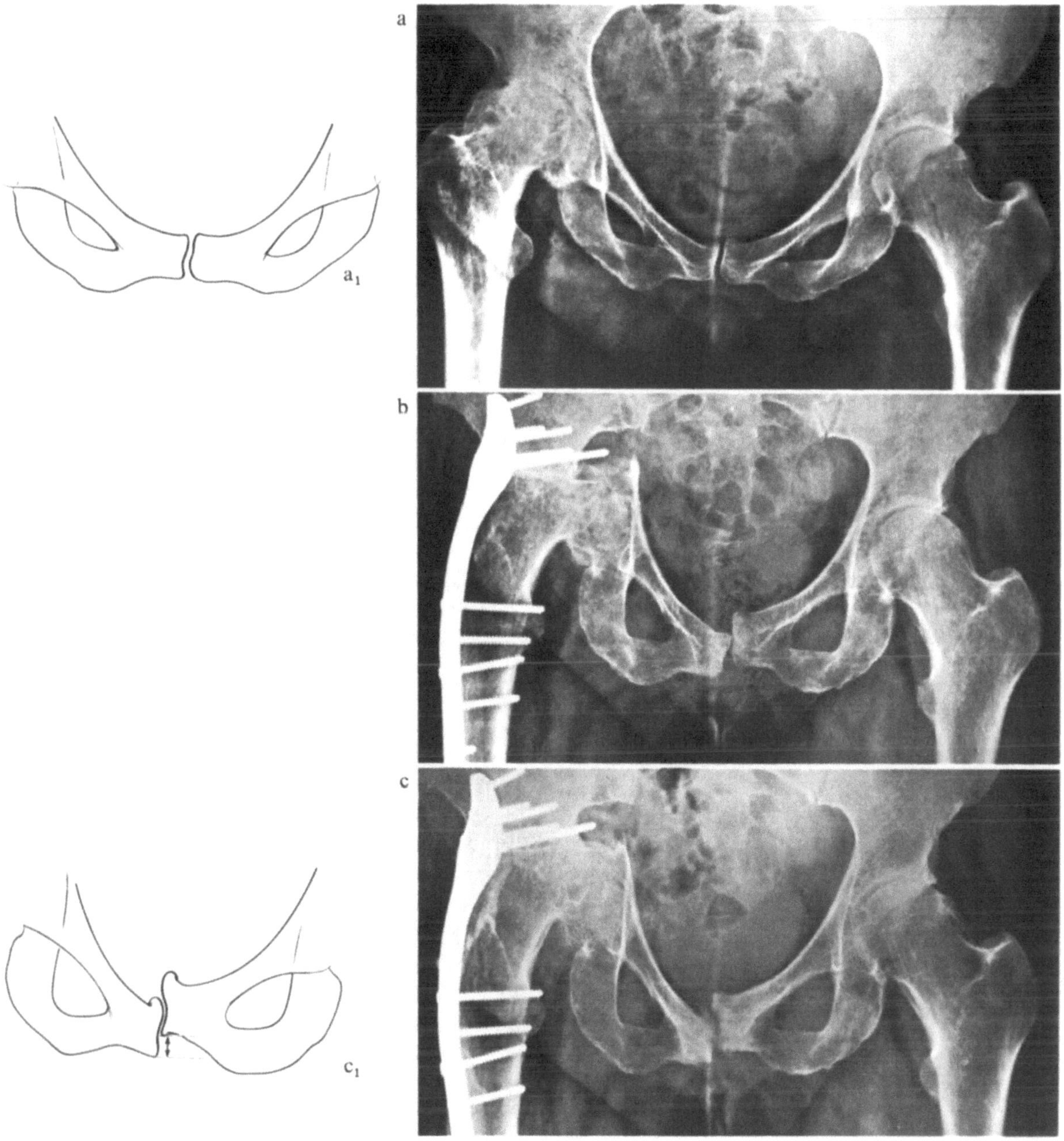

Fig. 265. *Dislocation of the symphysis following HA*. U. R., ♀, aged 52 years, No. 126413.

a^1, a^2) Preoperative radiograph.

b) Three months following Type IV HA with PO and severe medial displacement. Subluxation of the symphysis.

c^1, c^2) Three years later. Arthrotic changes at the symphysis. Patient completely complaint-free

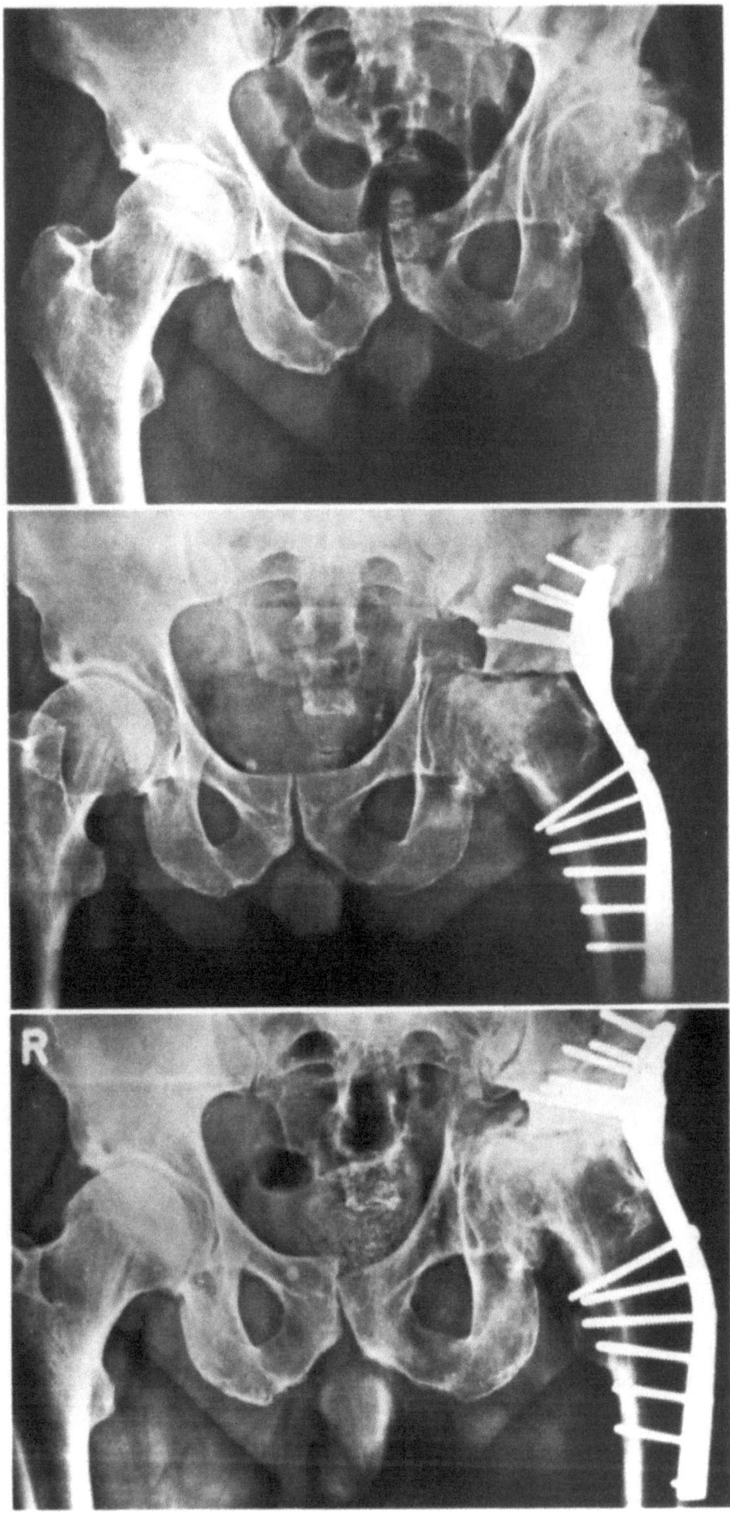

Fig. 266. *Dislocation of the symphysis following HA with PO and marked medial displacement*. L. H., ♂, aged 58 years, No. 153488.

a) Preoperative radiograph.

b) Immediately following operation. The symphysis seems to be intact.

c) Three months later. Marked dislocation. The patient is complaint-free

V. Summary of Part II (Specific Problems and Case Material)

In our clinic between 1961 and 1971, 583 HA were performed. Careful study of the case records and radiographs and of questionnaires sent to the patients was complemented by personal follow-up of more than 300 patients and careful critical evaluation of the data obtained. We came to the conclusion that HA still has a justifiable place in the operative treatment of hip disease.

Depending on the basic pathology, the extent of hip joint destruction may vary considerably with a correspondingly wide range of anatomical change. The nature of the hip disease should always be considered in choosing the HA procedure; in certain cases (particularly infected hips) it may be decisive. A classification of our HA by indication was obviously relevant. In cases of hip arthrosis and rheumatoid arthritis, cobra-head plate arthrodesis is with few exceptions the appropriate technique. Technical operative difficulties may occur in certain post-traumatic situations as well as in hip dysplasia, infected hips, NHF, GH and similar conditions. These problems require appropriate techniques for their solution.

In the last 10 years, considerable advances have been made in orthopedic surgery and particularly in hip surgery. For obvious reasons, procedures which retain or restore hip mobility are very attractive. Thus earlier techniques such as IO and particularly HA have been pushed into the background and have even fallen into disfavour. They are, however, certainly justified, at least until the TP has successfully withstood the test of time. There is frequently an unjustifiable tendency to associate HA exclusively with disadvantages and failure and TP exclusively with advantages and success. New operations should be judged on the basis of systematic follow-up. The present state of medical science is such that there is no excuse for unquestioning acceptance and advocacy of the latest novelty irrespective of whether the material or technique concerned has been tested for a sufficient length of time.

Under certain circumstances extremes may complement each other. Thus in the presence of bilateral hip joint disease the results of combining HA on one side with TP on the other side are surprisingly good.

It is known that the degenerative changes and increasing stiffness in the knee joints and LS seen in older patients create particularly severe problems for the patient whose hip is arthrodesed. The inability to compensate may cause intolerable back pain or knee pain. In such cases as well as in localised HA failure, there remains the possibility of converting the HA into a TP.

Following unsuccessful partial prosthetic replacement or an infected TP which is no longer suitable for replacement, HA may be performed instead of the unsatisfactory Girdlestone operation. This is particularly the case in younger patients who are more able to withstand the stress of the operation and the usually unavoidable prolonged immobilisation in a cast.

HA is an extensive operation which is not without risk and which requires a surgeon experienced in hip surgery (GERTSCH). It is noticeable that there is a considerable difference in the results achieved by different surgeons using the same operative technique. Failures such as PA and deformity demonstrate the considerable biomechanical load placed on the arthrodesed hip and the difficulty encountered in correct positioning of the leg at the time of operation. PA only occurs if the HA is unstable. The frequency of PA has been significantly reduced by the introduction of cobra-head plate arthrodesis (6.2%). Rearthrodesis with internal compression fixation, if necessary combined with a bone plasty, brings about union of the PA in the majority of cases. Thus, following reoperation of the cases in which primary bone union had failed to occur, only five PA (1.9%) remained following a total of 258 cobra-head plate arthrodeses. Infected PA following HA is treated by removal of the metal, débridement, cancellous bone plasty and drainage followed by application of a hip spica for 3 – 4 months.

Malposition occurs too frequently (13.8%) and can almost always be ascribed to incorrect intraoperative positioning of the leg. Corrective osteotomy had to be performed in a quarter of the cases with deformity.

Wound infection occurred in 24 cases (4.1%). This very frequently took the form of an infected hematoma. It should be possible to reduce this infection rate further by strict asepsis, shortening the duration of the operation and immediate wound revision if a hematoma occurs.

In cases of fresh postoperative infection the internal fixation material is not removed; further débridement is carried out and suction and perfusion drains are left in place.

If quiescent infection is present, the surgeon should wait for union of the HA before reoperating.

Fatigue fractures following HA are rare (1%). They are well vascularised and therefore tend to heal more rapidly than fresh fractures. They are treated by internal compression fixation.

An incidental radiological finding is the subluxation of the symphysis which follows marked medial displacement of the distal pelvic component following PO. It does not give rise to complaints and treatment is unnecessary.

Literatur

Abbott, L.C., Fischer, F.J.: Arthrodesis of the hip with special reference to the method of securing ankylosis in massive destruction of joint. Surg. Gynecol. Obstet. **52,** 863 (1931).

Abbott, L.C., Lucas, D.B.: Arthrodesis of the hip. A two-stage method for difficult cases. Surg. Clin. North Am. **36,** 1035 (1956).

Adams, J.C.: Vulnerability of the sciatic nerve in closed ischiofemoral arthrodesis by nail and graft. J. Bone Joint Surg. B **46,** 748 (1964).

Adams, J.C.: Ischio-Femoral Arthrodesis. Edinburgh-London: Livingstone 1966.

Adams, J.C.: Surgical treatment of osteoarthritis. The Practitioner **208,** 48 (1972).

Albee, F.H.: Arthritis deformans of the hip; a preliminary report of a new operation. J. Am. Med. Ass. **1,** 1977 (1908).

Albee, F.H.: Bone-Graft Surgery. Philadelphia: W.B. Saunders 1915.

Albert, E.: Einige Fälle von künstlicher Ankylosenbildung an paralytischen Gliedmaßen. Wien Med. Presse **23,** 725 (1882).

Allgöwer, M., Perren, S.M., Rüedi, Th.: Biophysikalische Aspekte der normalen und der heilenden Knochencorticalis. Langenbecks Arch. Chir. **328,** 109 (1971).

Alvik, I.: Arthrodesis of the hip. A method allowing weightbearing and walking postoperatively. Acta Orthop. Scand. **32,** 451 (1962).

Alvik, I.: Arthrodesis and arthroplasty of the hip joint. Acta Orthop. Scand. **33,** (1–4), 253 (1963).

Alvik, I.: Arthrodesis of the hip with early mobilization and rehabilitation. Sicot, XIe Congrès, Mexico, p. 866 (1969).

Apley, A.G., Denham, R.A.: Osteotomy as an aid to arthrodesis of the hip. J. Bone Joint Surg. B **37,** 185 (1955).

Axer, A.: Compression arthrodesis of the hip joint. J. Bone Joint Surg. A **43,** 492 (1961).

Banks, H.H.: Factors influencing the result in fractures of the femoral neck. J. Bone Joint Surg. A **44,** 931 (1962).

Bastos, D.M.: Arthrodesis de cadera en las secuelas poliomieliticas. Sicot, XIe Congrès Mexico, p. 873 (1969).

Baumann, F., Behr, O.: Elektromyographische Untersuchungen der Hüftmuskulatur nach Arthrodese. Arch. Orthop. Unfallchir. **66,** 1 (1969).

Beck, W.: Über Hüftarthrodesen mit der Kreuzplatte. Verh. DGOT 1968. Bücherei des Orthopäden, Vol. 3, Stuttgart: Enke 1969.

Becker, F.: Die Hüftarthrodese. In: Rütt: Die Therapie der Coxarthrose, p. 274. Stuttgart: Thieme 1969.

Bessler, W.: Resultate mit 85-Sr-Skelettszintigraphie. Radioisotope in der Lokalisationsdiagnostik (4th annual meeting. Ges. Nuklearmed. Heidelberg 1966), p. 431, Stuttgart: F.K. Schattauer 1967.

Bick, E.M.: Source Book of Orthopaedics, p. 349, Baltimore: Williams & Wilkins 1948.

Blaimont, P.: Libération d'une arthrodèse ancienne de la hanche par arthroplastie, pour traitement d'une arthrose du genou. Soc. Belge d'Orthop. Meeting of 23 Nov., p. 983, 1968.

Boitzy, A.: La Fracture du Col du Fémur Chez L'enfant et L'adolescent. Paris: Masson 1971.

Boitzy, A., Zimmermann, H.: Komplikationen bei Totalprothesen der Hüfte. Arch. Orthop. Unfallchir. **66,** 192 (1969).

Bosworth, D.M.: Femoro-ischial transplantation. J. Bone Joint Surg. **24,** 38 (1942).

Bosworth, D.M.: Blade-plate fixation. J. Am. Med. Ass. **141,** 1111 (1949).

Bouillet, R., Delchef, J.: L'arthrose du genou conséquence éloignée de l'ankylose de la hanche. Acta Orthop. Belg. **34** (6), 947 (1968).

Boyd, H.B., George, I.L.: Complication of fractures of the neck of the femur. J. Bone Joint Surg. **29,** 13 (1947).

Breitenfelder, J., Port, J.: Hat die Hüftgelenksarthrodese in der Kombination mit der totalen Endoprothese ihre Berechtigung? Z. Orthop. III, 237, (1973).

Brittain, H.A.: Ischiofemoral arthrodesis. J. Bone Joint Surg. B **29,** 93 (1941/42).

Brittain, H.A.: Architectural Principles in Arthrodesis, 2nd ed. Edinburgh-London: Livingstone 1952.

Buchholz, H.W.: Das künstliche Hüftgelenk. Materia Medica Nordmark **21,** 613 (1969).

Bucholz, H.W.: Personal communication, 1973.

Burkardt, A.: Statik und Dynamik der versteiften Hüfte. Lecture, Nr. 21, Schweiz. Ges. für Orthop., annual meeting Fribourg, 1973.

Burkardt, A.: Personal communication, 1973.

Burns, B.H.: Fixation of the osteo-arthritic hip by nailing. Lancet **236,** 978 (1939).

Carter, J., Wickstrom, J.: Arthrodesis of the hip: an assessment of results in one hundred patients. South. med. J. (Bgham, Ala.) **64,** 451 (1971).

Castaing, J., Douvion, J.C., Autret, J.: Technique de l'arthrodèse de la hanche avec ostéotomie intertrochantérienne non fixée. Rev. Chir. Orthop. **48,** (6), 757 (1962).

Čech, E., Stryhal, F., Čech, O.: Influence of Osteotomy of pelvis on pelvic diameters. Cs. Gynek. **36** (6), 329 (1971).

Chapchal, G.: Die Arthrodese des Hüftgelenkes. Chir. Praxis **65** (1959).

Chapchal, G.: Die Arthrodese bei der Hüftearthrose. Langenbecks Arch. Chir. **301**, 417 (1962).

Chapchal, G.: Orthopädische Chirurgie und Traumatologie der Hüfte, p. 192. Stuttgart: Enke 1965.

Charnley, J.: Compression Arthrodesis. Edinburgh-London: Livingstone 1953.

Charnley, J.: Stabilisation of the hip by central dislocation. J. Bone Joint Surg. B **37**, 514 (1955).

Charnley, J.: Treatment of mono-articular arthritis of the hip by the central dislocation operation. J. Bone Joint Surg. B **38**, 592 (1956).

Charnley, J.: Arthroplasty of the hip—A new operation. Lancet **1961 II**, 1129

Charnley, J.: Personal communication, 1970.

Ciuccarelli, C. Marchi, F.: L'artrodesi transarticolare con duo viti associata da osteotomia nel trattamento della coxartrosi. Chir. Organi Mov. **51**, 273 (1962).

Claffey, T.J.: Avascular necrosis of the femoral head. J. Bone Joint Surg. B **42**, 802 (1960).

Cleveland, M., Fielding, J.W.: Intracapsular fracture of neck. Am. Acad. Orthop. **12**, 35 (1955).

Conforty, B.: Bio-mechanical considerations on arthrodesis of the hip joint. Khirurgiya (Sofiya) **15**, 213 (1962).

Conforty, B.: Personal communication, 1973.

Cotta, H., Dreyer, J.: Die operative Behandlung arthrotischer Beschwerden an den unteren Gliedmassen. Z. Allgemeinmed. „Der Landarzt" (Stuttg.) **47**, 161 (1971).

Cotta, H., Schulitz, K.P.: Der totale Hüftgelenkersatz. Stuttgart: Thieme 1973.

Coventry, M.B.: Personal communication, 1973.

Crenshaw, A.H.: Campbells operative orthopaedics, 5th ed., Vol. II, p. 1141. Saint Louis: Mosby 1971.

Dahmen, G.: Zur Indikation schmerzlindernder und funktionsverbessernder Operationen am Hüftgelenk: Alloarthroplastik, Arthrodese, Umstellungsosteotomie. Orthopädie. **42**, (2), 246 (1971).

Danielsson, L.G.: Late results of Perthes' disease. Acta Orthop. Scand. **36**, 70 (1965).

Daraignez, BJ.E.: L'arthrodèse. Thèse, Bordeaux, 1891.

Daubenspeck, K.: Fixation of pressure-plates by means of screws in the arthrodesis of hip-joints. Sicot, IXe Congrès, Mexico, p. 855, 1969.

Davis, J.B.: The muscle-pedicle bone graft in hip fusion. J. Bone Joint Surg. A **36**, 790 (1954).

De Beule, F.: La résection de la Hanche suivie de Fixation de l'extrémité supérieure du fémur à la tubérosité ischiatique. J. Chir. (Brux.) **9**, 173 (1909).

Debeyre, J., Goutallier, D., Boucker, C.: Traitement chirurgical des coxites rhumatismales isolées. Rev. Rhum. **37**, 63 (1970).

Debeyre, J., Huchet, C.A.: La luxation interne trans-acétabulaire dans le traitement opératoire des arthroses de la hanche (Technique de Charnley) Rev. Chir. Orthop. **45**, 397 (1959).

Debrunner, H.U.: Orthopädisches Diagnostikum. Stuttgart: Thieme 1966.

Demigneux, F., Rainaut, J.J., Cedart, Cl.: Etude de la hanche opposée aux arthrodèses. Rev. Chir. Orthop. **54** (7), 649 (1968).

Des Brosses, J.: Les indications actuelles de l'arthrodèse de la hanche chez l'adulte. Thèse de Lyon; Bosc, éd. 1956.

Dimiccoli, N.: Reduction-arthrodesis in congenital unilateral inveterate dislocation of the hip. Arch. Putti **20**, 156 (1965).

Documenta Geigy: Durchschnitts- und Idealgewicht Erwachsener (Größe, Gewicht, Alter) In: Build and Blood Pressure Study, I, Society of Actuaries, Chicago (1959) und Statist. Bull. Metrop. Life Insur. Co., 40, Nov.-Dec. 1959. Wissenschaftliche Tabellen, 6th ed., p. 588, 1960.

Dollinger, J.: Arthrodesen bei der Kinderlähmung. Zbl. Chir. **18** (36), 689 (1891).

Dreyer, J., Pingel, P.: Unsere Erfahrungen bei der Hüftarthrodese mit Beckenosteotomie und Kreuzplatte. Arch. orthop. Unfallchir. **66**, 310 (1969).

Dupont, A., Charnley, J.: Low-Friction arthroplasty of the hip for the failures of previous operations. J. Bone Joint Surg. B **54**, 77 (1972).

Dustmann, H.O., Hamacher, P.: Modifikation der Kreuzplatte für Hüftarthrodesen. Z. Orthop. **109**, 182 (1971).

Dwyer, A.F.: Experience of a new method of hip arthrodesis. Aust N. Z. J. Surg. **34**, 105 (1964).

Dwyer, A.F., Cass, C.A.: Internal fixation in hip arthrodesis. Med. J. Aust. **49**, 977 (1961).

Elmendorff, H.F., v., Simmert, H., Hupfauer, W.: Über Brüche von metallischen Implantaten. Arch. Orthop. Unfallchir. **67**, 141 (1969).

Endström, G.: Destruction of hip joint in rheumatoid arthritis during long-term steroid therapy. Acta Rheumatol. Scand. **7**, 151 (1961).

Farkas, A.: A new operative treatment of tuberculosis coxitis in children. J. Bone Joint Surg. B. **21**, 323 (1939).

Faysse, R.: L'arthrodèse et les opérations mobilisatrices. Lyon Chir. **63**, 469 (1967).

Fielding, J.W., Wilson, H.J., Zickel, R.E.: A continuing end-result study of intracapsular fracture of the neck of the femur. J. Bone Joint Surg. A **44**, 965 (1962).

Fischer, O.: Der Gang des Menschen. Abh. d. K. S. Ges. d. Wiss. XXV – XXVII, 1896 – 1904.

Fiskin, V.J.: Compression arthrodesis of the hip joint. Orthop. Travmatol Protez **5**, 66 (1965).

Flatmark, A.L., Lone, T.: The prognosis of abduction fracture of the neck of the femur. J. Bone Joint Surg. B **44**, 324 (1962).

Francillon, M.R.: Orthopédie de la coxarthrose. Doc. Rheumatologica Geigy, Nr. 13 (1958).

Francon, F.: Coxarthrie. Doc. Rheumatologica Geigy, Nr. 9 (1956).

Friedebold, G.: Die klinische Bedeutung der Anpassungsvorgänge der Skelettmuskulatur. Verh. Dtsch. Orthop. Ges. 54. Kongr. **75**, 75 (1967).

Furlong, R.: The surgical treatment of rheumatoid disease. Practitioner **208**, 33 (1972).

Fürmaier, A.: Überlegungen zur Statik des arthrodesierten Hüftgelenkes. Arch. Orthop. Unfallchir. **51**, 28 (1959).

Gardiner, T.B.: Nail and graft arthrodesis of the hip. J. Bone Joint Surg. B **44**, 588 (1962).

GERTSCH, R.: Die Arthrodese des Hüftgelenkes mit Kreuzplatte und Beckenosteotomie. Helv. Chir. Acta **33,** 216 (1966).

GHORMLEY, R.K.: Use of anterior superior spine and crest of ilium in surgery of the hip joint. J. Bone Joint Surg. **13,** 784 (1931).

GILL, A.B.: Arthrodesis of the hip for ununited fractures. J. Bone Joint Surg. **29,** 305 (1947).

GIRDLESTONE, R.R.: The modern treatment of tuberculosis of the bones and joints. J. Bone Joint Surg. **6,** 519 (1924).

GIRDLESTONE, G.R.: Arthrodesis and other operations for tuberculosis of the hip. In: The Robert Jones Birthday Vol. London: Oxford University Press 1940.

GOEB, A.: Die operative Behandlung der Arthrosis deformans des Hüftgelenkes. Chir. Praxis **14,** 299 (1970).

GOERDES, W.: Erfahrungen mit der Technik der Hüftarthrodese nach Axer-Viernstein. Arch. Orthop. Unfallchir. **67,** 355 (1970).

GOERDES, W., HESSERT, G.R.: Indikationswandel bei Arthrodesen und Alloarthroplastiken des Hüftgelenkes. Arch. Orthop. Unfallchir. **69,** 264 (1971).

GOERDES, W., VIERNSTEIN, K., KLEMENT, J.: Erfahrungen mit Hüftarthrodese nach der AO-Technik. Arch. Orthop. Unfallchir. **70,** 304 (1971).

GOESSENS, H., PINGEL, P., DREYER, J.: L'arthrodèse de hanche par plaque en croix. Acta Orthop. Belg. **36** (3), 350 (1970).

GSCHWEND, N.: Eine wenig bekannte Komplikation der Hüftarthrodese oder die van Neecksche Krankheit des Erwachsenen. Arch. Orthop. Unfallchir. **62,** 263 (1967).

GSCHWEND, N.: Die operative Behandlung der progressiv chronischen Polyarthritis, p. 133. Stuttgart: Thieme 1968.

GSCHWEND, N.: Operation am polyarthritischen Hüftgelenk. Therapiewoche **20** (18), 746 (1970).

GSCHWEND, N.: Personal communication. Dec. 1973.

Gschwend, N., NACHACHAN, F., ZIPPEL. J.: Total hip replacement in rheumatoid arthritis. In: Chapchal. G.: Arthroplasty of the Hip. p. 241. Stuttgart: Thieme 1973.

GUILLEMINET, M., DESBROSSES, J.: Arthrodèse de la hanche pour d'arthroplastie avec interposition inerte. Lyon Chir. **49** (8), 897 (1954).

HACKENBROCH, M.: Arthrodese, Arthroplastik, Arthrolyse. Arch. Orthop. Unfallchir. **51,** 549 (1960).

HACKENBROCH, M.: Zur Frage der operativen Behandlung des femoral-funktionell defekten Hüftgelenkes. Z. Orthop. **92,** 610 (1960).

HACKENBROCH, M.: Zur normalen und pathologisch veränderten Mechanik des Hüftgelenks. In: Hohmann, G., Hackenbroch, M., Lindemann, K., Handbuch der Orthopädie, Vol. IV, part I, 1. Stuttgart: Thieme, 1961.

HAFFERL, A.: Lehrbuch der Topographischen Anatomie. Berlin-Göttingen-Heidleberg: Springer 1957.

HAFFERL, A.: Lehrbuch der Topographischen Anatomie. Neubearbeitet von Thiel, W. 3. Aufl. 1969.

HANSLIK, L., FRIEDEBOLD, G.: Die Indikationsstellung zur Hüftarthrodese nach Entwicklung stabiler Alloarthroplastiken. Arch. Orthop. Unfallchir. **68,** 325 (1970).

HARTLEY, J., SILVER, N.: Muscle-pedicle bone grafts. J. Bone Joint Surg. A **36,** 800 (1954).

HENDERSON, J.S.: Combined intra-articular and extra-articular arthrodesis for tuberculosis of the hip joint. J. Bone Joint Surg. A **15,** 51 (1933).

HERBERT, J.J.: Etude critique sur les arthrodèses de la hanche. Rev. Chir. Orthop. **46** (1), 3 (1960).

HERBERT, J.J., FOUCHER, J., FOUCHER, G., HERBERT, A.: Prothèses totales de hanches atypiques. Rev. Chir. Orthop. **59,** 523 (1973).

HETTINGER, TH.: Die maximalen Drehmomente im Hüft-Knie- und Fußgelenk bei verschiedenen Winkelstellungen. Arbeitsphysiol. **15,** 355 (1954).

HEUSNER, P.: Über Hüftresektion wegen angeborener Luxation. Zbl. Chir. **45,** 751 (1884).

HIBBS. A.R.: A preliminary report of twenty cases of hip joint tuberculosis treated by an operation devised to eliminate motion by fusing the joint. J. Bone Joint Surg. A **8,** 522 (1926).

HIRSCH, C.: Studies on the mechanism of low back pain. Acta Orthop. Scand. **20,** 261 (1950/51).

HOFMEISTER, F.: Die orthopädisch-chirurgische Behandlung der traumatisch bedingten Schenkelkopfnekrosen. Arch. Orthop. Unfallchir. **49,** 556 (1958).

HÖGER, P. M.: Röntgenologische Untersuchungen nach Hüftarthrodese bei Arthrosis deformans. Diss., Hamburg, 1964.

HOHMANN, D.: Untersuchungen zur Frage des Standbeines bei Hüftarthrodesierten. Arch. Orthop. Infallchir. **54,** 153 (1962).

HOLEVITCH, Y.: Arthrodèse allongeante de l'articulation de la hanche chez les poliomyélitiques. Rev. Chir. Orthop. **49** (3), 301 (1963).

HÖRDEGEN, K.M., TÖNNIS, D.: Der Einfluß der Hüftgelenks-Arthrodese auf die Wirbelsäule. Arch. Orthop. Unfallchir. **69,** 97 (1970).

HOWARD, R.C.: V-Arthrodesis of the hip. J. Bone Joint Surg. B **32,** 282 (1950).

HOWARD, R.C.: Stability of osteosynthesis in hip arthrodesis. Acta Orthop. Scand. **35,** 225 (1965).

HUGGLER, A.: Die Hüftarthrodese nach Charnley. Arch. Orthop. Unfallchir. **52,** 366 (1960).

HUGGLER, A.: Die Alloarthroplastik des Hüftgelenkes. Stuttgart: Thieme 1968.

HUGGLER, A.: Wandel in der Indikation zur intertrochanteren Osteotomie. In Morscher E., Die intertrochantere Osteotomie bei Coxarthrose, p. 122, Bern-Stuttgart-Vienna: Huber 1971.

JODOGNE, G.: La coxarthrose. Rev. Méd. Liège **25,** (20), 663 (1970).

JUDET, J.: A study of the arterial vascularisation of the femoral neck in the adult. J. Bone Joint Surg. A **37,** 663 (1955).

JUDET, R.: Traité de Thérapeutique Chirurgicale, Tome I, p. 451, Paris: Masson 1961.

JUDET, R., JUDET, J., ROY-CAMILLE, R.: La vascularisation des pseudarthroses des os longs d'après une étude clinique et expérimentale. Rev. Chir. Orthop. **44,** 381 (1958).

KALÉN, R.: Internal fixation in hip joint arthrodesis. Acta Orthop. Scand., Suppl. 112, 1 (1968).

KAPANDJI, J.A.: Physiologie Articulaire Fascicule II Membre Inférieur. Paris: Maloine 1965.

KATAYAMA, R., ITAMI, Y., MARUMO, E.: Treatment of hip and knee-joint tuberculosis: an attempt to retain motion. J. Bone Joint Surg. A **44,** 897 (1962).

KELLY, E.C.: Encyclopedia of Medical Sources. Baltimore: Williams & Wilkins 1948.

KELLY, P.J., MARTIN, W.J., COVENTRY, M.B.: Bacterial (suppurative) arthritis in the adult. J. Bone Joint Surg. A **52,** 1595 (1970).

KNIGHT, R.A., BLUHM, M.M.: Brittain ischiofemoral arthrodesis. J. Bone Joint Surg. **27,** 578 (1945).

KOCHER, TH., DE QUERVAIN, F.: Enzyklopaedie der gesamten Chirurgie, Vol. I, p. 582, Leipzig: Vogel 1901.

KOLBEL, R., WEIGERT, M.: Total alloarthroplasty following arthrodesis. Z. Orthop. **108,** 587 (1971).

KRAKOVITS, G.: Über die Auswirkung einer Beinverkürzung auf auf die Statik und Dynamik des Hüftgelenkes. Z. Orthop. **102** (3), 418 (1967).

KÜNTSCHER, G.: Die Technik der „geschlossenen" Hüftarthrodese. Chirurg **24,** 404 (1953).

LAGRANGE, M.: Résection orthopédique de la hanche pour luxation pathologique. Bull. Soc. Chirurgie Paris **32** (1892). Ref: Karlén A.: Acta Chir. Scand., Suppl. **96** (1944).

LAM, S.J.S.: Arthrodesis of the hip. With special reference to early mobilisation without external splintage. J. Bone Joint Surg. B **50,** 14 (1968).

LAMPUGNANI, C.: La decapitazione del femore nella lussazione congenita dell'anca; studio pratico di ortopedia chirurgica antisettica. G. Accad. Med. Torino **33,** 538 (1885).

LANGE, M.: Orthopädisch-Chirurgische Operationslehre, 2nd ed., p. 550. Munich: Bergmann 1962.

LANGE, M.: Review of a series of more than five hundred cases. J. Int. Coll. Surg. **29,** 638 (1958).

LANGENSKIÖLD, A., LAURENT, L. E.: Compression arthrodesis of the hip joint by the method of Axer. Acta Orthop. Scand. **38,** 359 (1967).

LETOURNEI, E.: Die operative Versorgung der Hüftgelenkpfannenbrüche. Langenbecks Arch. Chir. **316,** 423 (1966).

LIECHTI, R.: Hüftarthrodesen. Lecture, Schweiz. Ges. für Orthop., annual meeting, Chur, 1972.

LIECHTI, R.: Arthrodeses de la hanche sans „plaque en croix". Lecture Nr. 22, Schweiz. Ges. für Orthop. annual meeting, Fribourg, 1973.

LIECHTI, R.: Indikation und Technik der Kreuzplattenarthrodese. Orthop. Praxis **4,** 1974. (im (Druck)

LIECHTI, R., WEBER, B.G.: Beitrag zur Prophylaxe der operativen Infektionen. Unsere Erfahrungen nach vierjähriger Durchführung präventiver Impfung mit Staphylokokkenvaccine. Chirurg **44,** 269 (1973).

LINDAHL, O.: Hip-joint arthrodesis: to find the best position. Acta Orthop Scand. **37,** 317 (1966).

LINDSTRÖM, N.: Partial intra plus juxta articular arthrodesis with simultaneous nailing according to Watson-Jones. Acta Orthop. Scand. **25,** 255 (1956–57).

LIPSCOMB, P.R., MDCASLIN, F.E.: Arthrodesis of the hip. Review of 371 cases. J. Bone Joint Surg. A **43,** 923 (1961).

LOEFFLER, F., MATZEN, P.F., KNOEFLER, W.E., Orthopädische Operationen, Vol. I, p. 252 Berlin: VEB, Verlag Volk und Gesundheit 1971.

LÜHKEN, H.: Die Statik des menschlichen Beckens. Z. Anat. Entwickl.-Gesch. **104,** 729 (1935).

MAGERL, F., BLATTER, R.: Diagnostic du descellement des prothèses totales de la hanche. De Boitzy A.: Périarthrite, ostéogénèse, travaux divers, p. 296. Bern-Stuttgart-Vienna: Huber 1972.

MALGAIGNE, J.F.: Oeuvres complètes d'Ambroise Paré. Chez Baillière J.B., Libraire de l'Académie Royale de Médecine **54** (1840).

MAQUET, P.: Biomechanics and osteoarthrithis of the hip Sicot, XIe Congrès, Mexico, p. 882 (1969).

MARAGLIANO, D.: Nuovi punti di appoggio chirurgico nelle lussazione vere da coxite. Chir. Organi Mov. **5,** 225 (1921).

MARMOR, L.: Surgery for osteoarthritis. Geriatrics **27,** 89 (1972).

MARNEFF, R.: Intervention mobilisatrice de principe dans les ankyloses coxo-fémorales. Soc. Belge d'Orthop. Meeting of 23 Nov., p. 969, 1968.

MAY, V.R., JR., MAUCK, W.: Intra-articular hip fusion with the intramedullary nail. Clin. Orthop. **25,** 113 (1962).

McKEE, G.K.: Arthrodesis of the hip with a lag-screw. J. Bone Joint Surg. B **39,** 477 (1957).

McKEE, G.K.: Case presentations and results of total replacement prothesis. In: Rütt, A. Die Therapie der Koxarthrose. Stuttgart: Thieme 1969.

McKEE, G.K.: Personal communication, 1970.

MEEL, P.J.: Arthrodesis of the hip; with a description of an operative technique. Arch. Chir. Neerl. **23** (3), 225 (1971).

MERLE D'AUBIGNÉ, R.: Nécroses traumatiques de la tête fémorale Chir. Rép. Traum. **5,** 61 (1960).

MERLE D'AUBIGNÉ, R., CHABROL, J.: Les arthrodèses de la hanche par enclouage. Résultats. Indications. Techniques. Rev. Chir. Orthop. **71,** 293 (1952).

MERLE D'AUBIGNÉ, R., CORMIER: Nécrose traumatique de la tête du fémur en dehors des pseudarthroses. Revue Orthop. **42** (2), 246 (1956).

MERLE D'AUBIGNÉ, R., POSTEL, M.: Réinterventions après arthroplasties de la hanche. Rev. Chir. Orthop. **42** (3), 18 (1956).

MERLÉ D'AUBIGNÉ, R., RAMADIER, J.O., JUTEAU, B.: L'ARTHRODÈSE dans les luxations congénitales de la hanche chez l'adulte. Rev. Chir. Orthop. **48** (6), 685 (1962).

MERLE D'AUBIGNÉ, R., RAMADIER, J.O., POSTEL, M., MAZAS, F., VAILLANT, J.M.: L'arthrodèse de la hanche. Rev. Chir. Orthop. **50** (5), 789 (1964).

MEULI, H. CH.: Zur operativen Behandlung der polyarthritischen Hüfte. Dtsch. Med. Wochenschr. **91** (40), 1779 (1966).

MEULI, H. CH.: Moderne Aspekte der Operation von Hüftarthrosen. In: Arthritis-Arthrose, Arthritis Osteoarthrosis, p. 237, Bern-Stuttgart-Vienna: Huber 1969.

MITTAG, G.: Behandlung, Verlauf und Spätschicksal von 300 Schenkelhalsfrakturen. Chirurg **27,** 224 (1956).

MOREAU, P.F.: Observations pratiques relatives à la résection des articulations affectées de carie. Paris: Croullebois 1803.

MORRIS, J.B.: Charnley compression arthrodesis of the hip. J. Bone Joint Surg. B **48,** 260 (1966).

MORSCHER, E.: Die intertrochantere Osteotomie bei Coxarthrose. Bern-Stuttgart-Vienna: Huber 1971.

MORTENS, J., JENSEN, E.: Charnley stabilisation of the hip. J. Bone Joint Surg. B **42,** 466 (1960).

MÜLLER, B.S.: Kompressionsarthrodese des Hüftgelenkes. Beitr. Orthop. **15** (3), 149 (1968).

MÜLLER, G.: Girdlestone-Hüfte nach infizierter Totalprothese. Lecture, Schweiz. Ges. für Orthop. annual meeting, Chur, 1972.

MÜLLER, G.: Personal communication, 1972.

MÜLLER, M.E.: Ostéosynthèse externe de compression pour arthrodèses et ostéotomies. Réunion des orthopédistes suisses. St. Gall. Rev. Chir. Orthop. **39,** 531 (1953).
MÜLLER, M.E.: Die extraartikuläre ischiofemorale Hüftarthrodese. Helv. Chir. Acta **22** (2), 127 (1955).
MÜLLER, M.E.: Chirurgie de la hanche (12 interventions). Bulletin-AO, 1967.
MÜLLER, M.E.: Die Varisationsosteotomie bei der Behandlung der Koxarthrose. In: Rütt, A., Die Therapie der Koxarthrose. Stuttgart: Thieme 1969.
MÜLLER, M.E.: Hüftnahe Femurosteotomien, 2nd ed. Stuttgart: Thieme 1970.
MÜLLER, M.E., ALLGÖWER, M., WILLENEGGER, H.: Technik der Operativen Frakturbehandlung. Berlin-Göttingen-Heidelberg: Springer 1963.
MÜLLER, M.E., ALLGÖWER, M., WILLENEGGER, H.: Manual der Osteosynthese. Berlin-Heidelberg-New York: Springer 1969.
MÜLLER, M.E., ALLGÖWER, M., WILLENEGGER, H.: Manual of Internal Fixation. Berlin-Heidelberg-New York: Springer 1970.
NEFF, G.: Fehler und Gefahren bei Hüftoperationen. Langenbecks Arch. Chir. **284,** 693 (1956).
NIGST, H.: Spezielle Frakturen- und Luxationslehre. Vol. III (Hüftgelenk und proximaler Oberschenkel). Stuttgart: Thieme 1964.
NOESBERGER, B.: Biomechanische Grundlagen der Intertrochanteren Femurosteotomie bei Koxarthrose und ihre Mehrjahresresultate in einem Kollektiv von 100 Fällen. Schweiz. Med. Wochenschr. **100,** 101 (1970).
ONJI, Y., KURATA, Y., KINDO, HA.: A new method of hip fusion using an intramedullary nail. A preliminary report. J. Bone Joint Surg. B **47,** 690 (1965).
OSMOND-CLARKE, H.: Hip joint surgery in the twentieth century. Rheum. Phys. Med. **2,** 173 (1971).
OSTAPCUK, A.D.: Kompresivnij arthrodez tazobedernovo sustava. Ortop. Travmatol. Protez. **25,** (1), 59 (1964).
OTTE, P.: Die Arthrodese des Hüftgelenks bei Koxarthrose. In: Rütt, A., Die Therapie der Coxarthrose, p. 258. Stuttgart: Thieme 1969.
PADOVANI, P., JOLY, J.P.: Résultats éloignés de 308 arthrodèses de hanche. Rev. Chir. Orthop. **47** (1), 83 (1961).
PARK, H.: An Account of a New Method of Treating Diseases of the Knee and Elbow in a Letter to Mr. Percival Pott by H. Park of Liverpool. Anthology of Orthopaedics, 1781.
PAUL, J. P.: The biomechanics of the hip joint and its clinical relevance. Roy. Soc. Med. **59,** 943 (1966).
PAUL, J.P.: The effect of walking speed on the force actions transmitted at the hip and knee joints. Proc. Roy. Soc. Med. **63,** 200 (1970).
PAUWELS, F.: Beitrag zur Klärung der Beanspruchung des Bekkens, insbesondere der Beckenfugen. Z. Anat. Entwickl.-Gesch. **114,** 167 (1948).
PAUWELS, F.: Die Bedeutung der Bauprinzipien der unteren Extremität für die Beanspruchung des Beinskeletts. Z. Anat. Entwickl.-Gesch. **114,** 525 (1950).
PAUWELS, F.: Neue Richtlinien für die operative Behandlung der Koxarthrose. Verh. Dtsch. Orthop. Ges. **48,** 332 (1961).
PAUWELS, F.: Über die Bedeutung einer Zuggurtung für die Beanspruchung des Röhrenknochens. Verh. Dtsch. Orthop. Ges. **52,** 231 (1965).
PEASE, C.N.: Fusion of the hip in children. The Chandler method, J. Bone Joint Surg. A **29,** 874 (1947).
PERARD, V.S.: Anatomy and Drawing. 4th ed. New York-London: Pitman 1955.
PHEMISTER, D.B.: Treatment of necrotic head of femur in adults. J. Bone Joint Surg. A **31,** 55 (1949).
PIGGOT, J.: Charnley stabilisation of the hip. J. Bone Joint Surg. B **42,** 476 (1960).

RANG, M.: Anthology of Orthopaedics. Edinburgh-London: Livingstone 1966.
RATOMSKI, R., JESKE, W., ADAMCZEWSKI, J., HABRYCH, A.: Die operative Hüftarthrodese nach Müller. Beitr. Orthop. **17,** 113 (1970).
REICHELT, A., STALL, CHR.: Die kausalgenetische Bedeutung der Behandlungsart für die Entwicklung von Hüftkopfnekrosen nach Schenkelhalsfrakturen. Z. Orthop. **111,** 28 (1973).
RINALDI, E.: Possibilità di terapia chirurgica negli insuccessi di artroplastiche dell'anca. Arch. Putti Chir. Organi Mov. **23,** 134 (1968).
ROCHER, H.L.: Technique simplifiée pour l'arthrodèse extra-articulaire de la hanche par greffon tibial dans la coxalgie type. 37. J. Méd. Bordeaux **114,** (1969).
ROESLER, H., HAMACHER, P.: Die biostratische Analyse der Belastung des Hüftgelenkes Parts I and II. Z. Orthop. **110,** 67, 186 (1972).
ROSEN, H.: Personal communication, 1972.
RUCKDESCHEL, G., HESSERT, G.R., SCHÖLLHAMMER, TH.: Quantitative in vitro-Untersuchungen zur Folge der Gentamycinabgabe aus Polymethyl-methacrylat-Polymerisatblöcken. Arch. Orthop. Unfallchir. **74,** 291 (1973).
RUSSE, O.: Behandlung der Schenkelhalsfraktur. Zbl. Chir. **77,** 1063 (1952).
RÜTER, A., GANZ, R.: Totalprothesen nach Hüftarthrodesen. In: Cotta, H. Schulitz, K.P., Der Totale Hüftgelenkersatz, p. 72, Stuttgart: Thieme 1973.
RUTISHAUSER, E.: Les coxites rhumatismales. Doc Rheum. Geigy, Nr. 16, 1959.
RÜTT, A.: Die Therapie der Koxarthrose. Stuttgart: Thieme 1970.

SALEM, G.: Erfahrungen bei 798 Schenkelhalsfrakturen. Langenbecks Arch. Chir. **268,** 602 (1951).
SCHNEIDER, R.: Technik der Hüftarthrodese mit Beckenosteotomie. Langenbecks Arch. Chir. **316,** 233 (1966).
SCHNEIDER, R.: Hip arthrodesis with the Cobra head plate and pelvic osteotomy. Rec. Surg. and Traum. **14,** Basel, Munich: Karger (im Druck).
SCHNEIDER, R.: Reoperationen und Komplikationen der Totalprothesen der Hüfte. In Vorbereitung.
SCHNEIDER, R.: Personal communication, Sept. 1973.
SCHOERNER, R.: Vor- und Nachteile versteifender Operationen am Hüftgelenk. Arch. Orthop. Unfallchir. **45,** 230 (1952).
SCHUMM, H.C.: Extra-articular immobilization of the hip joint. Surg. Gynecol. Obstet. **48,** 112 (1929).
SEEWALD, K., DEBRUNNER, A.: Untersuchungen über die Veränderung des nicht erkrankten Hüftgelenkes bei Hüftankylosierten. Z. Orthop. **98** (3), 288 (1964).
SEGMÜLLER, G.: Funktionsdiagnostik der Pseudarthrose mittels 85-Sr-Szintimetrie. Ther. Umschau B **28** (5), 329 (1971).

SEGMÜLLER, G.: Ergebnisse und Indikation der Totalprothese bei der rheumatischen Coxitis. Verhandlungen. Privately published by: Vereinigung der Orthop. Österreichs, Vienna, 99, 1972.

SEGMÜLLER, G.: Orthopädische Fragestellungen und ihre Beantwortung durch die Skelettscintigraphie. Med. Neuheiten, **1/2,** 1 (72).

SLOOFF, T.J.J.H.: The unstable endoprothesis of the hip. Arch. Chir. Neerl. **23** (2), 205 (1971).

SOMERVILLE, E.W.: Two nail fixation of the hip. J. Bone Joint Surg. B **51,** 648 (1969).

SPRANGER, M.: Abdominelle Komplikationen nach Hüftgelenksarthrodesen und Schenkelhalsnagelungen. Arch. Orthop. Unfallchir. **69,** 351 (1971).

STEINDLER, A.: Kinesiology of the Human Body, p. 276. Springfield, Illinois USA: Thomas 1955.

STEVENS, J.: Osteoarthritis of the hip. A review with special consideration of the problem of bilateral malum coxae senilis. Clin. Orthop. Padova **71,** 152 (1970).

STEWART, M.J., COKER, T.P.: Arthrodesis of the hip. A review of 109 patients. Clin. Orthop. **62,** 136 (1969).

STEWART, M.J.· MILFORD, L.W.: Fracture dislocation of the hip and end result study. J. Bone Joint Surg. A **36,** 315 (1954).

STINCHFIELD, F.E., CAVALLARO, W.U.: Arthrodesis of the hip joint. A. Follow-up study. J. Bone Joint Surg. A **32,** 48 (1950).

STONE, M.M.: Arthrodesis of the hip. J. Bone Joint Surg. A **38,** 1346 (1956).

SYME, J.: Exarticulation of the Hip Joint in Scotland. Edinburgh, 1799, 1823.

TAITZ, J.: Arthrodesis of a prosthetic hip joint. J. Bone Joint Surg. A **43,** 555 (1961).

TEINTURIER, P.: Arthrodèse de la hanche. Lambeau pédiculé trochantérien avec vissage ischiofémoral. Rev. Chir. Orthop. **52,** 645 (1966).

TELESZYNSKI, M., FACZYNSKI, A., SZWALUK, F.: Ocena wplywu przeciazenia stawu biodrowego u jednostronnie amputowanych. Chir. Narzadow Ruchu **24,** 6, 547 (1959).

THOMPSON, F.R.: Combined hip fusion and subtrochanteric osteotomy allowing early ambulation. J. Bone Joint Surg. A **38,** 13 (1956).

THOMPSON, V.P., EPSTEIN, H.C.: Traumatic dislocation of the hip. A survey of 204 cases covering a period of 21 years. J. Bone Joint Surg. A **33,** 746 (1951).

THOMSEN, W.: Zur Problematik der Arthrodese des Hüftgelenks und des Knöchelgelenks. Supplement to Z. Orthop. **94,** 469 (1961).

TÖNNIS, D.: Elektromyographische Kontrollmöglichkeit und Befunde bei aktiver Übungsbehandlung. Verh. Dtsch. Orthop. Ges. **52,** 36 (1965).

TÖNNIS, D.: Elektromyographische und histologische Befunde bei aktiver Übungsbehandlung. Verh. Dtsch. Orthop. Ges. **54,** 104 (1967).

TROJAN, E., PERSCHL, A.: Die Behandlungsergebnisse von 79 frischen, traumatischen Hüftgelenksverrenkungen und Hüftgelenksverrenkungsbrüchen. Ergebn. Chir. Orthop. **40,** 90 (1956).

TRUETA, J., HARRISON, M.H.M.: The normal vascular anatomy of the femoral head in adult man. J. Bone Joint Surg. B **35,** 442 (1953).

TRUMBLE, H.C.: Method of fixation of the hip joint by means of an extraarticular bone graft. Aust. N. Z. J. Surg. **1,** 411 (1932).

VAINIO, K., PUKKI, T.: Rheumatoid arthritis of the hip. Relaz. al cong. della Lega Int. contra il Reumatismo, Roma, 1961.

VALENTIN, B.: Geschichte der Orthopädie. Stuttgart: Thieme 1961.

VAN NECK, M.: Osteochondritis of pubis. Arch. Franco-Belg. Chir. **27,** 238, (1924).

VAN NES, C.P.: L'arthrodèse de la hanche pour arthrite déformante. Bull. Soc. belge Orthop. **2** (6), 253 (1939).

VESELY, D.G.: Ischiofemoral arthrodesis. An end-result of forty-four cases. J. Bone Joint Surg. A **43,** 363 (1961).

VIERSTEIN, K.: Erfahrungen bei Hüftarthrodesen. Verh. Dtsch. Orthop. Ges. **44,** 93 (1956).

VON LANZ, T.: WACHSMUTH, W.: Praktische Anatomie Vol. I/4, 2nd ed. Bein und Statik, Berlin-Heidelberg-New York: Springer 1972.

WALCHER, K.: Die Arthrodese im Zeitalter der Alloplastik. Münch. Wochenschr. **8,** 345 (1972).

WATSON-JONES, R.: Arthrodesis of the osteoarthritic hip. J. Am. Med. Ass. **110,** (4), 278 (1938).

WATSON-JONES, R., ROBINSON, W.C.: Arthrodesis of the osteoarthritic hip joint. J. Bone Joint Surg. B **38,** 353 (1956).

WEBER, B.G.: Vermeidung und Behandlung der Folgen von Hüftgelenksverletzungen. Unfallchir. Meeting in Garmisch-Partenkirchen. Franz X. Seitz u. Val. Höfling, München, 35 (1965).

WEBER, B.G.: Die Risiken in der Orthopädie. Schweiz. Med. Wochenschr. **99** (1), (1969).

WEBER, B.G.: Die Rotations-Totalendoprothese des Hüftgelenkes. Z. Orthop. **107,** (2), 304 (1970).

WEBER, B.G.: Hip arthrodesis. In: Tronzo, R.G., Surgery of the Hip Joint, p. 759. Philadelphia: Lea & Febiger 1973.

WEBER, B.G., LIECHTI, R., STÜHMER, G., BLATTER, R.: Prévention d'infections opératoires. De: Boitzy, A. Périarthrite de l'épaule, ostéogénèse et compression, travaux divers, p. 299, Bern-Stuttgart-Vienna: Huber 1972.

WEINREICH, M.: Zur Statik der Hüftarthrodese. Verh. Dtsch. Orthop. Ges. **47,** 509 (1959).

WEIS, J., MÜLLER, H.: Die Verhütung der Oberschenkelkopfnekrose nach Schenkelhalsbrüchen. Mschr. Unfallhk. **58,** 18 (1955).

WIEDMER, U.: Ergebnisse der Hüftarthrodese mit Kreuzplatte und Beckenosteotomie. Diss., AO-Bulletin, 1969.

WILTSE, L.L., THOMPSON, W.A.L.: Technic for arthrodesis of the hip when the femoral head and neck are absent. Arch. Surg. **59,** 888 (1949).

WINIWARTER, A.: Lehrbuch der chirurgischen Operationen und der chirurgischen Verbände, p. 193. Stuttgart: Enke 1895.

WITT, A.N.: Die Hüftarthrodese beim ältere Menschen. Chirurg **29** (2), 73 (1956).

WITT, A.N.: Fortschritte in der Behandlung der Koxarthrose. Münch. Med. Wochenschr. **111** (45), 2325 (1969).

WITT, A.N., HACKENBROCH, M.H., HEPP, W.R.: Zur Operationstechnik bei Grenzindikationen der Hüftarthroplastik mit Totalprothesen. Arch. Orthop. Unfallchir. **69,** 148 (1970).

WOLFF, J.: Das Gesetz der Transformation der Knochen. Berlin: Hirschwald 1892.

Subject Index

MIX
Papier aus verantwortungsvollen Quellen
Paper from responsible sources
FSC® C105338

If you have any concerns about our products,
you can contact us on
ProductSafety@springernature.com

In case Publisher is established outside the EU,
the EU authorized representative is:
Springer Nature Customer Service Center GmbH
Europaplatz 3, 69115 Heidelberg, Germany

Printed by Libri Plureos GmbH
in Hamburg, Germany